Clinical Manual of Prevention in Mental Health

Clinical Manual of Prevention in Mental Health

Edited by

Michael T. Compton, M.D., M.P.H.

Assistant Professor, Department of Psychiatry and Behavioral Sciences
and Department of Family and Preventive Medicine,
Emory University School of Medicine
Assistant Professor, Department of
Behavioral Sciences and Health Education
Rollins School of Public Health of Emory University
Atlanta, Georgia

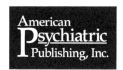

American Psychiatric Publishing, Inc.

Washington, DC
London, England

Note: The authors have worked to ensure that all information in this book is accurate at the time of publication and consistent with general psychiatric and medical standards, and that information concerning drug dosages, schedules, and routes of administration is accurate at the time of publication and consistent with standards set by the U.S. Food and Drug Administration and the general medical community. As medical research and practice continue to advance, however, therapeutic standards may change. Moreover, specific situations may require a specific therapeutic response not included in this book. For these reasons and because human and mechanical errors sometimes occur, we recommend that readers follow the advice of physicians directly involved in their care or the care of a member of their family.

If you would like to buy between 25 and 99 copies of this or any other APPI title, you are eligible for a 20% discount; please contact APPI Customer Service at appi@psych.org or 800-368-5777. If you wish to buy 100 or more copies of the same title, please e-mail us at bulksales@psych.org for a price quote.

Copyright © 2010 American Psychiatric Publishing, Inc.
ALL RIGHTS RESERVED

Manufactured in the United States of America on acid-free paper
13   12   11   10   09   5   4   3   2   1
First Edition

Typeset in Adobe's Formata and AGaramond.

American Psychiatric Publishing, Inc.
1000 Wilson Boulevard
Arlington, VA 22209-3901
www.appi.org

Library of Congress Cataloging-in-Publication Data
Clinical manual of prevention in mental health / edited by Michael T. Compton. — 1st ed.
    p. ; cm.
  Includes bibliographical references and index.
  ISBN 978-1-58562-347-1 (alk. paper)
  1. Preventive mental health services—Handbooks, manuals, etc. I. Compton, Michael T.
  [DNLM: 1. Mental Disorders—prevention & control. WM 140 C64075 2010]
  RA790.5.C547 2010
  362.2′0425—dc22
                                                                          2009028299

British Library Cataloguing in Publication Data
A CIP record is available from the British Library.

In honor of our patients, whose struggles we strive to alleviate; through them, we gain the insights necessary to advance the prevention of mental illnesses and the promotion of mental health.

Contents

Contributors xvii

Foreword xxiii
David Satcher, M.D., Ph.D.

Preface xxv
Michael T. Compton, M.D., M.P.H.

Acknowledgments xxxi

1 Prevention in Mental Health: An Introduction
From the Prevention Committee of the
Group for the Advancement of Psychiatry 1
Michael T. Compton, M.D., M.P.H., Carol Koplan, M.D.,
Christopher Oleskey, M.D., M.P.H., Rebecca A. Powers,
M.D., M.P.H., David Pruitt, M.D., and
Larry Wissow, M.D., M.P.H.
An Introduction to Prevention 1
Two Classifications of Prevention 2
Eight Principles in Considering Prevention in
Mental Health 9
Prevention-Minded Clinical Practice 21
Key Points 22
References 23

2 Identifying and Understanding Risk Factors and
Protective Factors in Clinical Practice 29
Anne Shaffer, Ph.D., and Tuppett M. Yates, Ph.D.
Risk Factors: Predicting Maladjustment and
Pathology 30

Protective Factors: Promoting Positive
Development and Health 34
Empirical and Clinical Implications 37
Conclusion 41
Key Points 42
References 43

3   **Prevention of Mood Disorders 49**

Christina P. C. Borba, M.P.H., and
Benjamin G. Druss, M.D., M.P.H.
Overview of the Epidemiology of
Mood Disorders 50
Risk Factors for Mood Disorders and
Implications for Prevention 52
Protective Factors for Mood Disorders and
Implications for Prevention 60
Primary Prevention of Mood Disorders 63
Secondary Prevention of Mood Disorders 65
Tertiary Prevention of Mood Disorders 67
What Practicing Psychiatrists Can Do in Routine
Practice to Promote the Prevention of Mood
Disorders 70
Conclusion 72
Key Points 72
References 73

4   **Prevention of Anxiety Disorders 83**

O. Joseph Bienvenu, M.D., Ph.D., Daniel J. Siegel, and
Golda S. Ginsburg, Ph.D.
Epidemiology of Anxiety Disorders 84
Risk Factors for Anxiety Disorders 85
Studies of Anxiety Disorders Prevention 87
Public and Provider Education as a
Prevention Tool 92

Important Considerations Pertaining to
Prevention of Anxiety Disorders 93
Conclusion 98
Key Points 98
References 99

5   **Complementary and Alternative Medicine in
    the Prevention of Depression and Anxiety 105**
    Ashli A. Owen-Smith, Ph.D., and Charles L. Raison, M.D.
    Definition of Complementary and
    Alternative Medicine 105
    Distinction Between "Complementary" and
    "Alternative" Medicine 107
    Complementary and Alternative Medicine
    Use in the United States 107
    Complementary and Alternative Medicine
    and Mental Illness Treatment 108
    Complementary and Alternative Medicine
    and the Prevention of Depressive and
    Anxiety Disorders 111
    Implications for Mental Health Practitioners 115
    Conclusion 117
    Key Points 118
    References 119

6   **Applying Prevention Principles to Schizophrenia
    and Other Psychotic Disorders 125**
    Michael T. Compton, M.D., M.P.H.
    Epidemiology of Schizophrenia 126
    Sequential Onset, Symptoms, Phenomenology,
    and Course of Schizophrenia 127
    Diagnostic Criteria and Course Specifiers 129
    Risk Factors and Risk Markers for
    Schizophrenia 132
    Schizophrenia and the Prevention Paradigm 138

Three Applications of Prevention Principles
to Schizophrenia 141
Conclusion: Advice for Clinicians. 146
Key Points 148
References 149

7 **Prevention of Alcohol and Drug Abuse 163**

Rebecca A. Powers, M.D., M.P.H.

Alcohol Use as a Problem and a Benefit:
The Paradox. 164
Drug Abuse and Dependence:
Always a Problem 169
Prevention Is Crucial 171
Prevention of Alcohol Abuse and
Dependence. 172
How Do Mental Health Professionals Assess and
Then Advise Patients About Problematic
Alcohol Use? 177
Prevention of Drug Abuse and Dependence 179
Relapse Prevention 191
Integrated Substance Abuse and
Mental Health Treatment 193
Evaluation of Prevention Efforts Is a Difficult Task . . . 194
Conclusion 195
Key Points 196
References 197
Appendix: Screening Tests for Alcohol-Related
Problems 204
  CAGE (Cut Down, Annoyed, Guilt, and
    Eye Opener) Questions. 204
  Alcohol Use Disorders Identification Test 205
  Michigan Alcohol Screening Test 207
  Tests for Alcohol Use. 209
  References 209

8 Suicide Prevention..........................**211**

Michael F. Grunebaum, M.D., and
Laili Soleimani, M.Sc., M.D.
Epidemiology of Suicidal Behavior:
A Brief Overview 212
Risk Factors for Suicide......................213
Protective Factors for Suicide.................217
Primary Prevention of Suicidal Behavior........217
Secondary Prevention.......................220
Tertiary Prevention 229
Adolescent Suicidality.......................231
Suicide Prevention Advice for Practitioners 232
Key Points 235
References 237

9 Prevention of Family Violence 243

Kenneth Rogers, M.D., M.S.H.S.,
Barbara Baumgardner, Ph.D., R.N.,
Kathleen Connors, L.C.S.W.-C., Patricia Martens, Ph.D.,
and Laurel Kiser, Ph.D., M.B.A.
Prevalence 244
Etiologies of Family Violence 246
Child Maltreatment..........................250
Domestic Violence...........................256
Principles of the Prevention of Family Violence
for Practicing Mental Health Professionals 261
Key Points 267
References 268

10 Prevention Principles for Adolescents in Psychiatric Practice: Preventing Conduct Disorder and Other Behavioral Problems 273

Kareem Ghalib, M.D., and Gordon Harper, M.D.

Normal Adolescence. 274
Conduct Disorder: A Brief Overview 274
Risk Factors for Conduct Disorder and
Other Behavioral Problems 276
Preventive Interventions. 277
Protective Factors and Health Promotion
Interventions 284
Translating the Research: Recommendations
for Preventing Harm and Promoting Strength
in Youth 290
Key Points 292
References. 292

11 Prevention Principles for Older Adults: Preventing Late-Life Depression, Dementia, and Mild Cognitive Impairment 297

*Joanne A. McGriff, M.D., M.P.H., William M.
McDonald, M.D., Paul R. Duberstein, Ph.D., and
Jeffrey M. Lyness, M.D.*

Definition of Terms. 298
Late-Life Depression 299
Dementia. 309
Mild Cognitive Impairment. 316
Key Points 321
References. 322

12 **Health Promotion and Prevention of Somatic Illnesses in Psychiatric Settings** **327**

Ann L. Hackman, M.D., Eric B. Hekler, Ph.D., and Lisa Dixon, M.D., M.P.H.

Scope of the Problem........................328
Health Promotion and Illness Prevention:
Definitions 334
Health Promotion Within the General
Population 335
Prevention and Health Maintenance in
People With Serious Mental Illnesses.........340
Conclusion and Future Directions............349
Key Points 353
References................................354

13 **Prevention of Cigarette Smoking: Principles for Psychiatric Practice** **365**

Rebecca A. Powers, M.D., M.P.H., and Michael T. Compton, M.D., M.P.H.

Smoking as an Efficient Means of
Nicotine Delivery..........................366
Smoking and Disease.......................367
Epidemiology of Cigarette Smoking 368
Risk and Protective Factors for
Cigarette Smoking.........................371
Prevention of Cigarette Smoking.............373
Recommendations for Clinical Practice........375
Conclusion................................382
Key Points 382
References................................383

Index **387**

List of Tables and Figures

Table 1–1	The traditional public health classification of prevention	4
Table 1–2	Institute of Medicine classification of prevention	7
Table 2–1	Examples of risk factors in multiple contexts	31
Table 2–2	Examples of protective factors in multiple contexts	35
Table 3–1	DSM-IV-TR diagnostic criteria for major depressive episode	51
Table 3–2	DSM-IV-TR diagnostic criteria for manic episode	53
Figure 4–1	The Coping and Promoting Strength program (CAPS) intervention model	96
Table 6–1	DSM-IV-TR diagnostic criteria for schizophrenia	130
Table 6–2	Select risk factors for schizophrenia	133
Table 6–3	Select risk markers for schizophrenia	136
Table 7–1	DSM-IV-TR diagnostic criteria for substance abuse	167
Table 7–2	DSM-IV-TR diagnostic criteria for substance dependence	168
Table 8–1	Evidence-based risk factors for suicide	214
Table 8–2	Stress-diathesis factors that may affect risk of suicidal behavior	215
Table 9–1	Etiological theories of family violence	247
Table 9–2	Risk factors for child abuse	249
Table 9–3	Risk factors for domestic violence	250
Table 9–4	Child maltreatment prevention efforts: summary of outcomes	251
Table 9–5	Practices to address the impact of domestic violence on children and parents: summary of outcomes	259

Table 10–1   Three stages of adolescent development
              across four domains: key features 275
Table 10–2   DSM-IV-TR criteria for conduct disorder 278
Table 10–3   "Risk factor matrix" for selected adolescent
              problem behaviors (as described by Hawkins
              and Catalano for Communities That Care). 280
Table 10–4   The Search Institute's 40 developmental assets
              for youths ages 12–18 years 285
Table 10–5   Positive youth developmental features and
              clinical applications 291
Table 11–1   DSM-IV-TR diagnostic criteria for dementia
              of the Alzheimer's type 310
Table 13–1   A summary of the Healthy People 2010
              U.S. health objectives pertaining
              to cigarette smoking 376

Contributors

Barbara Baumgardner, Ph.D., R.N.
Assistant Professor, Department of Psychiatry, University of Maryland School of Medicine, Baltimore, Maryland

O. Joseph Bienvenu, M.D., Ph.D.
Associate Professor, Department of Psychiatry and Behavioral Sciences, The Johns Hopkins University School of Medicine, Baltimore, Maryland

Christina P.C. Borba, M.P.H.
Doctoral Candidate, Department of Behavioral Sciences and Health Education, Rollins School of Public Health of Emory University, Atlanta, Georgia

Michael T. Compton, M.D., M.P.H.
Assistant Professor, Department of Psychiatry and Behavioral Sciences and Department of Family and Preventive Medicine, Emory University School of Medicine; Assistant Professor, Department of Behavioral Sciences and Health Education, Rollins School of Public Health of Emory University, Atlanta, Georgia

Kathleen Connors, L.C.S.W.-C.
Clinical Instructor, Department of Psychiatry, University of Maryland School of Medicine, Baltimore, Maryland

Lisa Dixon, M.D., M.P.H.
Professor and Director, Division of Health Services Research, Department of Psychiatry, University of Maryland School of Medicine; Associate Director of Research, VA Capitol Health Care Network MIRECC, Baltimore, Maryland

Benjamin G. Druss, M.D., M.P.H.
Professor and Rosalynn Carter Chair in Mental Health, Departments of Health Policy and Management and Behavioral Sciences and Health Education, Rollins School of Public Health of Emory University, Atlanta, Georgia

Paul R. Duberstein, Ph.D.
Professor, Director of the Laboratory of Personality and Development, and Director of the Rochester Program of Research and Innovation in Disparities Education, Department of Psychiatry, University of Rochester Medical Center, Rochester, New York

Kareem Ghalib, M.D.
Assistant Professor, Division of Child and Adolescent Psychiatry, Department of Psychiatry, College of Physicians and Surgeons, Columbia University; Medical Director, Children's Day Unit and Child and Adolescent Psychiatry Evaluation Service, New York State Psychiatric Institute, New York, New York

Golda S. Ginsburg, Ph.D.
Associate Professor, Department of Psychiatry and Behavioral Sciences, The Johns Hopkins University School of Medicine, Baltimore, Maryland

Michael F. Grunebaum, M.D.
Assistant Professor, Division of Molecular Imaging and Neuropathology, Department of Psychiatry, College of Physicians and Surgeons, Columbia University; Research Psychiatrist, New York State Psychiatric Institute, New York, New York

Ann L. Hackman, M.D.
Associate Professor, Department of Psychiatry, University of Maryland School of Medicine, Baltimore, Maryland

Gordon Harper, M.D.
Associate Professor, Department of Psychiatry, Harvard Medical School, and Medical Director, Child/Adolescent Services, Massachusetts Department of Mental Health, Chestnut Hill, Massachusetts

Eric B. Hekler, Ph.D.
Postdoctoral Research Fellow, Stanford Prevention Research Center, Stanford, California

Laurel Kiser, Ph.D., M.B.A.
Associate Professor, Department of Psychiatry, University of Maryland School of Medicine, Baltimore, Maryland

Carol Koplan, M.D.
Adjunct Assistant Professor, Department of Health Policy and Management and Department of Behavioral Sciences and Health Education, Rollins School of Public Health of Emory University, Atlanta, Georgia

Jeffrey M. Lyness, M.D.
Professor and Associate Chair for Education, and Director of the Geriatric Psychiatry Program, Department of Psychiatry, University of Rochester Medical Center, Rochester, New York

Patricia Martens, Ph.D.
Research Coordinator, The Family Center at the Kennedy Krieger Institute, Baltimore, Maryland

William M. McDonald, M.D.
J.B. Fuqua Chair in Late-Life Depression and Chief of the Division of Geriatric Psychiatry, Department of Psychiatry and Behavioral Sciences, Emory University School of Medicine, Atlanta, Georgia

Joanne A. McGriff, M.D., M.P.H.
Research Assistant, Department of Psychiatry and Behavioral Sciences, Emory University School of Medicine, Atlanta, Georgia

Christopher Oleskey, M.D., M.P.H.
Fellow in Child and Adolescent Psychiatry, Yale Child Study Center, New Haven, Connecticut

Ashli A. Owen-Smith, Ph.D.
Visiting Professor, Department of Behavioral Sciences and Health Education, Rollins School of Public Health of Emory University, Atlanta, Georgia

Rebecca A. Powers, M.D., M.P.H.
Adjunct Clinical Assistant Professor of Psychiatry, Stanford University School of Medicine, Los Gatos, California

David Pruitt, M.D.
Professor and Director of Child and Adolescent Psychiatry, Department of Psychiatry, University of Maryland School of Medicine, Baltimore, Maryland

Charles L. Raison, M.D.
Assistant Professor, Department of Psychiatry and Behavioral Sciences, Emory University School of Medicine, Atlanta, Georgia

Kenneth Rogers, M.D., M.S.H.S.
Assistant Professor, Department of Psychiatry, University of Maryland School of Medicine, Baltimore, Maryland

David Satcher, M.D., Ph.D.
Director, Satcher Health Leadership Institute, Poussaint-Satcher-Cosby Chair in Mental Health, Morehouse School of Medicine, Atlanta, Georgia; 16th U.S. Surgeon General

Anne Shaffer, Ph.D.
Assistant Professor, Department of Psychology, University of Georgia, Athens, Georgia

Daniel J. Siegel
Student, Political Science, Yale University, New Haven, Connecticut

Laili Soleimani, M.Sc., M.D.
Psychiatry Resident, Department of Psychiatry, Mount Sinai School of Medicine, New York, New York

Larry Wissow, M.D., M.P.H.
Professor, Department of Health, Behavior and Society, Johns Hopkins University, Bloomberg School of Public Health, Baltimore, Maryland

Tuppett M. Yates, Ph.D.
Assistant Professor, Department of Psychology, University of California, Riverside, Riverside, California

Disclosure of Competing Interests

The following contributors to this book have indicated a financial interest in or other affiliation with a commercial supporter, a manufacturer of a commercial product, a provider of a commercial service, a nongovernmental organization, and/or a government agency, as listed below:

Michael F. Grunebaum, M.D.—Principal investigator of a National Institute of Mental Health (NIMH)–supported clinical trial (K23 MH76049) comparing Paxil CR with Wellbutrin XL in depressed suicide attempters and ideators. In order to defray costs, the trial is using medication donated by GlaxoSmithKline.

William M. McDonald, M.D.—*Grant support:* Boehinger Ingelheim, Neuronetics; *Consultant/speaker honoraria:* Bristol-Myers Squibb, Janssen, Myriad. Dr. McDonald serves on the executive board of the Georgia Psychiatric Physicians Association and is director of the Fuqua Center for Late-Life Depression, both of which advocate for geriatric psychiatry. He is chair of the American Psychiatric Association (APA) Committee on Electroconvulsive Therapy and Other Electromagnetic Therapies and a member of the APA Council on Research. Dr. McDonald was an investigator in a trial sponsored by Janssen. He is presently principal investigator on an NIMH study that uses Neuronetics' transcranial magnetic stimulators. Dr. McDonald works for Emory University, which holds a patent for the transcranial magnetic stimulator used in the NIMH trial. He is also an investigator in a National Institute of Neurological Disorders and Stroke trial that is evaluating medication donated by GlaxoSmithKline (Paxil CR) and Wyeth (Effexor XR).

The following contributors to this book have no competing interests to report:

Barbara Baumgardner, Ph.D., R.N.
O. Joseph Bienvenu, M.D., Ph.D.
Christina P.C. Borba, M.P.H.
Michael T. Compton, M.D., M.P.H.
Kathleen Connors, L.C.S.W.-C.
Lisa Dixon, M.D., M.P.H.
Benjamin G. Druss, M.D., M.P.H.
Paul R. Duberstein, Ph.D.
Kareem Ghalib, M.D.
Golda S. Ginsburg, Ph.D.
Ann L. Hackman, M.D.
Gordon Harper, M.D.
Eric B. Hekler, Ph.D.
Laurel Kiser, Ph.D., M.B.A.
Carol Koplan, M.D.
Jeffrey M. Lyness, M.D.
Patricia Martens, Ph.D.
Joanne A. McGriff, M.D., M.P.H.
Christopher Oleskey, M.D., M.P.H.
Ashli A. Owen-Smith, Ph.D.
Rebecca A. Powers, M.D., M.P.H.
David Pruitt, M.D.
Charles L. Raison, M.D.
Kenneth Rogers, M.D., M.S.H.S.
Anne Shaffer, Ph.D.
Daniel J. Siegel
Laili Soleimani, M.Sc., M.D.
Tuppett M. Yates, Ph.D.

Foreword

In 1999, I issued *Mental Health: A Report of the Surgeon General* (http://www.surgeongeneral.gov/library/mentalhealth/home.html) to address the need to bring issues of mental health and mental illness to the forefront of our nation's health consciousness. At that time, and still today, we know a great deal more about treating mental illness than preventing mental illness and promoting mental health. A major course of action identified in the report focused on continuing to build the science base, especially evidence supporting strategies for mental health promotion and illness prevention.

In the 10 years since the report on mental health, significant progress has been made in the promotion of mental health and the reduction of stigma, as evident by the recent passage of the Paul Wellstone and Pete Domenici Mental Health Parity and Addiction Equity Act of 2008. However, although great strides have been made, there is still work to be done. Mental illness continues to be a major cause of morbidity and mortality throughout the world.

For this reason, *Clinical Manual of Prevention in Mental Health,* edited by Dr. Michael T. Compton, is timely and vital, as it serves to examine the new and emerging research on prevention in mental health. By providing practical suggestions for the implementation of preventive measures in the treatment of mood disorders, anxiety disorders, schizophrenia, and substance use disorders, this manual can help health care practitioners begin to move toward widespread adoption of mental illness prevention. This manual also addresses the significance of suicide and family violence prevention, an issue I highlighted in 1999 in the *Surgeon General's Call To Action To Prevent Suicide* (http://www.surgeongeneral.gov/library/calltoaction/). In addition, given the health disparities associated with individuals with severe mental illness, the focus on prevention of physical illness and disability among people with mental health problems is particularly important.

Disease prevention is one of the foundations of public health and is an essential component of all aspects of medicine. A comprehensive approach to the management of mental illness must take place in the context of a commitment to mental illness prevention and mental health promotion. *Clinical Manual of Prevention in Mental Health* will help to inform and guide practitioners to apply the principles of prevention to improve the mental health of their patients and communities. It is my hope that this manual can serve as a handbook to health care professionals, so that they might begin to practice evidence-based mental illness prevention and mental health promotion.

David Satcher, M.D., Ph.D.
Director, Satcher Health Leadership Institute,
Poussaint-Satcher-Cosby Chair in Mental Health,
Morehouse School of Medicine, Atlanta, Georgia;
16th U.S. Surgeon General

Preface

Psychiatrists and diverse other mental health and broader healthcare professionals are faced with many challenges in effectively evaluating and treating persons with psychiatric illnesses and substance use disorders. Resources are often stretched thin, especially for those with the most serious and disabling conditions, and many people who would benefit from treatment are untreated, undertreated, or treated only after extended delays for complex reasons. Clinicians clearly have difficulties and barriers in their efforts to provide comprehensive, efficacious, and timely treatment. Despite the challenges, this book encourages mental healthcare providers to expand their clinical practices, or the orientation or guiding principles of their practices, to include attention to *prevention* in addition to treatment.

Compared with our knowledge in some other areas of medicine, such as the prevention of infectious diseases, understandings of the prevention of mental illnesses remain in a relatively nascent state, especially in terms of how prevention can be incorporated into routine clinical practice. Yet, this book, *Clinical Manual of Prevention in Mental Health,* encourages readers to adopt what is currently known from prevention research, to the extent possible, in their practices. With this goal in mind, the authors of the various chapters have endeavored to balance reviewing the available research knowledge with providing guidance for practicing clinicians on how such knowledge can be incorporated into practice. This manual is exhaustive neither in reviewing prevention science nor in giving practical advice. However, it is my hope that a balance has been achieved so that the tenets of prevention become more accessible to mental health practitioners.

Compiling a "clinical" manual of "prevention" in mental health is inherently a difficult task given that the authors have been charged with writing for clinicians about a topic that is usually not viewed as the clinician's province. That is, at least in the older nomenclature (see the "traditional public health classification of prevention" defined and described in Chapter 1, "Prevention in Mental Health"), primary prevention is not explicitly about clinical treatment but is population-based (as is universal prevention in the newer nomenclature). If secondary and tertiary prevention are both related to treatment and rehabilitation, then one must naturally ask, "What is the added value of a manual on prevention for clinicians above and beyond available manuals on treatment and rehabilitation?" Indeed, some of the chapters address treatment-related issues, in the framework of secondary and tertiary prevention, to a large extent. However, given increasing emphasis on risk factor reduction and a growing body of research literature on prevention studies, the mental health professions are entering an era in which prevention principles can and should be integrated into treatment settings.

The science related to prevention in mental health is reviewed in this manual primarily for an audience of clinicians. There are pearls for practitioners about programs to try for their patients and clients, and it is my goal that mental health professionals' sensitivity to prevention concerns will be enhanced. The reviews and clinical pearls, however, are limited by the current developmental stage of psychiatric practice and research. For example, there are serious validity problems with psychiatric diagnoses and the current nosology of mental disorders. Because prevention depends partly on the science of etiology, a descriptive nosology that explicitly eschews causal explanations may be limited in its utility for prevention science. Nonetheless, for many readers, this manual will serve as their first relatively comprehensive review of prevention as it can be applied to psychiatric illnesses and substance use disorders.

Clinical Manual of Prevention in Mental Health had its genesis in discussions within the Prevention Committee of the Group for the Advancement of Psychiatry (GAP) during its semiannual meetings in White Plains, New York, in 2007. Our committee's objective during those discussions was to provide psychiatrists and other mental healthcare providers with a useful guide on becoming prevention-minded in routine clinical settings. Although much of the work of prevention is accomplished in nonclinical settings (e.g., through policy, legislation, and the structuring of healthcare organizations and insurance plans), we believe that there are many opportunities for practicing clinicians to promote mental health and move toward the prevention of mental illnesses in routine practice. In aiming to meet our objective, we had to make difficult decisions on what would and would not be included in this manual, given the space and scope constraints of a relatively concise text. We hope that the topics that were selected will be useful.

The manual begins with an introduction on incorporating prevention into mental health settings. This first chapter, written by the GAP Prevention Committee (myself, Carol Koplan, Christopher Oleskey, Rebecca Powers, David Pruitt, and Larry Wissow), presents two classifications of prevention (primary, secondary, and tertiary prevention; as well as universal, selective, and indicated preventive interventions). The GAP Prevention Committee also provides eight principles that we believe may help the reader form a foundation for the more specific topics presented in the chapters that follow. The second chapter ("Identifying and Understanding Risk Factors and Protective Factors in Clinical Practice"), provided by Anne Shaffer and Tuppett Yates, also serves as an introduction. The authors provide an in-depth overview of risk factors and protective factors, along with a presentation of how assessments of such factors can inform clinical practice.

In light of the remarkably high prevalence of mood and anxiety disorders, Chapters 3–5 focus on the prevention of these conditions. In Chapter 3 ("Prevention of Mood Disorders"), Christina Borba and Benjamin Druss present an overview of the prevention of mood disorders, and in Chapter 4 ("Prevention of Anxiety Disorders") O. Joseph Bienvenu, Daniel Siegel, and Golda Ginsburg contribute a similar overview pertaining to the prevention of anxiety disorders. In both chapters, the authors briefly review epidemiology and risk factors and discuss various forms of prevention that have been studied. Given the increasing use of complementary and alternative health practices in western cultures, Ashli Owen-Smith and Charles Raison review, in Chapter 5 ("Complementary and Alternative Medicine in the Prevention of Depression and Anxiety"), the potential uses of such practices in the prevention of depression and anxiety. As in other chapters, the authors discuss key implications for mental health practitioners.

In Chapter 6 ("Applying Prevention Principles to Schizophrenia and Other Psychotic Disorders"), I provide an overview of some of the ways that prevention principles can be applied to schizophrenia and other psychotic disorders. Although this area arguably remains in its infancy, promising recent research—especially research into the prodrome and early psychosis—suggests that some prevention applications are now feasible and others may be available in the near future. For example, in addition to early detection and phase-specific intervention, clinicians may be able to play a role in delaying, or even averting the onset of psychosis in particularly high-risk youth and young adults. In Chapter 7 ("Prevention of Alcohol and Drug Abuse"), Rebecca Powers gives a detailed account of alcohol and drug abuse prevention. She includes extensive information on the prevention of alcohol abuse and dependence, the prevention of illicit drug abuse and dependence, and, importantly, the prevention of substance abuse/dependence in adolescence, the developmental period during which addictive disorders typically begin. Other topics of particular relevance to practicing mental health professionals, such as relapse prevention and integrated substance abuse and mental health treatment for patients with dual diagnoses, are reviewed.

The prevention of internally and externally directed aggression and violence are the topics of the next two chapters. Michael Grunebaum and Laili Soleimani present, in Chapter 8 ("Suicide Prevention"), an overview of the epidemiology of suicidal behavior; risk factors for suicide; and primary, secondary, and tertiary suicide prevention strategies. They offer practical suicide prevention suggestions for clinicians. In their chapter on preventing family violence (Chapter 9, "Prevention of Family Violence"), Kenneth Rogers, Barbara Baumgardner, Kathleen Connors, Patricia Martens, and Laurel Kiser provide the reader with a review of the prevention of child physical abuse and neglect, child sexual abuse, and domestic violence. They too present a number of principles for the practicing mental health professional pertaining to the prevention of family violence.

The next two chapters focus on prevention principles for two particular age groups. In Chapter 10 ("Prevention Principles for Adolescents in Psychiatric Practice"), Kareem Ghalib and Gordon Harper give an overview of preventing conduct disorder and other behavioral problems among adolescents in psychiatric practice. In Chapter 11 ("Prevention Principles for Older Adults"), Joanne McGriff, William McDonald, Paul Duberstein, and Jeffrey Lyness review the prevention of late-life depression, dementia, and mild cognitive impairment among older adults. These two chapters focus on these select key topics, though other topics—such as the prevention of eating disorders in adolescence, the prevention of teenage pregnancy, and the prevention of delirium in ill older adults, for example—are admittedly crucial as well.

The final two chapters encourage mental health professionals to consider not only the prevention of mental illnesses but also physical health promotion and the prevention of physical illnesses among psychiatric patients. In Chapter 12 ("Health Promotion and Prevention of Somatic Illnesses in Psychiatric Settings"), Ann Hackman, Eric Hekler, and Lisa Dixon discuss health promotion and the prevention of physical illnesses in psychiatric settings. Rebecca Powers and I then give, in Chapter 13 ("Prevention of Cigarette Smoking"), an overview of the prevention of cigarette smoking, which is of great importance for mental health professionals in light of the astonishingly high rates of smoking among patients with serious mental illnesses.

In selecting these particular areas, we could not cover numerous other topics that may be of great interest and practical relevance to mental health professionals. For example, the manual does not review, or even mention, the prevention of many types of psychiatric illnesses, including adjustment disorders, personality disorders, sexual disorders, sleep disorders, somatoform disorders, and others. Additionally, a large array of topics that have broad social implications could not be covered. This absence of coverage is not due to a lack of importance or relevance to the mental health field, but to space and scope limitations. For example, the other authors and I have not discussed a number of critical complications that arise in applying prevention principles to mental health settings, in terms of politics, access to resources, resource distribution, and financing of prevention services. Numerous topics of great significance for social justice and population-based mental health—including the problem of poverty and other social determinants of disease; adverse health consequences of sexism, racism, and other forms of discrimination; the problem of violence, ranging from urban gang violence to war, torture, and genocide; and the interface between trade, commerce, economic structure and mental health—are not discussed. The integration of psychiatry and primary care is mentioned in some chapters, though this topic deserves a more comprehensive discussion given that prevention is likely to be advanced through such collaborations and integration. The manual also does not directly address the importance of infusing medical and residency education with a greater awareness of prevention principles. Nonetheless, this issue is of particular interest to the GAP Prevention Committee, and part of our objective in conceiving this book was that it would be a useful resource for psychiatry residents and other mental health trainees in addition to practicing mental health professionals.

I would like to point out two other important caveats, by way of introduction to this manual. First, some chapters use the term "patient," which historically, typically refers to a person who is seeking care from a doctor. Other terms, like "client" or "consumer," may be more appropriate, especially in light of recent conceptualizations of care such as the recovery paradigm and shared decision making. But for simplicity and ease of writing and reading, the manual often refers to individuals experiencing a psychiatric disorder as "patients." Second, some chapters make reference to a very important publication, the Institute of Medicine's 1994 report called *Reducing Risks for Mental Disorders: Frontiers for Preventive Intervention Research.* However, I wish to wholeheartedly acknowledge the fact that a new Institute of Medicine report on prevention in mental health was eagerly awaited as we compiled these chapters and as this manual was in production. The new report, *Preventing Mental, Emotional, and Behavioral Disorders among Young People: Progress and Possibilities,* will undoubtedly advance the field. Although the authors of this book did not have the good fortune of reading the report prior to writing their chapters, I recommend it, along with other related Institute of Medicine reports, to the readers of this manual.

My primary goal in the development of this book has been to encourage mental health professionals to adopt prevention-mindedness into their everyday practice with patients and in their collaborations with community organizations and agencies that may have a role to play in prevention efforts. I hope that *Clinical Manual of Prevention in Mental Health* will accomplish this goal and perhaps stimulate a much needed discussion within psychiatry and the other mental health professions of how we can consider prevention, in addition to treatment, in each and every patient we see.

Michael T. Compton, M.D., M.P.H.

Acknowledgments

The development and writing of this book were truly collaborative efforts, which seems particularly appropriate given that mental health promotion and the prevention of mental illnesses requires collaboration among numerous professionals. The 30 authors that I have worked with to develop the 13 chapters included here were exceptionally receptive, responsive, and giving of their time and tremendous expertise. Each of them played an important role in making this manual an informative and practical text for mental health professionals. It has also been a true pleasure to work with the experienced editorial staff at American Psychiatric Publishing, Inc., including Robert E. Hales, M.D., Editor-in-Chief; John McDuffie, Editorial Director of the Books Division; Greg Kuny, Managing Editor; and Bessie Jones, Acquisitions Coordinator.

I feel privileged to have developed this book with inspiration, and ongoing guidance and support, from my fellow members of the Prevention Committee of the Group for the Advancement of Psychiatry (GAP). I consider this entire book, beyond Chapter 1, their product, rather than mine. Also at GAP, I would like to thank Lois Flaherty, then President, for her kind support; David Adler and all of the members of the GAP Publications Board who reviewed and gave advice on Chapter 1; as well as other GAP members who provided helpful suggestions on the overall content and structure of the book.

Although not directly involved in the development of this book, Erica Frank, my residency training director during my second residency, in preventive medicine, deserves my special acknowledgment. During that critical training period, and since, she has been an advocate and mentor, pushing me to aim high and think big in my endeavor to bring together my two medical disciplines, psychiatry and preventive medicine. I also deeply appreciate the support and encouragement given by my partner, Kendrick Hogan, while I dedicated many extra hours to this project.

I appreciate Dr. David Satcher's willingness to provide a thoughtful foreword to the manual, and Ruth Shim's assistance with that process. I admire Dr. Satcher's past work (e.g., his issuing of the landmark *Mental Health: A Report of the Surgeon General*) as well as his current accomplishments in the arena of primary care, which address both prevention and mental health. Finally, I am very grateful to Beth Broussard, my close colleague and research team member, who generously gave of her time to provide unfaltering, highly professional, and thorough assistance in compiling and finalizing the various chapters. Her thoughtful advice, as well as practical help, while developing this manual has been especially meaningful to me, given that such work came at a very busy time when she and I were putting the finishing touches on our own book. I could not have met the deadlines or accomplished a satisfactory level of thoroughness without her.

Michael T. Compton, M.D., M.P.H.

1

Prevention in Mental Health

An Introduction From the Prevention Committee of the Group for the Advancement of Psychiatry

Michael T. Compton, M.D., M.P.H.

Carol Koplan, M.D.

Christopher Oleskey, M.D., M.P.H.

Rebecca A. Powers, M.D., M.P.H.

David Pruitt, M.D.

Larry Wissow, M.D., M.P.H.

An Introduction to Prevention

In recent decades, psychiatrists, psychologists, preventionists, and allied professionals have learned a great deal about risk and protective factors related to mental illnesses, as well as the development of evidence-based interventions

1

addressing such factors and disorders. These developments in the prevention of behavioral disorders, which parallel the medical profession's increased knowledge about preventing infectious diseases and chronic illnesses, were reviewed in detail in the 1994 Institute of Medicine (IOM) report titled *Reducing Risks for Mental Disorders: Frontiers for Preventive Intervention Research* (Institute of Medicine 1994). More recently, developments in the field and an overview of worldwide approaches have been described in two World Health Organization publications, *Prevention of Mental Disorders: Effective Interventions and Policy Options* (World Health Organization 2004a) and *Promoting Mental Health: Concepts, Emerging Evidence, Practice* (World Health Organization 2004b). These three resources are essential reviews of the expanding knowledge base on mental illness prevention and mental health promotion.

In the past, prevention has been the mainstay of the field of public health; however, this population-based approach is now being embraced by the general health sector and is becoming more widely accepted in the mental health field. Both general medicine and psychiatry are primarily involved in individual-level treatment, but with the widespread prevalence of chronic medical and psychiatric illnesses, and an aging population, there has been increased recognition of the importance of a population-based prevention approach. We have previously described what is meant by *prevention psychiatry* and discussed its historical context, recent epidemiological studies, evidence-based prevention practices, and the paradigm shift toward prevention (Koplan et al. 2007); in this chapter, we begin by providing an overview of two classifications of prevention: a traditional public health classification (primary, secondary, and tertiary prevention) and a newer classification put forth in the 1994 Institute of Medicine report (universal, selective, and indicated preventive interventions). We then give eight principles for mental health professionals to consider in their endeavor to become prevention-minded clinicians. It is our hope that this description of the two classifications, which are referred to throughout this book, and our eight principles, will provide a foundation for the reader to then delve more deeply into specific content areas addressed in the other chapters.

Two Classifications of Prevention

There are at least two ways of classifying prevention, and both are advantageous in framing the complex goals of prevention in mental health. The first is the traditional public health definitions of primary, secondary, and tertiary prevention (Table 1–1), and the second is the newer classification put forth in the aforementioned IOM report (Institute of Medicine 1994) (Table 1–2). The traditional public health classification encompasses a broad range of interventions that include routinely used treatments (i.e., tertiary prevention, or the treatment of established disease to reduce disability). However, the newer IOM classification focuses prevention on interventions occurring before the onset of a formal *Diagnostic and Statistical Manual of Mental Disorders* (DSM) disorder. In fact, the IOM report specifically states that the term *prevention* is reserved for those interventions that occur before the onset of the disorder, whereas *treatment* refers to interventions for individuals who meet or are close to meeting diagnostic criteria.

The Traditional Public Health Classification of Prevention

Primary prevention refers to keeping a disease or adverse outcome from occurring or becoming established by eliminating causes of disease or increasing resistance to disease (Katz 1997). As such, primary prevention seeks to decrease the number of new cases (incidence) of a disease, disorder, or adverse outcome (Institute of Medicine 1994). Thus, primary prevention refers to interventions occurring during the predisease stage and focusing on health promotion and specific protection (Katz 1997). Primary prevention protects health through personal and communal efforts and is generally the task of the field of public health (Last 2001). An example of primary prevention pertaining to infectious diseases is the prevention of influenza and other acute infections using vaccination. In mental health, examples of primary prevention are less numerous, partly because of the lack of understanding of discrete etiological factors. Thus, primary prevention in mental health tends to focus on the reduction of risk factors, such as adverse childhood experiences; such risk reduction is presumed to have primary prevention effects and, in some cases, to be strongly associated with decreased incidence. The success of primary prevention efforts in reducing mental disorders or adverse psychiatric outcomes is exemplified by the fact that many infectious diseases with psychiatric manifestations (e.g., syphilis, measles) have been eliminated or reduced in incidence. Mental hospitals once housed many people with the psychiatric sequelae of these and other disorders in addition to "primary" psychiatric illnesses. Suc-

Table 1–1.   The traditional public health classification of prevention

Type of prevention	Definition/key characteristics	Examples in medicine	Examples in psychiatry
Primary prevention	Keeps a disease or adverse outcome from occurring or becoming established by eliminating causes of disease or increasing resistance to disease; decreases the number of new cases (incidence); occurs during the predisease stage and focuses on health promotion and specific protection	Vaccination	Reduction of risk factors (e.g., adverse childhood experiences)
Secondary prevention	Interrupts the disease process before it becomes symptomatic; lowers the rate of established cases (prevalence); occurs during the latent stage of disease and focuses on presymptomatic diagnosis and treatment (early detection); controls disease and minimizes disability through the use of screening programs	Mammography; Papanicolaou smears, colonoscopy to detect early-stage cancers	Screening for depression and suicidal ideation
Tertiary prevention	Limits physical and social consequences or disability associated with existing, symptomatic disease, disorder, or adverse outcome; occurs during the symptomatic stage of disease and focuses on the limitation of disability and rehabilitation; softens the impact of long-term disease and disability by eliminating or reducing impairment, disability, or handicaps; minimizes suffering and maximizes potential years of useful life	Rehabilitation following a cerebrovascular accident	Relapse prevention; treatments to enhance psychosocial functioning

cessful prevention efforts have rendered mental disorders stemming from untreated infections and nutritional deficiencies relatively rare in the United States.

Secondary prevention refers to interrupting the disease process before it becomes symptomatic (Katz 1997). As such, secondary prevention ultimately lowers the number of established cases (prevalence) of the disease, disorder, or adverse outcome in the population (Institute of Medicine 1994). Thus, secondary prevention refers to interventions occurring during the latent stage of disease and focusing on presymptomatic diagnosis and treatment (early detection). Secondary prevention may control disease and minimize disability through the use of screening programs (Last 2001), and is generally the task of prevention-related as opposed to treatment-related aspects of the medical profession. If a disease is detected early it can be treated promptly and, ideally, resolved. Early detection and intervention decrease the time a person has a disease, thus reducing the number of individuals having the disease at any given time. From the medical field, examples of secondary prevention include mammography, Papanicolaou smears, colonoscopy, and other screening measures to detect the earliest stages of cancer, before overt symptoms develop. In psychiatry, an example of secondary prevention is screening for symptoms of depression or suicidal thinking to prevent the onset of full-syndrome depression and to prevent suicide attempts or completed suicides.

Tertiary prevention refers to limiting physical and social consequences or disability associated with an existing, symptomatic disease, disorder, or adverse outcome (Institute of Medicine 1994; Katz 1997). Thus, tertiary prevention refers to interventions that occur during the symptomatic stage of disease and focus on the limitation of disability and on rehabilitation (Katz 1997). Tertiary prevention softens the impact of long-term disease and disability by eliminating or reducing impairment or handicaps, minimizing suffering, and maximizing potential years of useful life (Last 2001), and is generally the task of the treatment- and rehabilitation-related aspects of the medical community. Of note, the traditional definition of tertiary prevention may be thought of as treatment, whereas the newer IOM classification presented in Table 1–2 limits the term *prevention* to refer to interventions occurring before the onset of disease. Nonetheless, tertiary prevention is an important consideration, especially given that most practicing mental health professionals mainly see patients with established disorders for whom tertiary prevention goals are crucial. In medicine, tertiary prevention is exemplified by rehabilitation after a cerebrovascular accident to minimize functional impairment. In psychiatry, tertiary prevention involves preventing relapse, reducing the likelihood of developing comorbidities, and providing treatments to enhance psychosocial functioning. For example, a number of evidence-based interventions have been studied in the context of severe and persistent mental illnesses—such as assertive community treatment, social skills training, and supported employment—to prevent relapse and rehospitalization, improve social interactions, and assist in obtaining competitive employment.

Institute of Medicine Classification of Prevention

The 1994 IOM report elaborated on the definition of primary prevention by emphasizing *the target population addressed by the intervention*, rather than by categorizing prevention based on the stage of disease during which an intervention occurs (the latter being the traditional public health classification; Institute of Medicine 1994). On the basis of the newer classification, primary prevention can be subdivided into universal, selective, and indicated preventive interventions depending on the target population receiving the intervention (Table 1–2).

Universal preventive interventions target a whole population or the general public. Such interventions are desirable for everyone in the eligible population (Institute of Medicine 1994), regardless of one's level of risk for the disease, disorder, or adverse outcome. In general medicine, universal preventive interventions include fluoridation of drinking water, fortification of food products, seat belt legislation, and routine childhood vaccinations. In the mental health field, such interventions may include public service announcements or media campaigns to prevent substance abuse or cigarette smoking, as well as legislation to increase the legal drinking age.

Selective preventive interventions target individuals or a subgroup of the population whose risk of developing a disease, disorder, or adverse outcome is significantly higher than average (Institute of Medicine 1994). A risk group may be identified based on psychological, biological, or social risk factors. In the field of medicine, an example of a selective preventive intervention is lifestyle modification and pharmacological management of hyperlipidemia to prevent cardiovascular disease. An example of a selective intervention in mental

Table 1–2. Institute of Medicine classification of prevention

Type of preventive intervention	Definition/key characteristics	Example in medicine	Example in psychiatry
Universal preventive intervention	Targets a whole population or the general public; such measures are desirable for everybody in the eligible population regardless of one's level of risk for the disease, disorder, or adverse outcome	Fluoridation of drinking water, fortification of food products, seat belt laws	Public service announcements, media campaigns, and drinking age limits to prevent substance abuse
Selective preventive intervention	Targets individuals or a subgroup of the population whose risk of developing a disease, disorder, or adverse outcome is significantly higher than average; a risk group may be identified based on psychological, biological, or social risk factors	Lifestyle modification and pharmacological management of hyperlipidemia	Group-based psychological treatments for children of depressed parents
Indicated preventive intervention	Targets particularly high-risk individuals (individuals who, on examination, are found to have a risk factor, condition, or abnormality that identifies them as being at high risk for the future development of the disease, disorder, or adverse outcome); such high-risk individuals may be identified as having minimal but detectable signs or symptoms foreshadowing a disease or disorder—or a biological marker indicating a predisposition to a disorder—although diagnostic criteria for the illness are not yet met	Detection and targeted treatment of the metabolic syndrome	Identification and treatment of individuals with symptoms consistent with the prodrome of schizophrenia

Source. Institute of Medicine: "New Directions in Definitions," in *Reducing Risks for Mental Disorders: Frontiers for Preventive Intervention Research.* Edited by Mrazek PJ, Haggerty RJ. Washington, DC, National Academy Press, 1994, pp. 19–29.

health care is psychological treatment for high-risk children who have a parent with a mental disorder such as major depression.

Indicated preventive interventions target particularly high-risk individuals—those who, on examination, are found to have a risk factor, condition, or abnormality that identifies them as being at high risk for the future development of a disease, disorder, or adverse outcome (Institute of Medicine 1994). Such high-risk individuals may be identified as having minimal, but detectable, signs or symptoms foreshadowing a disease or disorder—or a biological marker indicating a predisposition to a disorder—although diagnostic criteria for the illness are not yet met. An indicated preventive intervention relevant to both general medicine and psychiatry is the detection and targeted treatment of people with the metabolic syndrome, which is associated with an especially high risk of cardiovascular disease and diabetes. Another example in psychiatry that is currently being studied is the identification and treatment of individuals at ultra-high risk for schizophrenia (i.e., those with symptoms consistent with the prodrome), although they do not yet meet criteria for the diagnosis, as discussed in Chapter 6 ("Applying Prevention Principles to Schizophrenia and Other Psychotic Disorders"). Such prospective identification efforts are an important first step in developing targeted interventions to delay or avert the onset of the disorder.

Dr. Thomas Insel, Director of the National Institute of Mental Health, recently presented the notion of *preemption*, noting that preemptive interventions in psychiatry, which target individuals at greatest risk of a mental illness and those with subthreshold signs and symptoms, provide what has previously been labeled as selective or indicated prevention (Insel 2008). He notes that preemptive interventions can be directed best once an understanding of individual patterns of risk that predict a disorder are better elucidated. As the field advances, risk prediction is likely to rely on a combination of factors rather than a single biomarker. Such combinations are used in the prediction of risk for cardiovascular disease (e.g., the Framingham score) (Eichler et al. 2007).

The prevention of specific mental disorders or behavioral problems may be attainable using a variety of interventions. For example, in a meta-analysis of randomized, controlled trials of psychological interventions designed to reduce the incidence of depressive disorders, Cuijpers and colleagues (2008) examined data from 21 interventions, including 2 universal preventive interventions, 11 selective interventions, and 8 indicated interventions. These studies involved 5,806 participants, and follow-up periods ranged from 3 to 36 months. They found that the interventions reduced the incidence of depressive disorders by a mean of 22% in experimental groups compared with control groups, and that selective and indicated interventions had comparable prevention effects.

Eight Principles in Considering Prevention in Mental Health

With these classifications in mind, we propose eight principles that mental health professionals should consider in their efforts to become *prevention-minded* mental health professionals. The first two principles suggest that mental health professionals should have a basic understanding of epidemiology and risk and protective factors. The third, fourth, and fifth argue that evidence-based preventive interventions can in fact be applied in the clinical setting, and that such interventions involve patients as well as their family members. The sixth principle relates to the fact that primary and secondary prevention efforts often take place in venues outside of the clinical setting, such as schools, the workplace, and the community. The seventh and eighth suggest that mental health professionals have a role in efforts to reach broad prevention goals and in promoting overall health and awareness.

1. **The application of prevention efforts in mental health is based on epidemiological findings.** Prevention is typically population-focused, whereas treatment is usually oriented to an individual or a group. Thus, an understanding of prevention is informed by population-based understandings of mental illnesses. Two key epidemiological parameters are *incidence* and *prevalence*. Although both relate to the rate of occurrence of an illness in the population, the former refers to the number of new cases over a specified period of time (often measured in a year), whereas prevalence refers to the number of existing cases in a population at a given point in time or during a given time period. In the face of limited resources for prevention programs, more highly prevalent psychiatric conditions, such as depressive disorders, anxiety disorders, and substance use disorders, may be particu-

larly important targets of prevention efforts. Yet relatively low-incidence disorders or events, such as suicide, also call for prevention resources given the large associated costs and public health impacts. Further, an awareness of changing trends in incidence and prevalence allows mental health providers to more effectively target scarce prevention resources. For example, the demographic trends toward an aging American population suggest a need for further resources to study the prevention of late-life depression and suicide, cognitive decline, and dementia.

Epidemiological research also informs clinicians about *when* to intervene. Large-scale surveys indicate that half of all mental disorders begin by age 14, and three-quarters begin by age 24 (Kessler et al. 2005a, 2005b). Such studies demonstrate the early onset of mental disorders and support the importance of early intervention. Epidemiological studies also tell us that despite effective treatments, there are commonly long delays from the onset of psychiatric symptoms to the time when the patient seeks help and adequate treatment is initiated, often ranging from years to decades. Untreated psychiatric disorders are likely to be associated with elevated rates of school dropout and other academic problems, teenage pregnancy, unstable employment and poverty, involvement in the criminal justice system, problems in interpersonal relationships, and other psychosocial problems (National Institute of Mental Health 2005). Together, these facts highlight the need for earlier detection and intervention.

2. **Practicing prevention in the field of mental health requires an understanding of risk factors and protective factors.** Preventive interventions are commonly developed and guided by an understanding of both risk factors and protective factors. A *risk factor* is a characteristic that precedes a disorder and is statistically associated with that disorder. Some risk factors are *causal risk factors*, meaning that they have a known role in etiology. For example, a microdeletion involving the long arm of chromosome 22, at the 22q11.2 band—the velocardiofacial syndrome, characterized by variable features such as cleft palate, congenital heart anomalies, and immune disorders (Shprintzen et al. 2005)—is a risk factor for the development of psychosis. Other risk factors are *proxy risk factors* or markers of elevated risk (e.g., urbanicity of place of birth/upbringing and risk of psychosis). Furthermore, risk factors may be *malleable* or *nonmalleable*. That is, some risk factors—exemplified by family discord, deficits in parenting

skills, availability of firearms and other means of suicide, and poverty or socioeconomic deprivation—may be malleable through preventive interventions. Others may be nonmalleable risk factors. Though the latter are not likely to be altered through preventive interventions, they may be useful in terms of targeting early identification and intervention efforts. Having a history of adverse perinatal events (such as prenatal, labor, or delivery complications) and having a family history of a psychiatric illness are examples of nonmalleable risk factors. It is widely recognized that many risk factors for psychiatric illnesses, such as adverse childhood experiences (including child abuse and neglect, parental loss, or mental illness in a parent; Chapman et al. 2007), not only are highly prevalent in the population but also are risk factors for multiple adverse outcomes, not just one disorder (Durlak 1998; Felitti et al. 1998; Hawkins et al. 1999).

Equally important as risk factors are *protective factors*, which predate the associated disorder or adverse outcome and significantly reduce the risk of developing the disorder or outcome. Protective factors may prevent some stressors from occurring, protect against the adverse effects of stressors that do occur, decrease the likelihood of developing a disorder, and promote resiliency in the face of multiple stressors (Rutter 1979). Some examples of protective factors are support from a caring adult, such as a parent, relative, mentor, or therapist; good school performance; conflict resolution skills; positive peers; and clear and consistent discipline in the family. Chapter 2 ("Identifying and Understanding Risk Factors and Protective Factors in Clinical Practice") provides a more detailed overview of risk and protective factors.

3. **Evidence-based preventive interventions can be applied in the clinical setting.** Prevention research in recent decades has increased our knowledge of evidence-based practices that effectively prevent negative outcomes. However, how can a mental health professional apply this knowledge in routine practice? First, several practice guidelines and reviews that incorporate prevention principles are available, such as recommendations on the monitoring of metabolic indices in patients prescribed antipsychotic medications (American Diabetes Association et al. 2004; Casey et al. 2004; Nasrallah and Newcomer 2004). Second, well-validated screening tools, which can promote secondary prevention, are widely accessible for use in routine clinical settings. Third, prevention research has identified

risk factors, and these risk factors can be assessed in daily clinical practice; similarly, protective factors should be routinely evaluated. Thus, there exist a number of ways to bridge the gap from science (i.e., large, randomized, controlled trials of preventive interventions by prevention scientists) to clinical practice (i.e., routine, everyday, individual-level clinical care).

Prevention-minded clinical practice may have broad beneficial effects. For example, a study involving patients who smoke cigarettes found that as counseling interventions increased, patient satisfaction with care increased, and smoking decreased (Conroy et al. 2005). Surprisingly, smoking also decreased even in those *not* ready to quit smoking. This is an example of how routine prevention practices, including asking straightforward questions and performing brief counseling, can have a crucial effect on reducing unhealthy behaviors. When treating depressed and potentially suicidal patients, given that accessibility to lethal means is a proven risk factor for completed suicide, mental health professionals should routinely inquire about firearms in the household. Simply asking routine questions—for example, about substance use, cigarette smoking, availability of firearms, and comorbid medical conditions—is an important first step toward prevention-minded clinical care.

4. **For patients with established psychiatric illness, important goals include the prevention of relapse, substance abuse, suicide, and adverse behaviors that are associated with the development of physical illnesses.** An important principle of prevention in the clinical setting, when working with patients with psychiatric disorders, is a focus on relapse prevention. This is exemplified by the fact that more than 30% of those with a psychotic episode discontinue their treatment in the first year, and this increases the risk of relapse fivefold (Cooper et al. 2007; Robinson et al. 1999). Relapse prevention can be advanced in the clinical setting through psychoeducation and psychosocial methods of promoting medication adherence. Long-acting injectable antipsychotics can also be helpful with medication adherence in patients who prefer them. Regarding depression, continuation treatment is indicated for individuals with repeated episodes of depression in order to prevent relapse. As Dr. Thomas Insel (Director of the National Institute of Mental Health) noted: "While research develops transformative information and tools for preemption, we need more effective implementation of currently available treatments to

ensure the best outcomes. In the near-term, preventing relapse will have the greatest impact on public health." (Insel 2008, p. 14).

Every patient receiving mental health care should be screened for comorbid substance use disorders and should be periodically rescreened. Likewise, those in treatment for substance use disorders should be screened for comorbid psychiatric conditions, especially mood and anxiety disorders. Epidemiological research (Kessler et al. 2005b) shows that comorbidity is extensive, and patients often have multiple disorders, not just a single psychiatric disorder together with a single substance use disorder. In fact, approximately 45% of individuals with one mental disorder meet criteria for two or more disorders (National Institute of Mental Health 2005).

Obviously, given that an increased risk of suicide is associated with the presence of mental illnesses—including depression, bipolar disorder, psychotic disorders, personality disorders, and substance use disorders— ongoing screening for suicidality among psychiatric patients is of paramount importance. A detailed discussion of suicide prevention is provided in Chapter 8 ("Suicide Prevention").

Another important prevention goal is inquiring about, and then addressing, adverse behaviors that have physical health consequences. These include poor diet, physical inactivity, and cigarette smoking. This is particularly crucial given that many psychopharmacological agents can lead to weight gain and adversely affect metabolic indices. Guidelines are available for routine and regular screening of waist circumference, weight, body mass index, fasting lipid and glucose levels, and other laboratory measures (American Diabetes Association et al. 2004). Also important is the assessment of risky sexual behaviors, which are associated with human immunodeficiency virus infection (as is intravenous substance abuse) and other sexually transmitted diseases.

5. **Clinic-based prevention efforts should focus on family members of individuals with psychiatric illnesses in addition to established patients themselves.** Given the high heritability estimates for many mental illnesses, relatives of patients in psychiatric care can be considered an at-risk population deserving of prevention efforts. That is, many family members of patients with established mental illnesses or substance use disorders are at elevated risk for psychiatric disorders themselves. When working

with adult psychiatric patients who have children, it is critical to be aware of potentially evolving symptoms in the children that may warrant a referral to family therapy or a child and adolescent psychiatrist. Additionally, parenting skills is a topic of relevance for all adult patients with children. Evaluation of family dynamics should include an assessment of violence within the family (including intimate partner violence, child abuse, and elder abuse), a topic discussed in detail in Chapter 9, "Preventing Family Violence."

A growing body of research indicates that the children of depressed mothers may have improved outcomes by participating in a preventive intervention focused specifically on this high-risk group. For example, Clarke and colleagues (2001) conducted a randomized, controlled trial aimed at preventing depressive episodes in adolescent offspring of adults treated for depression in a health maintenance organization setting. Participants eligible for the intervention had subthreshold depressive symptoms but did not meet criteria for a past or present mood disorder. The 94 youths were randomly assigned to either receive usual care or receive usual care and participate in a 15-session, group-based cognitive therapy prevention program (the intervention condition), and results revealed a lower incidence of major depression at 12-month follow-up in the intervention condition group. Similarly, the Keeping Families Strong program, designed to promote resilience and reduce the risk of psychological disorders, also focuses on children of parents with depression. That program is conducted in outpatient mental health care settings and consists of 10 meetings, with a group for parents and a group for the children, which are conducted concurrently (Riley et al. 2008).

6. **Primary and secondary prevention often takes place in schools, the workplace, and community settings.**

Schools, colleges, and universities. Many prevention goals are best addressed during childhood and adolescence; school settings therefore serve as important sites for diverse prevention activities. Kellam and colleagues recently published a series of articles on their Good Behavior Game (GBG), a school-based preventive intervention (Kellam et al. 2008; Petras et al. 2008; Poduska et al. 2008; Wilcox et al. 2008). GBG is a universal preventive intervention implemented by teachers and directed toward entire first- and second-grade classrooms. Risk factors that are addressed include aggressive and disruptive classroom behavior. Recent studies by Kellam and colleagues were conducted in 41 classrooms in 19 schools in Baltimore, and another cohort was subsequently assessed (from the same classrooms in the subsequent academic year) to allow for replication. They found that male students with aggressive and disruptive behavior who had participated in GBG demonstrated long-term improvements (i.e., at ages 19–21) compared with those in standard setting (control) classrooms—lower rates of alcohol and drug use disorders, cigarette smoking, violent and criminal behaviors, antisocial personality disorder, and suicidal ideation.

Another example of an evidence-based prevention practice in the school setting is the Signs of Suicide (SOS) program, in which high school students are screened online and referred for help when appropriate (Aseltine et al. 2007). SOS incorporates two prominent suicide prevention strategies into a single program—a curriculum designed to raise awareness of depression, suicide, and related issues, and a brief screening for depression and other suicide risk factors, especially underlying mental illnesses and substance abuse. The curriculum includes a video, which depicts signs of depression and suicide and ways to respond to someone who may be depressed or suicidal, as well as a discussion guide. The brief screening tool is completed anonymously and scored by the student. The basic goal of the SOS program is to teach high school students to respond to signs of suicide in themselves and others and to follow appropriate steps to respond to those signs. SOS, the only universal school-based suicide preventive intervention that has demonstrated significant effects in a randomized, controlled trial, significantly lowers rates of suicide attempts and increases adaptive attitudes about depression and suicide in students.

Some colleges provide basic mental health education to selected students, such as resident assistants, to foster early identification of students with developing mental health problems and to facilitate referral to appropriate treatment. Other colleges and universities provide *gatekeeper training* to school personnel (i.e., individuals on campus who come into daily contact with students). A commonly used suicide prevention practice on college campuses is the Question, Persuade, and Refer (QPR) program, which teaches about the risk factors and signs of depression and suicide and recommends steps to take to refer someone who needs help. Such training has been shown to increase self-reported knowledge, appraisals of efficacy, and service access (Wyman et al. 2008). Although this program has not been rigorously evaluated to determine whether it actually decreases suicides or suicide attempts on campuses (a relatively rare event), the QPR program appears on the Best Practices Registry of the Suicide Prevention Resource Center (2008).

The workplace. Some prevention efforts are best suited for the workplace. For example, drug and alcohol use in the workplace can be a serious threat to health, safety, and productivity; PeerCare is a workplace-based peer intervention program that centers on substance use on the job or outside the job that affects job performance (Miller et al. 2007). This program effectively trains workers to recognize the signs of substance abuse and refer coworkers whom they suspect may have a problem with substances. Participation in the program was associated with a significant reduction in injury rates at the company where the program was studied (Spicer and Miller 2005). Employee Assistance Programs (Chan et al. 2004; Merrick et al. 2007; Teich and Buck 2003; Zarkin et al. 2000), another approach, initially addressed substance abuse in the workplace but have expanded their role to provide health education, reduce stress and depressive symptoms, and address aggression and violence in the workplace. Other examples of prevention in the workplace include a focus on disruptive physicians in the health care setting (Ramsay 2001; Wilhelm and Lapsley 2000) and programs to promote physical exercise among company employees (Proper et al. 2003; Sloan and Gruman 1988; Yancey et al. 2004).

The community. In many respects, prevention is an activity best accomplished in the community rather than in the clinic. Modern prevention science suggests that communities should implement prevention programs based on their own needs and goals. Communities That Care is a system that mobilizes community stakeholders to collaborate on implementing evidence-based prevention programs based on that community's profile of risk factors and needs (Hawkins et al. 2008). For example, programs aimed at reducing adolescent health and behavior problems are selected by the community coalition from a menu of proven school- and community-based interventions. The Communities That Care system works with communities (e.g., through training and technical assistance to mobilize a prevention coalition including diverse stakeholders) to select one or more evidence-based preventive intervention(s), implement the intervention(s) with fidelity, and measure related outcomes (Hawkins et al. 2008).

Many prevention activities take place in broad community settings or at the level of the entire population. For example, legislative and policy actions enforcing restrictions on selling alcohol to minors decrease their access to alcohol, thus limiting early initiation of drinking. After-school programs that promote extracurricular activities and engage positive role models can have positive impacts in the community (Roth and Brooks-Gunn 2003; Zaff et al. 2003). For the elderly population, social outlets and community centers decrease isolation, which may be a risk factor for depression. An evidence-based program, the Widows to Widows Program, provided support to new widows by pairing them with long-term widows. At 12 months, the new widows in the intervention group were significantly more likely to feel better than at the time of their husband's death, to have made new friends, to be engaged in new activities, and to feel less anxious than members of the control group (Vachon et al. 1980). For people with serious and persistent mental illnesses, drop-in centers that promote social engagement can have tertiary prevention effects outside of the clinical setting.

Mental health professionals can have an influential role in these diverse prevention activities outside of the clinical practice setting. Providers can support and promote prevention programs in schools, the workplace, and other community settings. They can serve as consultants in the development of such programs, by serving on advisory boards or planning committees. Mental health professionals can play an important role in providing mental health education in community venues and through the media. They can also advocate for prevention programs within their communities.

7. **Mental health professionals have a role in achieving broad prevention goals (beyond the prevention of mental illnesses), such as the prevention of delinquency, bullying, and behavioral problems; the prevention of unwanted pregnancy, especially teenage pregnancy; and the prevention of intentional and unintentional injuries.** A number of prevention programs have addressed delinquency, bullying, conduct disorder, and behavioral problems. Although we previously discussed the importance of school set-

tings for achieving many prevention goals (principle 6), here we emphasize that many prevention activities, such as those taking place in schools, target diverse outcomes—not necessarily mental illnesses per se—and that mental health professionals have a role in achieving these broader goals. Early intervention programs that include planning, social reasoning, and other social objectives, such as the High/Scope Perry Preschool Program curriculum designed for children born in poverty, have been associated with reduced rates of misconduct and even of felony arrests, in adolescence and early adulthood (Schweinhart and Weikart 1997). Research also indicates that participants in the program completed more schooling, had higher rates of employment, and earned a higher income than nonparticipants (Schweinhart and Weikart 1993). When program costs were compared against treatment impacts on educational resources, earnings, criminal activity, and welfare receipt, the High/Scope Perry Preschool Program was found clearly to be cost-effective, largely due to reduced criminality by male participants (Belfield et al. 2006). In the latter study, the authors found that higher tax revenues, lower criminal justice system expenditures, and lower welfare payments outweighed program costs, repaying $12.90 for every dollar invested.

The Incredible Years teacher classroom management program and the child social and emotion curriculum (the Dinosaur School)—two parts of a universal prevention program for children enrolled in the Head Start program, kindergarten, or first-grade classrooms in schools selected because of high rates of poverty—have been shown to enhance school protective factors and reduce child and classroom risk factors (Webster-Stratton et al. 2008). Extensive work by Webster-Stratton and colleagues indicates that this universal prevention program reduces risk factors leading to delinquency by promoting social competence and school readiness, while reducing conduct problems (Webster-Stratton 1998; Webster-Stratton et al. 2001). These programs achieve results through cognitive social learning theory methods such as videotape modeling, role play and practice of targeted skills, and reinforcement of targeted behaviors (Webster-Stratton et al. 2008). The prevention of conduct disorder and other behavioral problems is discussed in detail in Chapter 10 ("Prevention Principles for Adolescents in Psychiatric Practice: Preventing Conduct Disorder and Other Behavioral Problems").

Regarding bullying, the Olweus school-based intervention program (Olweus 1994, 2003) has been shown to be effective. The program works to create a school environment with warmth, positive interest, and involvement from adults; firm limits on unacceptable behavior; consistent use of nonpunitive, nonphysical sanctions for violations of rules; and adults who act as authorities and positive role models (Olweus 2003). Schools in Scandanavia implemented studies against bullying, based on the Olweus program, in a large number of primary and secondary schools (third to ninth grades). Some of the results included marked reductions in bully/victim problems for the period studied, a 50% reduction in the number of students reporting being bullied or bullying others, and a clear reduction in general antisocial behavior over the course of about 8 months to 2½ years (relative to baseline or to comparison schools) (Olweus 1994, 2003).

Another area of prevention to which mental health professionals may contribute is the issue of teenage pregnancy. Research shows that teenage pregnancy is associated with adverse socioeconomic and health outcomes in both the young mothers and their offspring (Chandra et al. 2002; Elfenbein and Felice 2003; Fraser et al. 1995; Jaffee et al. 2001) and a higher incidence of preterm birth, which is a risk factor for neonatal mortality (Olausson et al. 1999). Obtaining a thorough sexual history, including inquiry about birth control measures, is indicated for all adolescents as well as adults. Family planning should also be discussed. Given the importance of maternal health and prenatal care in terms of prevention of diverse adverse outcomes, pregnant patients and potentially pregnant patients need to be screened for adverse behaviors, such as prenatal tobacco, alcohol, and illicit drug use, and clinicians should counsel their patients accordingly. This is integral prevention-oriented work, even though prevention of psychiatric illnesses per se is not the ultimate goal.

Mental health professionals also have a role in the prevention of unintentional injuries such as those caused by motor vehicle accidents (in addition to addressing intentional injuries such as self-harm and suicide attempts). For example, it has been shown that untreated attention-deficit/hyperactivity disorder in adolescence and adulthood is associated with a much greater risk of problems related to driving, including increased traffic citations, motor vehicle crashes, and bodily injury related to such crashes (Barkley 2004). Furthermore, screening for alcohol use disorders, including inquiring about driving while under the influence of alcohol and the use of designated drivers, is not beyond the scope of discussion in routine psychiatric care. Many other examples could be given of ways in which mental health professionals can participate in broad prevention goals not necessarily tied to preventing particular mental illnesses.

8. **Mental health professionals can play a role in promoting mental health, overall health, and wellness.** According to the World Health Organization, the term *health* refers not just to the absence of disease, but to a "state of complete physical, mental and social well-being." *Mental health* is a "state of well-being in which the individual realizes his or her abilities, can cope with the normal stresses of life, can work productively and fruitfully, and is able to make a contribution to his or her community" (World Health Organization 2004b, p. 23). The term *mental health promotion* includes strategies and interventions that enable positive emotional adjustment and adaptive behavior. Thus, mental health promotion is somewhat different from mental illness prevention in that the former focuses on health, whereas the latter aims to avert onset of illness. Mental health promotion is a subset of health promotion more generally. In 1986, the Ottawa Charter for Health Promotion declared that *health promotion* is the process of enabling people to increase control over and improve their health (Ottawa Charter for Health Promotion 1986). The Charter describes fundamental conditions and resources that are prerequisites for health, including peace, shelter, education, food, income, a stable ecosystem, sustainable resources, and social justice and equity.

An authority in mental health promotion, the Victorian Health Promotion Foundation (VicHealth, in Victoria, Australia), aims to build the capabilities of organizations, communities, and individuals in ways that both 1) change social, economic, and physical environments so that they improve health for all, and 2) strengthen the understanding and the skills of individuals in ways that support their efforts to achieve and maintain health (VicHealth 2008). VicHealth's Mental Health Promotion Framework emphasizes the following determinants of mental health: social connectedness, freedom from discrimination and violence, and economic participation. Settings for promotion include: sports/recreational venues, the community, educational venues, the workplace, the arts/cultural/entertainment settings, and the health sector.

There are a number of ways that clinicians can promote mental health, overall health, and wellness. For example, proper sleep hygiene should be routinely encouraged, given evidence that inadequate sleep is associated not only with recurrent episodes of psychiatric illnesses, such as mania (Kasper and Wehr 1992; Wehr 1989), but also with being overweight or obese (Gangwisch et al. 2005) and with poor work performance (Davidhizar and Shearer 2000). In addition to promoting adequate sleep, mental health professionals should encourage routine exercise. Physical exercise is likely to improve mood (Lane and Lovejoy 2001; McLafferty et al. 2004; Timonen et al. 2002) in addition to having beneficial effects in terms of preventing chronic diseases such as cardiovascular disease, diabetes, and osteoporosis, as well as improving rehabilitation after injury or illness. Like encouraging adequate sleep and routine exercise, attention to stress reduction and patients' reactions to stressors is also a form of mental health promotion.

Prevention-Minded Clinical Practice

Given the existing challenges of psychiatric practice, is it really feasible to incorporate prevention principles into daily practice, thus becoming "prevention-minded"? We think so. Mental health professionals admittedly face challenges pertaining to the treatment of people with mental illnesses, especially in light of the fact that over a 12-month period, some 60% of those with a mental disorder get no treatment at all (National Institute of Mental Health 2005). Undertreatment is a particular problem in racial and ethnic minorities, the uninsured or underinsured, those living in poverty, the elderly, and other underserved groups. We recognize that challenges exist in terms of inadequate treatments and poor access to standard-of-care treatments for many psychiatric illnesses. Nonetheless, despite these ongoing challenges, we encourage mental health providers to actively seek to become prevention-minded. Incorporating the above eight principles into practice will promote a prevention-informed practice style.

Although mental health professionals typically provide treatment that can be thought of as tertiary prevention, these eight principles suggest ways to bring prevention into everyday practice. This work needs to be done in a developmentally and culturally informed manner. In primary care, recent trends have moved from a strictly treatment-focused approach to incorporating screening and prevention recommendations. The same should be true in the mental health arena. In daily practice, mental health professionals should inquire about risk factors and protective factors in patients' lives in addition to focusing on the presenting problem. Thus, mental health professionals should strive to be prevention-minded in all of their interactions with patients, their families, and the community.

Key Points

- The traditional public health classification of prevention, including primary, secondary, and tertiary prevention, can be applied in routine mental health care settings, as can the more recent Institute of Medicine classifications of selective and indicated preventive interventions.

- Universal preventive interventions occur primarily at the population level or in community settings, and mental health professionals can be involved in such programs through advocacy, policy making, public education, and community consultation. Schools, the workplace, and community settings are important arenas for prevention.

- Risk and protective factors should be assessed routinely in clinical practice.

- Psychiatrists and other mental health professionals have a role in achieving broad prevention goals, beyond the prevention of mental illnesses. These goals include the prevention of delinquency, bullying, and behavioral problems; the prevention of unintended pregnancy, especially teenage pregnancy; substance abuse prevention; and the prevention of intentional and unintentional injuries.

- Mental health professionals should consider screening, and providing preventive interventions when appropriate, for family members of patients with psychiatric illnesses.

- Every patient receiving mental health care should be screened for comorbid substance use disorders and physical illnesses, and rescreening should occur periodically. Likewise, those in treatment for substance use disorders should be screened for comorbid psychiatric conditions.

- Three ways that mental health professionals can promote mental health, overall health, and wellness—in addition to focusing on the treatment of mental illnesses—are: paying attention to their patients' sleep hygiene, encouraging regular physical activity, and aiding with stress reduction and coping skills.

- Mental health professionals should strive to be prevention-minded in all of their interactions with patients, their families, and the community.

References

American Diabetes Association, American Psychiatric Association, American Association of Clinical Endocrinologists, et al: Consensus development conference on antipsychotic drugs and obesity and diabetes. Diabetes Care 27:596–601, 2004

Aseltine RH Jr, James A, Schilling EA, et al: Evaluating the SOS suicide prevention program: a replication extension. BMC Public Health 7:161, 2007 DOI: 10.1186/1471-2458-7-161

Barkley RA: Driving impairments in teens and adults with attention-deficit/hyperactivity disorder. Psychiatr Clin North Am 27:233–260, 2004

Belfield CR, Nores M, Barnett S, et al: The High/Scope Perry Preschool Program: cost-benefit analysis using data from the age-40 follow-up. J Hum Resour 41:162–190, 2006

Casey DE, Haupt DW, Newcomer JW, et al: Antipsychotic-induced weight gain and metabolic abnormalities: implications for increased mortality in patients with schizophrenia. J Clin Psychiatry 65:4–18, 2004

Chan KK, Neighbors C, Marlatt GA: Treating addictive behaviors in the employee assistance program: implications for brief interventions. Addict Behav 29:1883–1887, 2004

Chandra PC, Schiavello HJ, Ravi B, et al: Pregnancy outcomes in urban teenagers. Int J Gynaecol Obstet 79:117–122, 2002

Chapman DP, Dube SR, Anda RF: Adverse childhood events as risk factors for negative mental health outcomes. Psychiatr Ann 37:359–364, 2007

Clarke GN, Hornbrook M, Lynch F, et al: A randomized trial of group cognitive intervention for preventing depression in adolescent offspring of depressed parents. Arch Gen Psychiatry 58:1127–1134, 2001

Conroy MB, Majchrzak NE, Regan S, et al: The association between patient-reported receipt of tobacco intervention at a primary care visit and smokers' satisfaction with their health care. Nicotine Tob Res 7 (suppl 1):S29–S34, 2005

Cooper D, Moisan J, Gregoire JP: Adherence to atypical antipsychotic treatment among newly treated patients: a population-based study in schizophrenia. J Clin Psychiatry 68:818–825, 2007

Cuijpers P, van Straten A, Smit F, et al: Preventing the onset of depressive disorders: a meta-analytic review of psychological interventions. Am J Psychiatry 165:1272–1280, 2008

Davidhizar R, Shearer R: Your best preparation for a good day's work: a good night's sleep. Health Care Manag 19:38–49, 2000

Durlak JA: Common risk and protective factors in successful prevention programs. Am J Orthopsychiatry 68:512–520, 1998

Eichler K, Puhan MA, Steurer J, et al: Prediction of first coronary events with the Framingham score: a systematic review. Am Heart J 153:722–731, 2007

Elfenbein DS, Felice ME: Adolescent pregnancy. Pediatr Clin North Am 50:781–800, 2003

Felitti VJ, Anda RF, Nordenberg D, et al: Relationship of childhood abuse and household dysfunction to many of the leading causes of death in adults: the Adverse Childhood Experiences (ACE) Study. Am J Prev Med 14:245–258, 1998

Fraser AM, Brockert JE, Ward RH: Association of young maternal age with adverse reproductive outcomes. N Engl J Med 332:1113–1118, 1995

Gangwisch JE, Malaspina D, Boden-Albala B, et al: Inadequate sleep as a risk factor for obesity: analyses of the NHANES I. Sleep 28:1289–1296, 2005

Hawkins JD, Catalano RF, Kosterman R, et al: Preventing adolescent health-risk behaviors by strengthening protection during childhood. Arch Pediatr Adolesc Med 153:226–234, 1999

Hawkins JD, Catalano RF, Arthur MW, et al: Testing communities that care: the rationale, design, and behavioral baseline equivalence of the community youth development study. Prev Sci 9:178–190, 2008

Insel TR: From prevention to preemption: a paradigm shift in psychiatry. Psychiatric Times 25:13–14, 2008

Institute of Medicine: Reducing Risks for Mental Disorders: Frontiers for Preventive Intervention Research. Edited by Mrazek PJ, Haggerty RJ. Washington, DC, National Academy Press, 1994

Jaffee S, Caspi A, Moffitt TE, et al: Why are children born to teen mothers at risk for adverse outcomes in young adulthood?: results from a 20-year longitudinal study. Dev Psychopathol 13:377–397, 2001

Kasper S, Wehr TA: The role of sleep and wakefulness in the genesis of depression and mania. Encephale 18:45–50, 1992

Katz DL: Epidemiology, Biostatistics, and Preventive Medicine Review. New York, WB Saunders, 1997

Kellam SG, Brown CH, Poduska JM, et al: Effects of a universal classroom behavior management program in first and second grades on young adult behavioral, psychiatric, and social outcomes. Drug Alcohol Depend 95 (suppl 1):S5–S28, 2008

Kessler RC, Berglund P, Demler O, et al: Lifetime prevalence and age-of-onset distributions of DSM-IV disorders in the National Comorbidity Survey Replication. Arch Gen Psychiatry 62:593–602, 2005a

Kessler RC, Chiu WT, Demler O, et al: Prevalence, severity, and comorbidity of 12-month DSM-IV disorders in the National Comorbidity Survey Replication. Arch Gen Psychiatry 62:617–627, 2005b

Koplan C, Charuvastra A, Compton MT, et al: Prevention psychiatry. Psychiatr Ann 37:319–328, 2007

Lane AM, Lovejoy DJ: The effects of exercise on mood changes: the moderating effect of depressed mood. J Sports Med Phys Fitness 41:539–545, 2001

Last JM (ed): A Dictionary of Epidemiology, 4th Edition. New York, Oxford University Press, 2001

McLafferty CL Jr, Wetzstein CJ, Hunter GR: Resistance training is associated with improved mood in healthy older adults. Percept Mot Skills 98 (3 pt 1):947–957, 2004

Merrick ES, Volpe-Vartanian J, Horgan CM, et al: Revisiting employee assistance programs and substance use problems in the workplace: key issues and a research agenda. Psychiatr Serv 58:1262–1264, 2007

Miller TR, Zaloshnja E, Spicer RS: Effectiveness and benefit-cost of peer-based workplace substance abuse prevention coupled with random testing. Accident Analysis and Prevention 39:565–573, 2007

Nasrallah HA, Newcomer JW: Atypical antipsychotics and metabolic dysregulation: evaluating the risk/benefit equation and improving the standard of care. J Clin Psychopharmacol 24 (suppl 1):S7–S14, 2004

National Institute of Mental Health: Mental illness exacts heavy toll, beginning in youth. June 6, 2005. Available at: http://www.nimh.nih.gov/science-news/2005/mental-illness-exacts-heavy-toll-beginning-in-youth.shtml. Accessed November 17, 2008.

Olausson PO, Cnattingius S, Haglund B: Teenage pregnancies and risk of late fetal death and infant mortality. Br J Obstet Gynaecol 106:116–121, 1999

Olweus D: Bullying at school: basic facts and effects of a school based intervention program. J Child Psychol Psychiatry 35:1171–1190, 1994

Olweus D: A profile of bullying at school. Educ Leadersh 60:12–17, 2003

Ottawa Charter for Health Promotion: First International Conference on Health Promotion, November 1986. Available at: http://www.who.int/hpr/NPH/docs/ottawa_charter_hp.pdf. Accessed July 14, 2009.

Petras H, Kellam SG, Brown CH, et al: Developmental epidemiological courses leading to antisocial personality disorder and violent and criminal behavior: effects by young adulthood of a universal preventive intervention in first- and second-grade classrooms. Drug Alcohol Depend 95 (suppl 1):S45–S59, 2008

Poduska JM, Kellam SG, Wang W, et al: Impact of the Good Behavior Game, a universal classroom-based behavior intervention, on young adult service use for problems with emotions, behavior, or drugs or alcohol. Drug Alcohol Depend 95 (suppl 1):S29–S44, 2008

Proper KI, Koning M, van der Beek AJ, et al: The effectiveness of worksite physical activity programs on physical activity, physical fitness, and health. Clin J Sport Med 13:106–117, 2003

Ramsay MAE: Conflict in the health care workplace. Proc (Bayl Univ Med Cent) 14:138–139, 2001

Riley AW, Valdez CR, Barrueco S, et al: Development of a family based program to reduce risk and promote resilience among families affected by maternal depression: theoretical basis and program description. Clin Child Fam Psychol Rev 11:12–29, 2008

Robinson D, Woerner MG, Alvir JM, et al: Predictors of relapse following response from a first episode of schizophrenia or schizoaffective disorder. Arch Gen Psychiatry 56:241–247, 1999

Roth JL, Brooks-Gunn J: Youth development programs: risk, prevention and policy. J Adolesc Health 32:170–182, 2003

Rutter M: Protective factors in children's responses to stress and disadvantage. Ann Acad Med Singapore 8:324–338, 1979

Schweinhart LJ, Weikart DP: Success by empowerment: the High/Scope Perry Preschool Study through age 27. Young Child 49:54–58, 1993

Schweinhart LJ, Weikart DP: The High/Scope Preschool Curriculum Comparison Study through age 23. Early Child Res Q 12:117–143, 1997

Shprintzen RJ, Higgins AM, Antshel K, et al: Velo-cardio-facial syndrome. Curr Opin Pediatr 17:725–730, 2005

Sloan RP, Gruman JC: Participation in workplace health promotion programs: the contribution of health and organizational factors. Health Educ Behav 15:269–288, 1988

Spicer RS, Miller TR: Impact of a workplace peer-focused substance abuse prevention and early intervention program. Alcohol Clin Exp Res 29:609–611, 2005

Suicide Prevention Resource Center: Best Practices Registry (BPR) for suicide prevention: Section III: Adherence to standards. Available at: http://www.sprc.org/featured_resources/bpr/standards.asp. Accessed November 29, 2008.

Teich JL, Buck JA: Datapoints: Mental health services in employee assistance programs, 2001. Psychiatr Serv 54:611, 2003

Timonen L, Rantanen T, Timonen TE, et al: Effects of a group-based exercise program on the mood state of frail older women after discharge from hospital. Int J Geriatr Psychiatry 17:1106–1111, 2002

Vachon ML, Lyall WA, Rogers J, et al: A controlled study of self-help intervention for widows. Am J Psychiatry 137:1380–1384, 1980

Victorian Health Promotion Foundation: VicHealth. Available at: http://www.vichealth.vic.gov.au. Accessed November 17, 2008.

Webster-Stratton C: Preventing conduct problems in Head Start children: strengthening parenting competencies. J Consult Clin Psychol 66:715–730, 1998

Webster-Stratton C, Reid MJ, Hammond M: Preventing conduct problems, promoting social competence: a parent and teacher training partnership in head start. J Clin Child Psychol 30:283–302, 2001

Webster-Stratton C, Jamila Reid M, Stoolmiller M: Preventing conduct problems and improving school readiness: evaluation of the Incredible Years Teacher and Child Training Programs in high-risk schools. J Child Psychol Psychiatry 49:471–488, 2008

Wehr TA: Sleep loss: a preventable cause of mania and other excited states. J Clin Psychiatry 50(suppl):8–16, discussion 45–47, 1989

Wilcox HC, Kellam SG, Brown CH, et al: The impact of two universal randomized first- and second-grade classroom interventions on young adult suicide ideation and attempts. Drug Alcohol Depend 95 (suppl 1):S60–S73, 2008

Wilhelm KA, Lapsley H: Disruptive doctors: unprofessional interpersonal behaviour in doctors. Med J Aust 173:384–386, 2000

World Health Organization: Prevention of Mental Disorders: Effective Interventions and Policy Options. Summary Report. Geneva, World Health Organization, 2004a. Available at: http://www.who.int/mental_health/evidence/en/prevention_of_mental_disorders_sr.pdf. Accessed July 14, 2009.

World Health Organization: Promoting Mental Health: Concepts, Emerging Evidence, Practice. Summary Report. Geneva, World Health Organization, 2004b. Available at: http://www.who.int/mental_health/evidence/en/promoting_mhh.pdf. Accessed July 14, 2009.

Wyman PA, Brown CH, Inman J, et al: Randomized trial of a gatekeeper program for suicide prevention: 1-year impact on secondary school staff. J Consult Clin Psychol 76:104–115, 2008

Yancey AK, McCarthy WJ, Taylor WC, et al: The Los Angeles Lift Off: a sociocultural environmental change intervention to integrate physical activity into the workplace. Prev Med 38:848–856, 2004

Zaff JF, Moore KA, Papillo AR, et al: Implications of extracurricular activity participation during adolescence on positive outcomes. J Adolesc Res 18:599–630, 2003

Zarkin GA, Bray JW, Qi J: The effect of Employee Assistance Programs use on healthcare utilization. Health Serv Res 35:77–100, 2000

2

Identifying and Understanding Risk Factors and Protective Factors in Clinical Practice

Anne Shaffer, Ph.D.

Tuppett M. Yates, Ph.D.

Historically, psychiatry, psychology, and related disciplines have focused on disease mitigation, deficit reduction, and health restoration, to the relative exclusion of competence promotion and health maintenance. Similarly, early efforts to understand the development of psychopathology emphasized sources of risk and vulnerability for disorders, rather than those of strength and protection. This chapter adds to the growing effort to restore this balance by reviewing the extant literature on risk factors and protective factors in development and psychopathology, with the ultimate aim of informing emerging models of strengths-based, integrative approaches to clinical practice. Our review is not specific to a particular mental health outcome (e.g., depression, anxiety, antisocial behavior) or prevention effort (i.e., primary, secondary, or tertiary prevention, or universal, selective, or indicated preventive interventions; see Cowen 2000; Institute of Medicine 1994). Instead, we provide a conceptual introduction to the study of risk and protection, and we conclude with suggestions regarding the applications of these concepts in clinical practice.

Risk Factors: Predicting Maladjustment and Pathology

The field of mental health is plagued by the manifold challenges of uncovering the causes of psychiatric disorders and of predicting low-base-rate phenomena such as individual mental illnesses. Early efforts in this vein focused on the identification of *high-risk individuals*, those for whom the probability of a particular disorder was heightened as a function of identifiable (and quantifiable) risk factors. Research on the offspring of schizophrenic parents exemplifies this model, wherein youth deemed to be at risk due to parental psychopathology were followed across time to identify factors associated with the appearance (or avoidance) of schizophrenia (Garmezy 1974; Sameroff et al. 1987; Watt et al. 1984).

Risk factors are variables that are associated with an increased probability of negative outcomes. These are characteristics of individuals, environments, or communities that directly or indirectly contribute to maladaptation. In addition, the same risk factor may have both direct and indirect effects. Low birth weight, for example, is directly associated with a number of physical health problems, but the effects of low birth weight on psychosocial maladaptation may be indirect, mediated by the effects that such infants' difficulty being soothed may have on parents' behaviors toward their infants. *Vulnerability factors* are similar to risk factors in that, they too, increase the probability of negative outcomes, but the negative influence of vulnerability factors interacts with context, such that their strength is magnified in contexts of risk or adversity (Masten and Garmezy 1985). For example, poor emotion regulation skills may be especially likely to lead to maladaptation in stressful or chaotic environments.

Risk factors have been identified and studied at multiple levels of analysis, including at the individual level, at the family level, and in broader social/cultural context (Table 2–1). Common individual-level risk factors include low IQ, premature birth, high stress reactivity, and low educational attainment (i.e., school dropout). Some of these factors represent inherent vulnerabilities (e.g., genetic polymorphisms) that are not likely targets for intervention due to the difficulties or impossibilities of altering them. However, from an intervention and prevention perspective, it is important to be aware of risk factors, even those that are not likely to respond to intervention. These factors can indicate individuals who are most in need of prevention efforts, or who may require modification of interventions to address their particular vulnerabilities. Other risk factors are reflective of life experiences that may themselves be preventable (e.g., school dropout, unemployment), but engender risk of further maladaptation once they have occurred.

Table 2–1. Examples of risk factors in multiple contexts

Individual-level risk factors

Low educational attainment

Stress reactivity

Cognitive disabilities; below-average intelligence

History of premature birth

Genetic liabilities

Family-level risk factors

Maternal age at birth of child

Loss of caregiver or disruption of care

Maltreatment; poor parenting quality

Single parenthood

Parental substance abuse or psychopathology

Intrafamilial conflict

Sociocultural-level risk factors

Neighborhood violence or disorder

Poverty, unemployment, or homelessness

War, political violence

Discrimination

Family-level factors that are associated with an increased risk of mental health problems are numerous and well documented and include parenting quality (Harnish et al. 1995), family violence and maltreatment (Cicchetti and Lynch 1995; Yates et al. 2003a), and parental mental illness or substance abuse (Field 1998; Luthar et al. 1998), among others. Again, many of these so-called risk factors are also the target of some prevention efforts themselves, such as programs designed to prevent maltreatment or to support the early identification of postpartum depression. Beyond individual and family factors, aspects of the individual's broader social or cultural context may enhance the risk of negative outcomes, including associations with deviant peers (Patterson et al. 2000; Snyder et al. 2005), neighborhood violence or deprivation (Leventhal and Brooks-Gunn 2000; Limber and Nation 1998), and political unrest or war (Pine et al. 2005).

As suggested by the interactions of risk and vulnerability factors, contemporary risk research emphasizes the dynamic nature of risk across time and context. Risk factors rarely occur in isolation, and their meaning may change across the developmental continuum. Although there are some examples of specificity in the relations between risk factors and later psychopathology, such as the experience of early and extensive trauma with dissociative disorders, or high familial expressed emotion and schizophrenia (Butzlaff and Hooley 1998; Goodwin and Sachs 1996), most disorders do not evidence such specificity in causal risk factors. Thus, early efforts to identify individual, disease-specific risk factors were quickly supplanted by cumulative risk models, which incorporate the natural comorbidity of risk and attend to the consistent lack of specificity between specific risk factors and individual negative outcomes. Cumulative risk indices reflect the total number of risk and vulnerability factors affecting the development and functioning of an individual, family, or population (Sameroff 2006; Werner and Smith 1982; Zeanah et al. 1997). These models consistently reveal *risk gradients*, wherein the number of risk factors robustly predicts negative outcomes, including mental health disorders (Appleyard et al. 2005; Rutter 1979; Sameroff and Chandler 1975). These risk gradients reflect the well-recognized nature of risk factors—that they tend to co-occur rather than to exist in isolation—and understanding risk in context is critical to effective interventions. Furthermore, contextualizing patients' problems requires a recognition of the multiple levels at which risk occurs, including the community level and the systems involved (e.g., education, social services), as well as sociocultural variations in the impact of risk factors.

Issues of measurement and definition are central to the accurate and effective specification of risk status. As can be seen in Table 2–1, some risk factors appear readily quantifiable because they are naturally dichotomous (e.g., premature birth, homelessness, death of a parent or other caregiver). Yet even these seemingly straightforward risks may exert differential effects on development depending on their timing, context, and duration. For example, the death of a parent in childhood is readily determined as present or absent, but a more nuanced understanding of risk acknowledges that the impact of this risk factor may vary as a function of the age at which the loss occurred, the nature of the relationship with the deceased caregiver, the quality of the relationship with the remaining caregiver(s), and the surrounding familial and cultural context within which the loss occurred; the importance of considering developmental timing in particular is discussed later in the chapter (in the "Developmental Timing" section). If seemingly dichotomous risks prove nuanced, the challenge is even more striking for risks that can have a range of values (e.g., maternal age at the birth of a child, family income). In these instances, cut points frequently define the threshold for risk. Specifying a cut point may be informed by normative or objective data, such as known levels at which certain factors carry higher risk. Alternatively, cut points may be established based on individual samples, by a median split or a particular percentile rank, which is common practice in research studies. Cut points that are specific to samples are less preferable, due to issues with generalizability to other samples, but are often unavoidable (Obradovic et al., in press).

Despite multiple challenges in the identification and quantification of risk, cumulative risk indices afford multiple advantages in understanding the processes by which risk factors affect development, both by capturing the reality of co-occurring risk factors and by creating a statistically powerful way of measuring risk in natural environments (Bronfenbrenner 1994; Masten and Coatsworth 1998). Just as the accumulation of risk and vulnerability factors increases the likelihood of maladaptation, the elimination or reduction of such factors reduces the probability of negative outcomes. Thus, the identification of risk factors is critical to effective prevention, as knowledge regarding what increases the likelihood of a certain (negative) outcome, such as a mental health disorder, is the first step toward preventing that outcome (Durlak 1998).

Clinicians must attend to risk factors, in terms of both the broad developmental risks described above and the individual risks that may be salient for a given evaluation (e.g., expressed emotion in evaluating schizophrenia, loss or stressful life events in evaluating depression, prior behavior in evaluating suicidality). Yet, as alluded to earlier, contemporary clinical practice needs to advance beyond risk- and deficit-based models of maladaptation to integrate and embrace asset- and competence-based models of adaptation. For clinicians to attend *only* to risk factors is to miss a large part of the story of how psychopathology does, or does not, develop, which is often just as readily explained by the presence of strengths, or protective factors.

Protective Factors: Promoting Positive Development and Health

The study of strength and protection grew out of traditional risk research, in which a significant minority of individuals was observed to attain positive adjustment despite exposure to numerous risks and adverse experiences (Luthar 2006; Werner and Smith 1982). These individuals' developmental trajectories typify *resilience*, the dynamic developmental process wherein the individual is able to utilize resources within and outside of the self to negotiate current challenges adaptively and, by extension, to develop a foundation on which she or he can rely in the face of future challenges (Yates et al. 2003b). The growth of resilience research has fueled interest in understanding and facilitating positive developmental outcomes, in addition to predicting and ameliorating negative outcomes (Yates and Masten 2004a). Factors that are associated with positive development may include *assets*, which are generally positive influences for all individuals (e.g., high intelligence, good parenting quality) and are sometimes referred to as *promotive factors*. *Protective factors*, which are especially important for counteracting the deleterious impact of risk factors (e.g., positive adult role models outside the family, such as mentors), may also be called *compensatory factors* (Masten and Shaffer 2006).

Like risk and vulnerability factors, assets and protective factors operate across multiple contexts and levels of analysis (Table 2–2). Individual capacities such as emotion regulation, humor, and empathy (Eisenberg et al. 1997; Kestenbaum et al. 1989; Masten 1986) are complemented by family cohesion

Table 2–2.   Examples of protective factors in multiple contexts

Individual-level protective factors

Cognitive abilities; above-average intelligence

Positive self-perceptions, self-esteem

Sense of humor

Self-regulation skills (impulse control, coping, emotion regulation)

Family-level protective factors

Warm and supportive parenting or family relationships

Mentors or other adult role models

Sociocultural-level protective factors

High-quality educational opportunities

Socioeconomic advantage

Supportive relationships with peers or nonfamilial adults

and social influences such as peer relationships (Chen et al. 2003; Cumsille and Epstein 1994), as well as community-level influences such as school quality and neighborhood resources (Leventhal and Brooks-Gunn 2000; Ozer and Weinstein 2004; Pleibon and Kliewer 2001). Furthermore, a powerful but often overlooked protective factor is a history of prior positive adaptation. Development is cumulative such that current positive adaptation with respect to salient developmental issues will engender later competence (Yates et al. 2003b), and many domains of adaptation show evidence of continuity over time (Burt et al. 2008; Masten et al. 2005). In this way, the strength of protective processes (and also of risk processes) may be magnified across time by virtue of the cumulative nature of development (Sroufe 1979).

Identifying and evaluating assets and protective factors bring challenges that are similar to those already discussed with respect to risk and vulnerability factors. For example, some of the factors identified as assets or protective factors, such as parenting quality or IQ, exist on continua. In some cases, we may conceptualize one end of the continuum as risk and the other as protection, yet the meaning of the various points on the continuum may change with context (e.g., developmental timing, culture). Thus, assets and protective factors are more than mirror images of vulnerability factors and risk factors. Indeed, the very same construct may operate as a vulnerability factor in one context and as a protective factor in another. Determining whether a given variable operates as a risk factor, a protective factor, or both, can be a conceptual distinction but is often also an empirical question; by investigating how a variable relates to outcomes of interest at both high and low levels, its influence can be better understood (Stouthamer-Loeber et al. 2002). For example, the "action" of SES, as it relates to adjustment outcomes, may only be at low levels (i.e., poverty) or may occur along the entire SES gradient.

Contemporary research has revealed that individual factors (and their developmental impact) transact with developmental contexts (e.g., age, gender, culture) and levels of analysis (e.g., genetic, physiological, relational, cognitive, emotional) (Cicchetti and Curtis 2007). As knowledge and techniques in the fields of genetics and neuroimaging have improved, we have gained a better understanding of risk and protective processes that were previously considered difficult to detect or to change (Hanson and Gottesman 2007; Rutter 2006). For example, genes were once thought to be static and unidirectional markers of risk, as in adoption and twin studies that have shown a higher risk of disorders such as alcoholism among individuals more closely genetically related to someone with that disorder (e.g., Heath et al. 1997).

However, more recent findings from the field of behavioral genetics provide a more nuanced understanding of the dynamic interplay between genes and environment. For example, the work of Suomi (2000) with rhesus monkeys provides evidence of gene-environment interactions in allelic variations of the serotonin (5-hydroxytryptamine) transporter gene (*5-HTT*). Whereas individuals with a short allele *5-HTT* polymorphism were originally thought to be at higher risk of later problems, due to expected inefficiency in serotonergic function, Bennett and colleagues (1998) showed that the impact of the allelic variation was dependent on rearing environment. That is, in contexts of positive rearing by mothers, the polymorphism was associated with *higher* social status and lower aggression, whereas those reared by peers only (in contexts simulating neglectful care) showed *increased* aggression and *lower* social status. Other researchers have confirmed that the meaning of a given factor as compromising or promotive varies as a function of the caregiving milieu; this research has included studies with human populations (Caspi et al. 2002, 2003).

Similar variation may be seen across community and cultural contexts. For example, authoritarian, restrictive parenting has long been viewed as a risk factor in traditional family systems research (Baumrind 1968; Darling and Steinberg 1993). Yet research reveals that restrictive parenting operates as a protective factor in a high-risk setting, although it is negatively related to competence in a low-risk setting (Baldwin et al. 1990). Similarly, data suggest that the optimal level of maternal psychological and behavioral control varies as a function of the level of problem behaviors in the peer groups of African American adolescents (Mason et al. 1996). Extending this pattern to cross-cultural research, deVries's (1984) study of temperament and adaptation among Masai infants in East Africa provides an excellent example of the intersection of context and protection. Contrary to the widely held belief in Western cultures that an "easy" temperament is adaptive, a highly reactive temperament was found to be more successful in eliciting the care needed to foster survival in a sample of Masai infants. Although a comprehensive discussion of interaction effects is beyond the scope of this chapter, it is important to recognize that the influence of a given factor as either protective or vulnerability enhancing is moderated by the context in which it is embedded, and the developmental stage at which it is introduced. Amid these many challenges, the natural question becomes: How can we integrate our knowledge of risk and protective factors into contemporary clinical practice?

Empirical and Clinical Implications

As risk research has emphasized the multiplicative salience of cumulative risks, so too has intervention research begun to recognize the power of cumulative protection for mitigating the negative effects of risk and promoting wellness (Wyman et al. 2000; Yoshikawa 1994). These wellness-promotion models, as well as their risk-reduction counterparts, have clear applicability to clinical practice. Thus, clinicians are encouraged to attend to both presenting complaints and *presenting competencies*—that is, the individual strengths of each patient that are likely to influence the onset and course of a psychiatric disorder. These efforts will provide the clinician with a more comprehensive view of the patient's presenting problem in context, and may offer leverage to enhance positive adaptation and stave off negative outcomes.

However, the leading edge of these efforts rests at the translation point between research and practice, and between efforts to identify discrete predictors of subsequent outcomes and efforts to identify the developmental processes that mediate such outcomes. Despite the challenges of translating research into practice, prevention science remains an applied field that is explicitly tied to its basis in theoretical and empirical science (Cicchetti and Hinshaw 2002). From this foundation, several clear applications to the science and practice of prevention and intervention warrant mention.

Cause, Correlate, or Consequence?

Sometimes it may not be clear whether risk factors are correlates (proxies for other experiences) that relate to negative outcomes, or whether they are causal risk factors that actually engender the outcomes of interest (Kraemer et al. 2001). Prevention scientists have encouraged researchers who study risk and protective factors not to settle with mechanistic descriptions of which variables are statistically predictive of outcomes, but to develop more thorough contextual accounts of the factors that are evidently influential or causal (Biglan 2004). As noted above, this is particularly relevant for clinicians, who typically work with patients on an individual basis and can work to understand the specific context of risk and protection for each patient, recognizing that even the most statistically significant of risk factors may operate differently for each person.

It can also be difficult to ascertain whether risk factors represent actual experiences that are detrimental to development, or whether they serve as markers for the underlying or mediating processes by which the factors influence adaptation (Obradovic et al., in press). For example, economic strain in a family is often associated with poor outcomes for children, and thus is a commonly identified risk factor. However, studies that have focused more closely on the processes by which this factor leads to a child's maladaptation have found that the effects are actually mediated by the intervening effect that economic strain has on parental stress, which leads to lower parenting quality, in turn affecting the child's adaptation (Conger et al. 1994). Findings such as these emphasize that, beyond identifying factors associated with the increased likelihood of various outcomes, we must carefully consider the *processes* by which these associations occur.

Process-Oriented Research and Developmental Timing

An emphasis on the processes by which risk and protective factors influence the development of psychopathology has represented a large step forward from earlier correlational research that simply sought to detect associations among variables. In focusing on process in prevention science, the integration of developmental theory has been of primary importance (Cicchetti and Hinshaw 2002; Institute of Medicine 1994). Understanding developmental norms, understanding the processes by which risk and protective factors lead to developmental outcomes, and consideration of the timing and importance of developmental transitions are all critical in designing and implementing effective prevention programs (Cicchetti and Hinshaw 2002). Methodological advances, such as the implementation of large-scale, longitudinal studies and the availability of newer statistical methods such as multilevel modeling, have increased our understanding of how risk and protective factors work, and that they often work through intervening or indirect mechanisms. For clinicians, the implications of this research indicate that it is not enough to identify risk and protective factors, but to discover *how* these factors are influencing adaptation for a patient. The process by which risk and protective factors operate for each individual can vary, due to interactions with other environmental variables, the developmental stage of the patient, and the patient's history of prior adaptation in basic domains such as relationships, cognitions (i.e., patterns of thinking and sources of bias), and emotions (i.e., positive or negative affectivity and emotion regulation).

An awareness of developmental theories and norms is crucial to the implementation of prevention efforts. Certainly, a central tenet of prevention science holds that intervention and prevention efforts are more likely to be effective when they take place early, prior to the establishment of maladaptive pathways. Thus, developmental timing cannot be ignored in providing clinical services with maximal effectiveness (Farmer and Farmer 2001).

The targets of intervention and prevention efforts also change across development (Yates and Masten 2004b). During infancy and early childhood, clinical prevention efforts are focused largely on primary prevention. These prevention efforts seek to avert developmental pathways toward maladaptation. Areas of intervention in this developmental period may include bolstering parenting skills, improving the child's nutrition, and achieving school readiness. In middle childhood, many prevention efforts are school-based, because this is a primary context for development and functioning during this age period. Because academic achievement and peer relations are both highly salient domains during this age period, prevention strategies often focus on early identification of peer problems (such as bullying or aggression) or problems that interfere with school performance (such as attention-deficit/hyperactivity disorder or learning disorders). These prevention strategies may be characterized more as secondary prevention, initiated by the early identification of problems. As noted previously, these secondary prevention strategies may be most effective if they capitalize on existing protective factors or other areas of strength in prior development.

By adolescence, peers have become an even more dominant social influence and during this time preventive interventions may frequently focus on preventing delinquency or substance abuse by reducing negative peer influences. In addition, new developmental tasks, such as early romantic relationships and preparation for jobs or higher education, begin in adolescence. Following the transition to adulthood, prevention is more likely to be secondary or tertiary in nature, working to minimize incipient problems or prevent the relapse of psychopathology. However, the transition to parenting is one new context for many adults that may warrant the implementation of primary prevention efforts.

A consideration of developmental timing also draws attention to the windows of opportunity that can occur as particularly effective points for prevention or intervention. Developmental systems theory posits that, during times of change, a system is more unstable as it seeks a new homeostasis (Ford and Lerner 1992; Smith and Thelen 2003). These transitions result in a system that is vulnerable to outside influence, which includes the (presumably positive) influence of clinical interventions. Such transition points may be normative, such as starting school, or specific to individuals already treated for psychopathology, such as discharge from inpatient treatment.

Risk- and Resilience-Informed Intervention

In applying knowledge of risk and protective factors to intervention and clinical practice, several points bear additional emphasis. First, it is important to be cognizant of the differences between distal and proximal risk factors (Cicchetti and Hinshaw 2002). In general, there are more likely to be opportunities for intervention or amelioration when targeting proximal risk factors, which are "nearer" to the individual, such as cognitive/behavioral coping strategies, educational attainment, or emotion regulation skills. However, certain prevention efforts may choose to focus on more distal factors at the level of the social environment, such as the Head Start program (Garces et al. 2002) or the Abecedarian Project (Campbell et al. 2002), which seek to improve educational opportunities for children living in poverty. These projects are designed to yield "more bang for the buck," by targeting many individuals at once. However, as noted above, many distal risk or protective factors work through their indirect influence on intervening factors; careful consideration must therefore be given to the processes by which these factors effect change.

From resilience research, there is also a reminder that prevention efforts should focus not only on reducing negative outcomes but also on promoting competence and positive adaptation (Cicchetti and Hinshaw 2002; Cowen 2000). Adaptation occurs in multiple domains, although clinicians are too often trained to focus on domains in which their patients are not doing well. Identifying areas of strength will not only promote an individual's sense of self-worth but also likely mitigate the impact of risks. In addition, emphasizing wellness-promotion aspects of prevention efforts may be less stigmatizing than identifying at-risk populations for targeted interventions, which may increase the acceptance by communities and consumers that is necessary for program implementation.

Conclusion

Much of this chapter has reviewed the ways that science has informed clinical practice, yet it is important to mention that clinical practice can inform science as well. The complicated nature of human development and functioning in various contexts can be highly individualized, and a great deal about risk and resilience can be learned from case examples (Biglan 2004; Masten et al. 1990). As clinicians learn more about the lives-in-context of the individuals they are treating, they gain information and insight that can be used to refine the scientific findings and theories that were derived from broad samples and generalizable results.

The key points that we wish to emphasize in this chapter, regarding the nature of risk and resilience, unfortunately do not readily condense into quick lists that are easily memorized. Instead, the most enduring, and vexing, truth about the processes of risk and resilience is that they are immensely complicated and questions about how these processes work lack simple answers.

Mechanisms of risk and protection cannot be understood without capturing the context in which these processes unfold. Furthermore, contexts are dynamic and change over time, with the course of development or according to changing circumstances. Thus effective prevention efforts must focus not only on reducing risk factors and promoting protective factors, but on the *processes* by which these factors exert their influence on development and adaptation.

Key Points

- Clinicians must recognize that risk and protective factors exist and operate at multiple levels of analysis, including at the individual level, at the family level, and in broader social/cultural context. Furthermore, the influences and interactions between levels are frequently bidirectional in nature, as well as dynamically changing over time.

- Understanding context is critical to effective interventions—when clinicians learn about patients' presenting complaints, they must be understood in the broader context of risk and protection within which those complaints are embedded. This requires cultural competence and sensitivity to diversity, as well as understanding of the community and the various systems (e.g., social services, specialty medical care, educational systems) in which the patient is involved.

- Clinicians should attend to both presenting complaints *and* presenting competencies. That is, by asking patients and their families about their strengths, clinicians may gain a better, more useful picture of the presenting problem in context, and may open up avenues of change through intervention.

- *Processes* are key; it is critical to identify not only what is going on in patients' lives, but *how* it is going on. The *how* is critical to effective intervention, and these processes are often related to basic adaptive processes (relationships, cognitions, emotions). To the extent that we can restore, protect, or foster these processes, our practice will be improved.

- Consideration of developmental timing is necessary in understanding the context in which risk and protective factors operate. Risk and protective factors, as well as the processes by which they exert their effects, may vary over time. Similarly, the most appropriate targets of intervention and prevention efforts are likely to change across developmental stages.

References

Appleyard K, Egeland B, van Dulmen MHM, et al: When more is not better: the role of cumulative risk in child behavior outcomes. J Child Psychol Psychiatry 46:235–245, 2005

Baldwin AL, Baldwin C, Cole RE: Stress-resistant families and stress-resistant children, in Risk and Protective Factors in the Development of Psychopathology. Edited by Rolf J, Masten AS, Cicchetti D, et al. New York, Cambridge University Press, 1990, pp 257–280

Baumrind D: Authoritarian vs. authoritative parental control. Adolescence 3:255–272, 1968

Bennett AJ, Lesch KP, Heils A, et al: Serotonin transporter gene variation, strain, and early rearing environment affect CSF 5-HIAA concentrations in rhesus monkeys (*Macaca mulatta*). Am J Primatol 45:168–169, 1998

Biglan A: Contextualism and the development of effective prevention practices. Prev Sci 5:15–21, 2004

Bronfenbrenner U: Ecological models of human development, in The International Encyclopedia of Education, 2nd Edition. Edited by Husen T, Postlewhaite TTN. New York, Elsevier, 1994, pp 1643–1647

Burt KB, Obradovic J, Long JD, et al: The interplay of social competence and psychopathology over 20 years: testing transactional and cascade models. Child Dev 79:359–374, 2008

Butzlaff RL, Hooley JM: Expressed emotion and psychiatric relapse. Arch Gen Psychiatry 55:547–552, 1998

Campbell FA, Ramey CT, Pungello E, et al: Early childhood education: young adult outcomes from the Abecedarian Project. Applied Developmental Science 6:42–57, 2002

Caspi A, McClay J, Moffitt TE, et al: Role of genotype in the cycle of violence in maltreated children. Science 297:851–853, 2002

Caspi A, Sugden K, Moffitt TE, et al: Influence of life stress on depression: moderation by a polymorphism in the 5-HTT gene. Science 301:386–389, 2003

Chen X, Chang L, He Y: The peer group as a context: mediating and moderating effects on relations between academic achievement and social functioning in Chinese children. Child Dev 74:710–727, 2003

Cicchetti D, Curtis WJ (eds): Development and Psychopathology, Special Issue: A Multilevel Approach to Resilience, Vol 19. New York, Cambridge University Press, 2007

Cicchetti D, Hinshaw SP: Editorial: prevention and intervention science: contributions to developmental theory. Dev Psychopathol 14:667–671, 2002

Cicchetti D, Lynch M: Failures in the expectable environment and their impact on child development: the case of child maltreatment, in Developmental Psychopathology: Risk, Disorder, and Adaptation, Vol 12. Edited by Cicchetti D, Cohen D. New York, Wiley, 1995, pp 32–71

Coie JD, Watt NF, West SG, et al: The science of prevention: a conceptual framework and some directions for a national research program. Am Psychol 48:1013–1022, 1993

Conger RD, Ge X, Elder GH, et al: Economic stress, coercive family process, and developmental problems of adolescents. Child Dev 65:541–561, 1994

Cowen E: Now that we all know that primary prevention in mental health is great, what is it? J Community Psychol 28:5–16, 2000

Cumsille PE, Epstein N: Family cohesion, family adaptability, social support, and adolescent depressive symptoms in outpatient clinic families. J Fam Psychol 8:202–214, 1994

Darling N, Steinberg L: Parenting style as context: an integrative model. Psychol Bull 113:487–496, 1993

deVries MW: Temperament and infant mortality among the Masai of East Africa. Am J Psychiatry 141:1189–1194, 1984

Durlak JA: Common risk and protective factors in successful prevention programs. Am J Orthopsychiatry 68:512–520, 1998

Eisenberg N, Guthrie IK, Fabes RA, et al: The relations of regulation and emotionality to resiliency and competent social functioning in elementary school children. Child Dev 68:295–311, 1997

Farmer TW, Farmer EMZ: Developmental science, systems of care, and prevention of emotional and behavioral problems in youth. Am J Orthopsychiatry 71:171–181, 2001

Field T: Maternal depression effects on infants and early intervention. Prev Med 27:200–203, 1998

Ford DH, Lerner RM: Developmental systems theory: an integrated approach. Newbury Park, CA, Sage, 1992

Garces E, Thomas D, Currie J: Longer-term effects of Head Start. American Economic Review 92:999–1012, 2002

Garmezy N: The study of competence in children at risk for severe psychopathology, in The Child in His Family: Children at Psychiatric Risk, Vol 3. Edited by Anthony EJ, Koupernik C. New York, Wiley, 1974, pp 77–97

Goodwin J, Sachs R: Child abuse in the etiology of dissociative disorders, in Handbook of Dissociation: Theoretical, Empirical, and Clinical Perspectives. Edited by Michelson LK, Ray WJ. New York, Plenum, 1996, pp 91–105

Hanson DR, Gottesman II: Choreographing genetic, epigenetic, and stochastic steps in the dances of developmental psychopathology, in Multilevel Dynamics in Developmental Psychopathology: Pathways to the Future. Edited by Masten AS. Mahwah, NJ, Erlbaum, 2007, pp 27–43

Harnish JD, Dodge KA, Valente E: Mother-child interaction quality as a partial mediator of the roles of maternal depressive symptomatology and socioeconomic status in the development of child behavior problems. Child Dev 66:739–753, 1995

Heath AC, Bucholz KK, Madden PAF, et al: Genetic and environmental contributions to alcohol dependence risk in a national twin sample: consistency of findings in women and men. Psychol Med 27:1381–1396, 1997

Institute of Medicine: Reducing Risks for Mental Disorders: Frontiers for Preventive Intervention Research. Washington, DC, National Academy Press, 1994

Kestenbaum R, Farber E, Sroufe LA: Individual differences in empathy among preschoolers: concurrent and predictive validity, in Empathy and Related Emotional Responses: No. 44: New Directions for Child Development. Edited by Eisenberg N. San Francisco, CA, Jossey-Bass, 1989, pp 51–56

Kraemer HC, Stice E, Kazdin AE, et al: How do risk factors work together?: mediators, moderators, and independent, overlapping, and proxy risk factors. Am J Psychiatry 158:848–856, 2001

Leventhal T, Brooks-Gunn J: The neighborhoods they live in: the effects of neighborhood residence on child and adolescent outcomes. Psychol Bull 126:309–337, 2000

Limber SP, Nation MA: Violence within the neighborhood and community, in Violence Against Children in the Family and the Community. Edited by Trickett PK, Schellenbach CJ. Washington, DC, American Psychological Association, 1998, pp 171–209

Luthar SS: Resilience in development: a synthesis of research across five decades, in Developmental Pyschopathology: Risk, Disorder, and Adaptation, 2nd Edition, Vol 3. Edited by Cicchetti D, Cohen D. New York, Wiley, 2006, pp 739–795

Luthar SS, Cushing G, Merikangas KR, et al: Multiple jeopardy: risk and protective factors among addicted mothers' offspring. Dev Psychopathol 10:117–136, 1998

Mason CA, Cauce AM, Gonzales N, et al: Neither too sweet nor too sour: problem peers, maternal control, and problem behavior in African American adolescents. Child Dev 67:2115–2130, 1996

Masten AS: Humor and competence in school-age children. Child Dev 57:461–473, 1986

Masten AS, Coatsworth JD: The development of competence in favorable and unfavorable environments. Am Psychol 53:205–220, 1998

Masten AS, Garmezy N: Risk, vulnerability, and protective factors in developmental psychopathology, in Advances in Clinical Child Psychology, Vol 8. Edited by Lahey BB, Kadin AE. New York, Plenum, 1985, pp 1–52

Masten AS, Shaffer A: How families matter in child development: reflections from research on risk and resilience, in Families Count: Effects on Child and Adolescent Development. Edited by Clarke-Stewart A, Dunn J. Cambridge, UK, Cambridge University Press, 2006, pp 5–25

Masten AS, Morison P, Pellegrini D, et al: Competence under stress: risk and protective factors, in Risk and Protective Factors in the Development of Psychopathology. Edited by Rolf J, Masten AS, Cicchetti D, et al. Cambridge, UK, Cambridge University Press, 1990, pp 236–256

Masten AS, Roisman GI, Long JD, et al: Developmental cascades: linking academic achievement and externalizing and internalizing symptoms over 20 years. Dev Psychol 41:733–746, 2005

Ozer EJ, Weinstein RS: Urban adolescents' exposure to community violence: the role of support, school safety, and social constraints in a school-based sample of boys and girls. J Clin Child Adolesc Psychol 33:463–476, 2004

Patterson GR, Dishion TJ, Yoerger K: Adolescent growth in new forms of problem behavior: macro- and micro-peer dynamics. Prev Sci 1:3–13, 2000

Pine DS, Costello J, Masten A: Trauma, proximity, and developmental psychopathology: the effects of war and terrorism on children. Neuropsychopharmacology 10:1–12, 2005

Pleibon LE, Kliewer W: Neighborhood types and externalizing behavior in urban school-age children: tests of direct, mediated, and moderated effects. J Child Fam Stud 10:419–437, 2001

Rutter M: Protective factors in children's responses to stress and disadvantage, in Primary Prevention of Psychopathology: Social Competence in Children. Edited by Kent MW, Rolf JE. Hanover, NH, University Press of New England, 1979, pp 49–74

Rutter M: How does the concept of resilience alter the study and understanding of risk and protective influences on psychopathology? Ann N Y Acad Sci 1094:1–12, 2006

Sameroff A: Identifying risk and protective factors for healthy child development, in Families Count: Effects on Child and Adolescent Development. Edited by Clark-Stewart A, Dunn J. Cambridge, UK, Cambridge University Press, 2006, pp 53–76

Sameroff AJ, Chandler MJ: Reproductive risk and the continuum of caretaking casualty, in Review of Child Development Research, Vol 4. Edited by Horowitz FD, Hetherington M, Scarr-Salapatek S, et al. Chicago, IL, Chicago University Press, 1975, pp 187–243

Sameroff AJ, Seifer R, Zax M, et al: Early indicators of developmental risk: Rochester Longitudinal Study. Schizophr Bull 13:383–394, 1987

Smith LB, Thelen E: Development as a dynamic system. Trends Cogn Sci 7:343–348, 2003

Snyder J, Schrepferman L, Oeser J, et al: Deviancy training and association with deviant peers in young children: occurrence and contribution to early onset conduct problems. Dev Psychopathol 17:397–413, 2005

Sroufe LA: The coherence of individual development: early care, attachment, and subsequent developmental issues. Am Psychol 34:834–841, 1979

Stouthamer-Loeber M, Loeber R, Wei E, et al: Risk and promotive effects in the explanation of persistent serious delinquency in boys. J Consult Clin Psychol 70:111–123, 2002

Suomi SJ: A biobehavioral perspective on developmental psychopathology: excessive aggression and serotonergic dysfunction in monkeys, in Handbook of Developmental Psychopathology, 2nd Edition. Edited by Sameroff AJ, Lewis M, Miller SM. New York, Kluwer Academic/Plenum, 2000, pp 237–256

Watt N, Anthony EJ, Wynne L, et al (eds): Children at Risk for Schizophrenia. New York, Cambridge University Press, 1984

Werner EE, Smith RS: Vulnerable But Invincible: A Longitudinal Study of Resilient Children and Youth. New York, McGraw-Hill, 1982

Wyman PA, Sandler I, Wolchik S, et al: Resilience as cumulative competence promotion and stress protection: theory and intervention, in The Promotion of Wellness in Children and Adolescents. Edited by Cicchetti D, Rappaport J, Sandler I, et al. Washington, DC, Child Welfare League of America, 2000, pp 133–184

Yates TM, Masten AS: Fostering the future: resilience theory and the practice of positive psychology, in Positive Psychology in Practice. Edited by Linley PA, Joseph S. Hoboken, NJ, Wiley, 2004a, pp 521–539

Yates TM, Masten AS: The promise of resilience research for practice and policy, in What Works? Building Resilience: Effective Strategies for Child Care Services. Edited by Newman T. Ilford, UK, Barnardo's, 2004b, pp 6–15

Yates TM, Dodds MF, Sroufe LA, et al: Exposure to partner violence and child behavior problems: a prospective study controlling for child physical abuse and neglect, child cognitive ability, socioeconomic status, and life stress. Dev Psychopathol 15:199–218, 2003a

Yates TM, Egeland B, Sroufe LA: Rethinking resilience: a developmental process perspective, in Resilience and Vulnerability: Adaptation in the Context of Childhood Adversities. Edited by Luthar SS. New York, Cambridge University Press, 2003b, pp 234–256

Yoshikawa H: Prevention as cumulative protection: effects of early family support and education on chronic delinquency and its risks. Psychol Bull 115:28–54, 1994

Zeanah CH, Boris NW, Larrieu JA: Infant development and developmental risk: a review of the past 10 years. J Am Acad Child Adolesc Psychiatry 36:165–178, 1997

3

Prevention of Mood Disorders

Christina P.C. Borba, M.P.H.

Benjamin G. Druss, M.D., M.P.H.

This chapter addresses the prevention of mood disorders, which are disturbances of emotion that affect an individual's life. The term *depression* is an umbrella term that encompasses many different forms of affective or mood disorders. All of them share certain characteristics. However, *unipolar depression* or *major depression* is manifested only by symptoms of depression, whereas *bipolar depression* represents depression in the context of a history of hypomania or mania (National Institute of Mental Health 2007). Unipolar depression can also encompass dysthymic disorder and depressive disorder not otherwise specified. Bipolar disorder is also known as manic-depressive disorder or sometimes bipolar affective disorder (National Institute of Mental Health 2007).

Epidemiology is the study of the distribution of disorders in the population but it also examines the etiology and course of diseases. The distribution of disorders is reported as *incidence* and *prevalence*, the former referring to the rate at which new cases of a disorder arise, and the latter meaning the proportion of the population with the disorder at a given point in time. Preventive interventions are directed toward reducing the incidence of a disorder, whereas treatment interventions seek to reduce the prevalence (Institute of Medicine 1994). Knowledge of the age at onset of a specific disorder is required in order to time an intervention appropriately—specifically, before the onset of the disorder—and these decisions can be guided by epidemiological data.

Overview of the Epidemiology of Mood Disorders

Major depressive disorder is a mood disorder characterized by one or more episodes of a depressed mood, lack of interest in activities normally enjoyed, changes in appetite or weight, sleep disturbances, fatigue, feelings of worthlessness and guilt, difficulty concentrating, and thoughts of death or suicide. The DSM-IV-TR criteria for a major depressive episode are presented in Table 3–1 (American Psychiatric Association 2000a). Depression is a common, serious illness, and most people who experience depression need treatment to get better. There is no single known cause of depression; rather, it likely results from a combination of genetic, biochemical, environmental, and psychological factors (National Institute of Mental Health 2007). As noted above, the term *unipolar depression* is used to distinguish it from depression that occurs within the context of bipolar disorder.

Depression is a leading cause of disability, accounting for 8% of the total disability-adjusted life years in the United States and being the fourth leading contributor to the global burden of disease in the year 2000 (Usdin et al. 2004). By the year 2020, depression is projected to become the second leading contributor to the global burden of disease for all ages and both sexes (Ustun et al. 2004). Depression is also associated with an increased mortality risk. In a meta-analysis, Cuijpers and Smit (2002) found that major depression was associated with a 1.81-fold increase in the odds of mortality across a range of community surveys. The Epidemiologic Catchment Area (ECA) study estimated the 1-month prevalence of a major depressive disorder to be between 1.7% and 3.4% across the five sites (Regier et al. 1988). The first National Comorbidity Survey (NCS), conducted from 1990 to 1992, reported a 1-month prevalence of a major depressive disorder of 4.9% in the national sam-

Table 3–1. DSM-IV-TR diagnostic criteria for major depressive episode

A. Five (or more) of the following symptoms have been present during the same 2-week period and represent a change from previous functioning; at least one of the symptoms is either (1) depressed mood or (2) loss of interest or pleasure.

Note: Do not include symptoms that are clearly due to a general medical condition, or mood-incongruent delusions or hallucinations.

(1) depressed mood most of the day, nearly every day, as indicated by either subjective report (e.g., feels sad or empty) or observation made by others (e.g., appears tearful).   **Note:** In children and adolescents, can be irritable mood.

(2) markedly diminished interest or pleasure in all, or almost all, activities most of the day, nearly every day (as indicated by either subjective account or observation made by others)

(3) significant weight loss when not dieting or weight gain (e.g., a change of more than 5% of body weight in a month), or decrease or increase in appetite nearly every day.   **Note:** In children, consider failure to make expected weight gains.

(4) insomnia or hypersomnia nearly every day

(5) psychomotor agitation or retardation nearly every day (observable by others, not merely subjective feelings of restlessness or being slowed down)

(6) fatigue or loss of energy nearly every day

(7) feelings of worthlessness or excessive or inappropriate guilt (which may be delusional) nearly every day (not merely self-reproach or guilt about being sick)

(8) diminished ability to think or concentrate, or indecisiveness, nearly every day (either by subjective account or as observed by others)

(9) recurrent thoughts of death (not just fear of dying), recurrent suicidal ideation without a specific plan, or a suicide attempt or a specific plan for committing suicide

B. The symptoms do not meet criteria for a Mixed Episode.

C. The symptoms cause clinically significant distress or impairment in social, occupational, or other important areas of functioning.

D. The symptoms are not due to the direct physiological effects of a substance (e.g., a drug of abuse, a medication) or a general medical condition (e.g., hypothyroidism).

E. The symptoms are not better accounted for by bereavement, i.e., after the loss of a loved one, the symptoms persist for longer than 2 months or are characterized by marked functional impairment, morbid preoccupation with worthlessness, suicidal ideation, psychotic symptoms, or psychomotor retardation.

Source. Reprinted from American Psychiatric Association: *Diagnostic and Statistical Manual of Mental Disorders,* 4th Edition, Text Revision. Washington, DC, American Psychiatric Association, 2000. Copyright 2000, American Psychiatric Association. Used with permission.

ple of 8,098 persons ages 15–54 years (Blazer et al. 1994). The NCS replication, conducted from 2001 to 2002, found a 12-month prevalence of 6.6% in
the national sample (Kessler et al. 2003).

Symptoms of mania include increased energy, increased activity, restlessness, excessively euphoric mood, extreme irritability, racing thoughts, distractibility, aggressive behavior, increased sexual drive, and substance abuse.
These symptoms can result in strained personal relationships, poor job or school
performance, and even suicide. The DSM-IV-TR criteria for a manic episode
are presented in Table 3–2. Bipolar disorder is treatable, and people with this
illness can lead full and productive lives (National Institute of Mental Health
2001).

About 5.7 million U.S. adults, or about 2.6% of the population ages 18 years
and older, in any given year have bipolar disorder (Kessler et al. 2005). Bipolar
disorder typically develops in late adolescence or early adulthood. However,
some people have their first symptoms during childhood, and some develop
them late in life. These symptoms are often not recognized as an illness, causing people to deal with them alone for years before the disorder is properly diagnosed and treated. Bipolar disorder causes dramatic mood swings that
repeatedly fluctuate from overly high and irritable to sad and hopeless and back,
often with periods of normal mood in between. These changes in mood are
often accompanied by severe changes in energy and behavior (National Institute of Mental Health 2001).

Risk Factors for Mood Disorders and Implications for Prevention

In any attempt to understand the etiology of mood disorders, the best explanation according to current research is the diathesis-stress model. This theory,
originally introduced as a means to explain some of the causes of schizophrenia (Zubin and Spring 1977), generally indicates that each person inherits
certain physical vulnerabilities to problems that may or may not appear,
depending on what stresses occur in his or her life. The model suggests that
people have varying degrees of vulnerabilities or predispositions for developing mood disorders. Having a propensity toward developing a mood disorder
alone is not enough to trigger the illness—an individual's diathesis must in-

Table 3–2. DSM-IV-TR diagnostic criteria for manic episode

A. A distinct period of abnormally and persistently elevated, expansive, or irritable mood, lasting at least 1 week (or any duration if hospitalization is necessary).

B. During the period of mood disturbance, three (or more) of the following symptoms have persisted (four if the mood is only irritable) and have been present to a significant degree:

  (1) inflated self-esteem or grandiosity

  (2) decreased need for sleep (e.g., feels rested after only 3 hours of sleep)

  (3) more talkative than usual or pressure to keep talking

  (4) flight of ideas or subjective experience that thoughts are racing

  (5) distractibility (i.e., attention too easily drawn to unimportant or irrelevant external stimuli)

  (6) increase in goal-directed activity (either socially, at work or school, or sexually) or psychomotor agitation

  (7) excessive involvement in pleasurable activities that have a high potential for painful consequences (e.g., engaging in unrestrained buying sprees, sexual indiscretions, or foolish business investments)

C. The symptoms do not meet criteria for a mixed episode.

D. The mood disturbance is sufficiently severe to cause marked impairment in occupational functioning or in usual social activities or relationships with others, or to necessitate hospitalization to prevent harm to self or others, or there are psychotic features.

E. The symptoms are not due to the direct physiological effects of a substance (e.g., a drug of abuse, a medication, or other treatment) or a general medical condition (e.g., hyperthyroidism).

Note: Manic-like episodes that are clearly caused by somatic antidepressant treatment (e.g., medication, electroconvulsive therapy, light therapy) should not count toward a diagnosis of bipolar I disorder.

Source. Reprinted from American Psychiatric Association: *Diagnostic and Statistical Manual of Mental Disorders,* 4th Edition, Text Revision. Washington, DC, American Psychiatric Association, 2000. Copyright 2000, American Psychiatric Association. Used with permission.

teract with stressful life events or environmental risk factors to evoke the onset of the illness (Durand and Barlow 2000). According to the model, the greater a person's inherent vulnerability for developing a mood disorder, the less environmental stress will be required to cause the person to become ill. Someone with less vulnerability for becoming ill may require greater levels of external risk factors to develop a disorder.

Genetic Vulnerability

Family, twin, and adoption studies have examined the role of genetic vulnerability for the development of mood disorders. It has been shown that the greater the proportion of genes that a person shares with an individual who has a mood disorder, the higher the risk of developing the disorder (Tsuang and Faraone 1990). For example, the monozygotic concordance rate for depression ranges from 0.39 to 0.50 (Kendler and Prescott 1999; Tsuang and Faraone 1990), and for bipolar disorder, from 0.40 to 0.70 (Kieseppa et al. 2004; Tsuang and Faraone 1990). The lifetime risk of depression has been reported as 16.6% in the first-degree relatives of affected individuals, compared with 5.8% in first-degree relatives of unaffected control subjects (Gershon et al. 1982). Another family study, with 335 probands and 2,003 first-degree relatives (Weissman et al. 1984), reported a lifetime rate of depression of 14.7 per 100 in the relatives of probands with mild depression, and a rate of 16.4 per 100 in the relatives of probands with severe depression. The rate of depression in the relatives of control subjects was 5.1 per 100, which was comparable to the rate in the general population. The risk of depression is higher among the relatives of probands with early-onset, recurrent depression. A study conducted by Bland and colleagues (1986) reported a morbidity rate of 17.4% in relatives of probands with early-onset, recurrent depression. This contrasted with a 3.4% rate in relatives of probands with a single episode of depression and later age at onset.

Family studies consistently show a threefold greater risk of depression in the children of depressed parents (Hammen et al. 1990; Warner et al. 1999; Weissman et al. 1997). When parental divorce, parental depression, parent-child bonding, and relationships were examined, parental depression remained the only significant risk factor in the children of depressed parents; in the offspring of nondepressed parents, these factors were predictive of depression but the rates of depression were lower (Fendrich et al. 1990).

Regarding bipolar disorder, studies have also shown an increased risk in the relatives of people with bipolar disorder. A meta-analysis (Craddock and Jones 1999) of eight family studies of bipolar disorder showed that the illness was seven times more likely among relatives of bipolar disorder probands than among relatives of control subjects. Earlier age at onset and a higher number of ill relatives increased the risk of illness in one's relatives, but other variables such as the type of relative did not appear to affect the risk of bipolar disorder (Craddock and Jones 1999). However, another study found the risk in siblings to be greater than that in parents and offspring (Gershon et al. 1975). Also, the lifetime risk of mood disorders in relatives of a proband with bipolar disorder does not appear to vary with the sex of the relative or of the proband (Rice et al. 1987).

Sociodemographic Characteristics

Depression

There are sex differences in rates of depression, with women having higher rates of depression than men. However, prior to puberty there are no sex differences in rates of depression. Following puberty there is a dramatic shift in the prevalence rates, with twofold greater rates among women compared with men (Angold et al. 1998). Studies suggest that sex hormones may play a role in this higher prevalence in women, especially because some women report depressed mood associated with the use of hormone replacement therapy (Zweifel and O'Brien 1997) or oral contraceptives (Cullberg 1972), or with menopause (Hunter et al. 1986). Regarding age, the mean age at onset for depression is 27 years (Regier et al. 1990), with a typical range of about 25 to 35 years (Eaton and Kessler 1981; Weissman 1996).

Marital status has been found to be associated with the onset and prevalence of depression. In the ECA study (Regier et al. 1988) and the NCS (Blazer et al. 1994; Kessler et al. 2003), married or never married people were found to have lower rates of depression than those who were divorced, separated, or widowed. For example, in the ECA study (Regier et al. 1988), divorced or separated individuals had a greater than two-fold increase compared to those who were married or never married (Coryell et al. 1992).

In the NCS (Blazer et al. 1994), the risk of depression was significantly higher for individuals earning less than $20,000 per year. The risk declined as income increased. Regarding employment status, homemakers had a very high risk of depression compared with women who were employed, with an odds ratio of 2.8. In the ECA study (Regier et al. 1988), no association was found between socioeconomic status and depression.

The prevalence of depression does not vary significantly with race or ethnicity, beyond the effects of socioeconomic and educational factors. Both the

ECA study (Regier et al. 1988) and the NCS (Blazer et al. 1994; Kessler et al. 2003) controlled for socioeconomic status and education, and both showed that race was not a significant predictor of depression. Particularly, in the NCS (Blazer et al. 1994; Kessler et al. 2003), the lifetime prevalence of depression was lower overall among African Americans, except for African Americans 35–44 years of age. The highest prevalence, however, was in African American women 35–44 years of age. No significant association was found in terms of adjusted odds ratios for race/ethnicity in the study, which is consistent with the ECA study (Regier et al. 1988).

In contrast to fixed risk factors such as age and sex, personality, which is not fixed, may interact with depression. Methodological issues have complicated the study of personality traits as risk factors for depression. For example, when depressed, people may not provide valid reports of their premorbid functioning (Hirschfeld et al. 1997). A study compared patients' self-report personality measures during their depressive episode and then again following complete recovery 1 year later and found that the depressed state significantly influenced assessment of emotional strength, interpersonal dependency, and extraversion (Hirschfeld et al. 1983). The most methodologically clear approach is to evaluate a person before she or he develops a depressive disorder. This assessment was conducted with a large study sample of subjects at risk for developing depression ($N = 1,179$) (Hirschfeld et al. 1989). The researchers found that the personality features most predictive of first onset of depression among middle-age adults were decreased emotional strength (referring to emotional stability and resiliency, characterized by assertiveness, caring, coping, and stress-management skills) and increased interpersonal dependency (meaning a complex relationship of thoughts, beliefs, feelings, and behaviors revolving around needs to associate closely with valued people). Among younger adults, no personality features were associated with later development of depression. The authors concluded that this could be due to the fact that psychosocial factors may become more important in late-onset depression, whereas genetic factors are more important in early-onset depression (Hirschfeld et al. 1989).

Bipolar Disorder

In contrast to depression, bipolar disorder has shown no significant sex differences in rates of occurrence (Kessler et al. 1997; Weissman et al. 1988). The

NCS (Kessler et al. 1997) reported no sex difference in the mean number of total episodes of mania and depression combined and no significant sex difference in the median number of total episodes. Regarding age, the mean age at onset for bipolar disorder is younger than for depression, typically ranging from 18 to 27 years, with a mean age at onset of 21 years of age (Kessler et al. 1997).

Initially, it was thought that bipolar disorder occurred more frequently among individuals with a higher socioeconomic status (Weissman and Myers 1978). However, other studies have not replicated this finding. For example, in the ECA study (Weissman et al. 1982), neither occupation nor income nor educational level was found to influence the prevalence of bipolar disorder. In the NCS, individuals with a diagnosis of bipolar disorder were more likely to have annual incomes of less than $20,000 compared with those without a diagnosis of bipolar disorder (Kessler et al. 1997). In the ECA study (Weissman et al. 1982), bipolar disorder occurred much less frequently among married people, as contrasted with divorced or never-married people. Bipolar disorder was also more prevalent among those with multiple divorces. In the NCS (Kessler et al. 1997), bipolar disorder was more frequent among people who were unmarried and those with less than 12 years of education.

Environmental Factors

Depression

Clinicians have long described a relationship between life events and the onset of depression. Between 1960 and 1990, several studies found evidence of a relationship between stressful life events and the onset of depression. For example, a study reported that events involving loss, such as divorce or death, are associated with depression (Jenaway and Paykel 1997). Another study (Kendler et al. 1995) investigated, in 2,164 female twins, how genetic liability to depression and stressful life events interact in the etiology of depression. The researchers found that the incidence of depression increased significantly in the month of occurrence of 13 stressful events. Four of the events were termed severe, including death of a close relative, assault, serious marital problems, and divorce and/or breakup, and these predicted the incidence of depression, with an odds ratios of greater than 10. Genetic liability also had a significant impact on the onset of depression. The lowest probability of onset of depression was found in individuals with the lowest genetic liability, exemplified by being a monozygotic co-twin of an individual unaffected by depression, regardless of whether they had been exposed to a severe event. Probabilities of the onset of depression were significantly higher in individuals with the highest genetic liability, such as a monozygotic co-twin of someone with depression. Kendler and colleagues (1995) concluded that genetic factors influence the risk of depression in part by influencing the susceptibility of individuals to the depressive effects of life events.

Trauma in early life has been considered a risk factor for depression. Several studies have examined this relationship (Bifulco et al. 1991, 1998). In one study with 286 working-class mothers, 9% reported childhood sexual abuse (Bifulco et al. 1991). Of these women, 64% experienced depression over the course of 3 years. Another study (Bifulco et al. 1998) found that childhood neglect or abuse was strongly associated with early-onset depression. This same association was found in a study by McCauley et al. (1997), in which childhood physical or sexual abuse was predictive of a variety of adult afflictions, including depression. Numerous studies have shown that negative experiences such as the ones described above can lead to the development of low self-esteem, helplessness, and hopelessness, which can predispose an individual to the development of depression (Kendler et al. 1993, 1998).

Bipolar Disorder

Stressful life events have been shown to increase the risk of recurrence of bipolar disorder (Ellicott et al. 2001). Severe social disruptions, such as moving or losing a job, were associated with the onset of a manic episode, but not depression, in a study of patients with bipolar disorder (Malkoff-Schwartz et al. 1998). Also, disturbances of the sleep-wake cycle and other circadian rhythm disturbances are core symptoms of bipolar episodes, both manic and depressive. Some researchers have hypothesized that disruption in social demands that set the biological clock can lead to instability in circadian rhythms, which can in turn trigger bipolar episodes (Ehlers et al. 1988). Sleep deprivation has been found to be a proximal cause of mania (Wehr et al. 1987). In another study, triggers of mania included biological causes such as drugs and hormones; psychosocial factors such as separation and bereavement; and direct disturbances of sleep schedules, caused by newborn infants, shift work, and travel (Wehr et al. 1987). This study speculated that sleep deprivation is both a cause and a consequence of mania, and thus mutually self-reinforcing sleep loss perpetuates the manic state.

General Medical Illnesses

Depression

Increased rates of depression have been reported among patients with several general medical illnesses; these illnesses include cardiovascular disease, AIDS, respiratory disorders, cancer, and several neurological conditions such as Parkinson disease and stroke (Evans et al. 1999; Stoner et al. 1998). The relationship is most evident in patients with cardiovascular disease. In a review of 13 prospective studies, Musselman et al. (1998) found a strong association between depression and subsequent cardiovascular morbidity and mortality. An association between a brain injury and an increased risk of depression in children has also been found (Rutter et al. 1983). Research has shown that learning difficulties and problems with self-esteem in children with brain injuries can predispose these children to depression (Rutter et al. 1983).

Bipolar Disorder

Bipolar disorder has been linked to both thyroid hypofunction and autoimmune thyroiditis (Valle et al. 1999). Evidence also suggests that patients, particularly women, may be at higher risk of having low thyroid levels regardless of which medications they use. Hypothyroidism may be a risk factor for bipolar disorder in some patients (Thomsen et al. 2005). A study of Danish patients found that those discharged from the hospital with a diagnosis of hypothyroidism were at greater risk of being subsequently hospitalized with a mood disorder such as bipolar disorder, compared with patients discharged from the hospital with a different diagnosis such as osteoarthritis (Thomsen et al. 2005). The risk of hospitalization with a mood disorder was greater in the first year following initial hospitalization with hypothyroidism, compared with the risk in the remaining period of the patient's lifetime.

Implications for Prevention

The interaction of psychosocial and other environmental factors with a person's biological predisposition is becoming increasingly recognized in physical disorders ranging from heart and lung disease to diabetes. Accumulating evidence suggests that environmental stressors work in conjunction with genetic vulnerabilities to produce a wide spectrum of psychiatric disorders, including mood disorders. For example, research has confirmed the substantial genetic contribution to vulnerability for bipolar disorder (Kieseppa et al. 2004). Earlier, a study of 680 female-female twin pairs demonstrated that major depression in women is a multifactorial disorder in which the four strongest predictors of depression are stressful life events, genetic factors, a previous history of major depression, and neuroticism (Kendler et al. 1993).

A recent study significantly extended the exploration of gene-environment interactions by demonstrating a gene-gene interaction with childhood maltreatment (Kaufman et al. 2006). A functional polymorphism in the promoter region of the serotonin transporter gene (5-HTTLPR) and a polymorphism of the brain-derived neurotrophic factor gene, in association with childhood maltreatment, increased the vulnerability to depression in children. This study also found that the higher the level of social support received by children, the lower the risk of depression, showing that genetic risk can be ameliorated by positive environmental factors. These findings have powerful implications for future prevention research.

The study of gene and environment interactions opens up new possibilities for identifying particularly vulnerable subpopulations and thus increases the likelihood that targeted interventions will produce significant results (Fishbein 2000). Prevention researchers are now in a better position to target children at high environmental risk, having an increased understanding of the role of various psychosocial stressors at the individual, family, and community levels. Prevention efforts can be much more targeted based on increased recognition of crucial periods in development and the importance of early intervention for shaping neurodevelopment and neurochemistry and providing the basis for later social, emotional, and cognitive development (Teicher et al. 2003).

Protective Factors for Mood Disorders and Implications for Prevention

Protective factors are conditions that can build resilience to a disease and can serve to buffer the negative effects of risk factors. It is when risk factors outweigh protective factors that the likelihood of developing a disorder such as depression or bipolar disorder is high (Rolf et al. 1990).

Factors such as a supportive social network and an easy temperament (adjusting easily and quickly to new situations and changes in one's routine, readily adapting to new experiences, and generally displaying positive moods and emotions) have been shown to protect against psychopathology including both depression and bipolar disorder. In some individuals whose parents suffer from depression, resiliency in late adolescence is associated with good outcomes (Beardslee and Podorefsky 1988). Most studies have found that children of parents with mood disorders do function well. However, it is the complex interaction between both risk and protective factors that activates the onset of a mood disorder. Therefore, a clear understanding of both risk and protective factors across the life span is crucial for the prevention of mood disorders.

Certain coping styles are considered a protective factor for mental health. Some coping styles protect an individual from stressful life events, whereas other coping styles enhance an individual's vulnerability to mental health problems. A study of adolescents showed that depressive symptomatology is accompanied by higher levels of passive and avoidant coping but lower levels of active and approach coping (Herman-Stahl and Petersen 1996; Herman-Stahl et al. 1995). *Active coping* refers to taking a direct and rational approach to dealing with a problem, whereas *approach coping* refers to one's tendency to attend to a stressor by seeking information or closely monitoring the stressor (Herman-Stahl and Petersen 1996; Herman-Stahl et al. 1995). In addition, evidence from the adult literature suggests that depression is negatively associated with problem-focused coping (i.e., attempts to do something constructive about a stressful situation) but positively associated with emotion-focused coping (i.e., efforts to regulate emotions experienced because of a stressful event) (Turner et al. 1992). A negative attributional style plays a key role in the formation of depressive symptoms (Garber and Hilsman 1992). For example, children and adolescents develop a negative cognitive style due to modeling of significant others, criticism, rejection, and experiences with uncontrollable stressful life events. When confronted with stressful life events, the negative cognitive style triggers negative coping styles and a low sense of self-efficacy, ultimately resulting in an increased vulnerability to developing depressive symptoms in adolescence and later on in life (Hilsman and Garber 1995).

Perceived self-efficacy refers to confidence in one's capabilities of performing in a certain manner to attain certain goals (Bandura 1997). For example, it has been shown that individuals with low academic self-efficacy are at risk for developing depression versus those with higher academic self-efficacy (*academic self-efficacy* refers to one's perceived capability to fulfill academic demands—one's belief in his or her efficacy to manage learning activities, master different academic subjects, and fulfill personal, parental, and teachers' academic expectations). A study examined the effects of low academic self-efficacy in an adolescent population. Results indicated that low levels of academic self-efficacy were associated with high levels of concurrent and subsequent depression (Bandura et al. 1999).

High levels of social support have been associated with positive outcomes following a wide variety of stressors (Resick 2001). The relationship between good social support and positive mental and physical health outcomes has been observed in inner-city children, college students, blue-collar workers, unemployed workers, business executives, new mothers, widows, and parents of children with serious medical illnesses (Resick 2001). Higher levels of social support have been associated with a lower risk of developing depression and bipolar disorder (McPherson et al. 1993; Travis et al. 2004). To be helpful in the prevention of depression, social support must be positive rather than negative, and the best source of support may vary depending on a person's developmental stage. For example, in early adolescence, parental support is usually more important than peer support (Stice et al. 2004). Social networks and emotional support may enhance mental and physical health by fostering effective coping strategies (Holahan et al. 1995), offsetting feelings of loneliness (Bisschop et al. 2004), and increasing feelings of self-efficacy (Travis et al. 2004). Optimism has also been associated with greater life satisfaction as well as with increased psychological well-being and health (Affleck and Tennen 1996).

Strong role models and mentors serve an important educational and developmental function for the development of resilient individuals. In the lives of children and adolescents, nonparental adults can play formative roles in development by conveying knowledge and skills, challenging youth with new perspectives, providing dependable support, motivating and inspiring hard work, promoting moral values, nourishing self-esteem, and facilitating occupational ambitions (Hirsch et al. 2002). In addition, having a nonparental mentor can help to buffer against the development of depression. Among 129 young African American mothers, those with natural mentors had lower levels of depression and benefited more from social support than did mothers without natural mentors (Rhodes et al. 1992). Having a mentor moderated the relationship between depression and social support, as well as between depression and relationship problems. From resilient role models one may learn a host of strategies to diminish the likelihood of developing stress-induced depression and/or to manage symptoms if they do develop. Such strategies include the fostering of psychosocial resilience factors such as positive emotions, cognitive flexibility, optimism, social support, and active coping (Southwick et al. 2005).

Primary Prevention of Mood Disorders

Primary prevention can be targeted toward high-risk groups, such as children who have experienced parental neglect or abuse or who have a parent with a mood disorder. Genetic counseling, a form of primary prevention, is another possible strategy for the prevention of mood disorders; however, currently there is a lack of clarity on the inheritance of these disorders and genetic markers remain unavailable. Reviews of various community-based initiatives have shown that primary prevention interventions have considerable promise when they address multiple risk factors, focus on multiple settings, and target neighborhoods or communities with a high level of need and risk (Institute of Medicine 1994). Such primary prevention interventions encourage families and communities to work together to reduce their exposure to the more stressful aspects of their lives that put them at high risk for developing a mood disorder. These interventions also assist individuals and families in building relationships that enhance social support and resilience. However, public health initiatives that target mood disorders have typically emphasized secondary and tertiary prevention, such as encouraging appropriate treatment seeking and educating health professionals about illness recognition and management. Primary prevention strategies have been explored only to a lesser extent.

However, recent prevention studies are showing promising results for reducing mental health disorders and increasing protective factors in young people at risk. Also, primary prevention interventions can be targeted to high-risk populations at different developmental stages. For example, home-visit programs by nurses for women during their pregnancy and through their children's infancy have been shown to be effective at decreasing behavior problems and significantly improving the well-being of women and children who are socioeconomically disadvantaged (Izzo et al. 2005). One example of such a home-visit program is the Prenatal/Early Infancy Project (Olds et al. 1988), a comprehensive program intended to prevent a range of maternal and pediatric problems. The program targeted a geographical area with high rates of poverty and child abuse and was able to enhance parenting skills, give social support, and help mothers achieve educational and occupational goals. Although such programs appear to reduce risk factors associated with mood disorders, their efficacy in actually preventing the onset of mood disorders remains to be clarified.

Childhood and adolescence is a period of rapid cognitive and social development and is a critical time for the implementation of programs aimed at preventing mood disorders. With this in mind, a family-based prevention program was developed and evaluated, targeting nonsymptomatic early adolescents at risk for future depression because of the presence of a significant mood disorder in one or both parents (Beardslee et al. 1997). Greater parental benefit from the intervention (in terms of changes in illness-related behaviors and attitudes) was associated with significant change among the children, including enhanced understanding of parental illness and improved communication with their parents. An example of a prevention program targeting children is the Families and Schools Together Program, a comprehensive community-based program focusing on high-risk children that has been shown to significantly strengthen social, emotional, and learning skills in both parents and children (Cummings et al. 2000). Another exemplary program, the Family Bereavement Program (Sandler et al. 1992), sought to improve the mental health of children who experienced the death of a parent. Children who participated in the program improved on symptoms of depression and conduct disorders.

Despite the fact that the risk of developing depression increases during adolescence (Petersen et al. 1993), few primary prevention studies have targeted this age group. The majority of research has focused on secondary and tertiary prevention efforts. In adulthood, psychosocial risk factors increase the likelihood of developing a mood disorder. However, enhancing protective factors such as problem-solving skills, increasing the availability of medical services, increasing social support from family and friends, and improving the ability to cope with one's emotions are all associated with decreasing the risk of developing a mood disorder (Institute of Medicine 1994). The University of Colorado Separation and Divorce Program (Bloom et al. 1985) was aimed at newly separated people. Results showed that those who participated in the program rated significantly higher in adjustment and had fewer separation problems; they also reported lower levels of psychiatric symptoms such as depression (Bloom et al. 1985).

Another primary preventive intervention study focused on an educational intervention that utilized cognitive-behavioral therapy (Muñoz et al. 1995). Medical outpatients from primary care clinics serving low-income and minority patients were chosen as the selected population at high risk for depression. This high-risk population was screened for already meeting diagnostic criteria for major depression or dysthymia. Those not clinically depressed were provided with an intervention intended to reduce the likelihood of clinical episodes of depression occurring. The intervention focused on keeping symptom levels low in this high-risk population by teaching individuals self-control approaches to the management of their own mood states; this was hypothesized to decrease the number of individuals who would eventually cross the threshold into a clinical episode of depression. The results showed that the cognitive-behavioral intervention significantly reduced the incidence of clinical episodes of depression in the nondepressed group (Muñoz et al. 1995). Two additional studies, one in a high school setting (Clarke et al. 1995) and one involving members of a health maintenance organization (Clarke et al. 2001), have shown that cognitive-behavioral therapy can prevent the onset of diagnosable disorders in at-risk adolescents selected on the basis of having subsyndromal depressive symptoms. These studies suggest that prevention is feasible and ought to be pursued (Muñoz et al. 2002). However, although such programs reduce risk factors, more research is needed to assess their impact on reducing the incidence of mood disorders.

Secondary Prevention of Mood Disorders

The U.S. Preventive Services Task Force's Guide to Clinical Preventive Services (DiGuiseppi et al. 1996) describes secondary prevention measures as those that are aimed at early disease detection, thereby increasing opportunities for intervention to prevent progression of the disease. Screening tests are a component of secondary prevention activities; however these need to be coupled with treatment to be effective. With early case finding, the natural history of disease, or how the course of an illness unfolds over time without treatment, can often be altered to maximize well-being and minimize suffering (DiGuiseppi et al. 1996).

Because of stigma, financial barriers, lack of knowledge regarding symptoms, inadequate availability of treatments for mood disorders, and underrecognition by health care providers, most people do not receive appropriate treatment for mood disorders (Institute of Medicine 1994; Regier et al. 1993). Regarding depression, estimates vary. In the ECA study, only 37% of persons with depression reported using mental health services in the previous 6 months (Leaf et al. 1986). In the NCS, for those with depression, only 21% received mental health treatment in a 12-month interval (Blazer et al. 1994). In the ECA study at 1-year follow-up, it was found that 28% of individuals with depression had received no treatment and 49% had had a general medical contact without a mental health care component during the year (Marino et al. 1995). Regarding individuals with bipolar disorder, based on the ECA study it is estimated that nearly 40% are untreated (Regier et al. 1993).

Secondary prevention efforts focus on the early detection and treatment of mood disorders to prevent disease progression, but the distinction between secondary prevention and tertiary prevention is not always clear because there are elements of tertiary prevention in interventions that are referred to as secondary prevention efforts. In regard to depression, multiple programs that aim at improving the provision of care to those experiencing recognized symptoms of depression have been studied. These programs incorporate both patient education and shared care involving primary care physicians, psychiatrists, and psychologists. They have been found to be successful for improving treatment adherence and patients' recovery from depression (Katon et al. 1995, 1996). This collaborative care approach resulted in a lower overall cost for each patient successfully treated for depression (Von Korff et al. 1998). Another study on improving the provision of care offered enhanced care with a combination of patient education, clinician educational meetings, automated pharmacy data, and enhanced collaborative management by a psychiatrist in a primary care setting (Gerrity et al. 1999). This resulted in enhanced medication adherence and recovery from depression at 6 months. Persistent benefits were seen at 28 months for those with moderately severe depression.

A similar type of program has been implemented for people with bipolar disorder (Simon et al. 2005). This population-based care program included initial assessment and care planning; monthly telephone monitoring, including brief symptom assessment and medication monitoring; feedback to and coordination with the mental health treatment team; and a structured group psychoeducational program, all of which were provided by a nurse care manager. The interim results of this program at 12 months indicated that it had a significant effect on the severity of mania and that program participants had a decline in depression ratings over time (Simon et al. 2005). The complete follow-up data showed that this systematic care management program reduced the frequency and severity of manic symptoms (Simon et al. 2006). The mean mania ratings decreased in the treatment group over time and the number of weeks during which patients had significant manic symptoms was approximately 25% lower in patients assigned to the intervention program. During the first 12 months, patients receiving the intervention had more medication management visits and more frequently used atypical antipsychotic drugs, but these differences were not statistically significant at 24 months (Simon et al. 2005).

Tertiary Prevention of Mood Disorders

Tertiary prevention encompasses activities that involve the care of established disease, with attempts made to restore the individual to his or her highest level of functioning, minimize the negative effects of disease, and prevent disease-related complications (DiGuiseppi et al. 1996). There are serious consequences to the undertreatment of mood disorders, including a major impact on a person's quality of life and economic productivity (Wells et al. 1989).

Several types of treatments have been efficacious for patients with depression. These include antidepressant medications, cognitive-behavioral therapy, and other forms of psychotherapy (American Psychiatric Association 2000b). Antidepressant medications are the most widely used treatment and the majority of studies have proven their efficacy. One of the major problems compromising the potential effectiveness of pharmacotherapy is that people often stop taking their medication too soon, before it is possible to fully assess the efficacy of the treatment. Although medication side effects are the primary reason for attrition, other factors include inadequate education of patients, patients' ambivalence about seeing a psychiatrist or taking a psychiatric medication, and the cost and accessibility of services (Depression Guideline Panel 1993). Another problem is failure of the prescribing physician to monitor how symptoms respond to treatment and to change treatments in a timely manner (Depression Guideline Panel 1993). Even successful acute-phase antidepressant pharmacotherapy should almost always be followed by at least 6 months of continuation treatment for the purpose of preventing relapse (American Psychiatric Association 2000b).

Some approaches have been shown to be efficacious in the tertiary prevention of depression (Hollon et al. 2002). Preliminary evidence suggests that psychosocial interventions may function as protective interventions against relapse and recurrence of depression. Research suggests that the greater the number of past depressive episodes, the greater a person's vulnerability for future depressive episodes (Kendler et al. 2001). In contrast to the palliative effect of maintenance medication, psychosocial treatments appear to grant protective effects beyond active treatment. It appears that treatment with psychosocial interventions such as cognitive-behavioral therapy may be particularly efficacious in providing protection against relapse (Hollon et al. 2005) because it has an enduring effect that extends beyond the end of treatment (Hollon and Shelton 2001). As a result of cognitive-behavioral therapy, patients acquire skills, or changes in thinking, that confer some protection against future onsets. Depression is associated with substantial impairment in domains including occupational functioning (Eaton et al. 1990), and adequate relapse prevention can substantially reduce these impairments (Mintz et al. 1992).

The Coping with Depression Course (Lewinsohn et al. 1989) is an example of a psychosocial intervention (i.e., a cognitive-behavioral group program that addresses specific target behaviors assumed to contribute to the maintenance of the disorder). One study showed that this type of intervention is efficacious as a cost-effective program for preventing short-term relapses during a 6-month period of treatment (Kühner et al. 1996). Another study examining cognitive-behavioral therapy (Fava et al. 1998) showed a substantially lower relapse rate than with routine clinical management in patients with major depressive disorder. The results of this study showed that long-term drug treatment is not the only tool to prevent relapse in patients with recurrent depression. Although maintenance pharmacotherapy seems to be necessary in some patients, cognitive-behavioral therapy does offer an alternative for others.

The primary goal of pharmacotherapy in persons with bipolar disorder is to prevent recurrence of both mania and depression (El-Mallakh and Karippot 2002). Recommended pharmacotherapy of bipolar disorder typically begins with lithium, divalproex, or an alternative mood stabilizer (American Psychiatric Association 2002). Mood stabilizers reduce the risk of cycling rapidly between episodes of mania and depression (Sachs and Thase 2000). For bipolar depression that does not respond to therapy with a mood stabilizer, an antidepressant typically is added (Sachs and Thase 2000). Nonadherence with a medication regimen in patients with bipolar disorder is a major concern. Patients with bipolar disorder may be nonadherent with their medications for several reasons. These include impaired insight pertaining to the illness and the appropriate course of treatment; drug-related side effects, such as weight gain, hair loss, and sedation; the dislike of the medication controlling or dampening a manic mood; wanting to stop treatment as soon as they feel well; and inadequate treatment management, such as insufficient information or lack of support from family and friends (American Psychiatric Association 2002).

The literature suggests that psychosocial interventions serve an important role in the tertiary prevention of bipolar disorder. However, it is recommended that psychotherapy be used in conjunction with medication (Craighead and Miklowitz 2000). Psychosocial interventions typically focus on better illness awareness and, importantly, daily symptom monitoring (Leverich and Post 1998). Also, psychosocial programs that deal with the management of stressors that may be particularly pertinent to an individual's vulnerable areas should be emphasized (Vieta and Colom 2004). Data have shown the important role that stress has in the progression of bipolar disorder, and data also support the advantage of systematic psychoeducational approaches (Scott and Colom 2005). It has also been found that ongoing daily assessments of the patient's mood by the patient or a family member provide a tool for evaluating drug and psychotherapeutic interventions on a much more precise and targeted time frame. Such careful monitoring provides the basis for developing an early warning system pertinent to each individual (Post and Leverich 2006). In instances of symptom development, particular degrees of altered mood or sleep are specified in advance to trigger actions from the individual, family members, and clinicians, such as medication dose modifications, calls to the physician or therapist, or related therapeutic maneuvers. These efforts are directed at maintaining a remission and attempting to avoid a major manic or depressive episode occurrence in which immediate intervention is needed on an emergency basis (Post and Leverich 2006).

What Practicing Psychiatrists Can Do in Routine Practice to Promote the Prevention of Mood Disorders

Because mood disorders are prevalent and responsive to treatment, and because they are generally underdiagnosed and undertreated, primary care physicians and mental health professionals alike should consider routinely screening for depressive and manic symptoms and treating or referring patients for psychiatric care as appropriate. For example, several studies have shown that there is a high prevalence of major depression in primary care settings, ranging from 6% to 10% (Katon and Schulberg 1992; Ormel et al. 1994). Evidence also suggests that more intensive, organized treatment that integrates mental health practitioners into primary care improves outcomes for depressed patients (Katon et al. 1995, 1996).

A collaborative care approach aims to improve patient education and integrates mental health professionals into the primary care clinic as consultants and partners (Coulehan et al. 1997). Collaborative care models have been shown to improve outcomes for patients in both secondary and tertiary prevention domains. The term *collaborative care* has been used to describe how mental health providers work with a group of primary care providers to treat common psychiatric disorders, such as mood disorders, in the community or in primary care clinics (Hedrick et al. 2003; Katon et al. 1995, 1996). A multidisciplinary team can provide clinical support to primary care providers. The team is designed to do the following (Hedrick et al. 2003; Katon et al. 1995, 1996):

- Enable screening, evaluation, and stabilization of psychiatric patients.
- Improve the ability of the primary care providers to deliver ongoing management of these disorders.

- Improve the education of clinical staff and trainees on topics related to primary care psychiatry.
- Increase the number of referrals to specialty mental health care providers.

In regard to patients with bipolar disorder, building a medical team and support network has been shown to be efficacious (Miklowitz 2002). Inherent in this process is the development of a careful longitudinal monitoring strategy, such that small symptom variations can directly feed back into therapeutic decisions, not only for modified psychopharmacological interventions but also for additional psychotherapeutic ones.

In addition, in practice, psychiatrists can play an important role in minimizing disability via tertiary prevention. The National Institute of Mental Health Strategic Plan for Mood Disorders focuses on enabling clinicians to detect mood disorders whenever they are present, to offer the best initial treatments to attain rapid recovery, to apply the best subsequent treatments to those whose disorder does not remit with their first treatment, and to prevent relapse in those who have recovered from a mood disorder (Frank et al. 2002).

According to the National Advisory Mental Health Council's Clinical Treatment and Services Research Workgroup, "all too often, clinical practices and service system innovations that are validated by research are not fully adopted in treatment settings and service systems for individuals with mental illness" (p. 1) (Hyman 1999). The message of this report is that mental health services need to be improved by focusing on the continuum of knowledge. That is, knowledge and understanding of mood disorders run from the basic sciences to the development of new treatments, then from treatment development to clinical trials, and ultimately from clinical trials to everyday practice (Hyman 1999).

Finally, combined treatments that include both psychotherapy and pharmacotherapy have been recommended for the tertiary prevention of mood disorders. A reexamination of existing research data on combined treatments for mood disorders showed that psychosocial interventions have significant benefit when combined with pharmacotherapy for some patients with mood disorders (Jindal and Thase 2003). The added benefit of combined treatment has been best established for severe, recurrent, and chronic depressive disorder and bipolar disorder (Jindal and Thase 2003). However, future research is needed to determine whether combined treatment by a single provider offers additional advantages for patients with a mood disorder (Jindal and Thase 2003).

Conclusion

Increased knowledge and application of public health approaches have led to a new recognition of the importance and effectiveness of more comprehensive interventions, rather than just focusing on a single individual in a single context (Cummings et al. 2000). In addition, new and improved assessment methods are now available for identifying early warnings signs in populations at high risk for the development of mood disorders (Carter et al. 2004). Therefore, if the public health goal is to reduce the prevalence and severity of mood disorders, then researchers need to shift away from searching solely for biogenetic causes and treatments and place more emphasis on investigating public health interventions that target vulnerable populations (Southwick et al. 2005). More time and funding should go toward researching interventions that reduce environmental stress, particularly childhood abuse and neglect, and strengthen competencies in populations that are genetically, psychosocially, and developmentally predisposed to the development of mood disorders. Also, a collaborative care approach aims to integrate mental health professionals into primary care (Coulehan et al. 1997) and has been shown to improve outcomes (Hedrick et al. 2003; Katon et al. 1995, 1996). In this model, a multidisciplinary team is designed to enable screening, evaluation, and stabilization of psychiatric patients, ultimately enabling us to provide more comprehensive preventive and treatment interventions for patients with a mood disorder.

Key Points

- The diathesis-stress model offers an explanation for understanding the etiology of mood disorders. This model suggests that each person inherits certain physical vulnerabilities to problems that may or may not appear, depending on the stressors that occur in his or her life. Therefore, the requirement to produce a disorder such as depression or bipolar disorder involves both an inherited tendency and specific stressful life conditions.

- Prevention efforts for mood disorders should target high-risk individuals such as children who have a parent with a mood disorder and/or have experienced abuse or neglect.

- High levels of social support have been associated with a decreased risk of developing depression and bipolar disorder. Therefore, prevention efforts aimed at increasing social networks and emotional support may enhance mental and physical health by fostering effective coping strategies. Also, strong role models and mentors serve an important educational and developmental function for the nurturance of resilient individuals.

- Community-based initiatives have shown that primary prevention interventions have considerable promise when they address multiple risk factors, focus on multiple settings, and target communities with a high level of risk and need.

- A collaborative care program incorporates both patient education and shared care involving primary care physicians, psychiatrists, and psychologists to aid in the prevention of disease progression. This approach integrates mental health professionals into primary care to enable the screening, evaluation, and treatment of patients with mood disorders.

- Long-term drug treatment in combination with psychosocial interventions such as cognitive-behavioral therapy is necessary for the prevention of relapse in patients who have recovered from a mood disorder.

References

Affleck G, Tennen H: Construing benefits from adversity: adaptational significance and dispositional underpinnings. J Pers 64:899–922, 1996

American Psychiatric Association: Diagnostic and Statistical Manual of Mental Disorders, 4th Edition, Text Revision. Washington, DC, American Psychiatric Association, 2000a

American Psychiatric Association: Practice guideline for the treatment of patients with major depressive disorder (revision). Am J Psychiatry 157 (suppl 4):1–45, 2000b

American Psychiatric Association: Practice guideline for the treatment of patients with bipolar disorder (revision). Am J Psychiatry 159 (suppl 4):1–50, 2002

Angold A, Cossello EJ, Worthman CW: Puberty and depression: the roles of age, pubertal status, and pubertal timing. Psychol Med 28:51–61, 1998

Bandura A: Self-efficacy: the exercise of control. New York, Freeman, 1997

Bandura A, Pastorelli C, Barbaranelli C, et al: Self-efficacy pathways to childhood depression. J Pers Soc Psychol 76:258–269, 1999

Beardslee WR, Podorefsky D: Resilient adolescents whose parents have serious affective and other psychiatric disorders: importance of self-understanding and relationships. Am J Psychiatry 145:63–69, 1988

Beardslee WR, Versage EM, Wright E, et al: Examination of preventive interventions for families with depression: evidence of change. Dev Psychopathol 9:109–130, 1997

Bifulco A, Brown GW, Adler Z: Early sexual abuse and clinical depression in adult life. Br J Psychiatry 159:115–122, 1991

Bifulco A, Brown GW, Moran P, et al: Predicting depression in women: the role of past and present vulnerability. Psychol Med 28:39–50, 1998

Bisschop MI, Kriegsman DMW, Beekman ATF, et al: Chronic diseases and depression: the modifying role of psychosocial resources. Soc Sci Med 4:721–733, 2004

Bland RC, Newman SC, Orn H: Recurrent and nonrecurrent depression: a family study. Arch Gen Psychiatry 43:1085–1089, 1986

Blazer DG, Kessler RC, McGonagle KA, et al: The prevalence and distribution of major depression in a national community sample: the National Comorbidity Survey. Am J Psychiatry 151:979–986, 1994

Bloom BL, Hodges WF, Kern MB, et al: A preventive intervention program for the newly separated: final evaluations. Am J Orthopsychiatry 55:9–26, 1985

Carter AS, Briggs-Gowan MJ, Davis NO: Assessment of young children's social-emotional development and psychopathology: recent advances and recommendations for practice. J Child Psychol Psychiatry 45:109–134, 2004

Clarke GN, Hawkins W, Murphy M, et al: Targeted prevention of unipolar depressive disorder in an at-risk sample of high school adolescents: a randomized trial of a group cognitive intervention. J Am Acad Child Adolesc Psychiatry 34:312–321, 1995

Clarke GN, Hornbrook MC, Lynch F, et al: A randomized trial of a group cognitive intervention for preventing depression in adolescent offspring of depressed parents. Arch Gen Psychiatry 58:1127–1134, 2001

Coryell W, Endicott J, Keller M: Major depression in a nonclinical sample: demographic and clinical risk factors for first onset. Arch Gen Psychiatry 49:117–125, 1992

Coulehan JL, Schulberg HC, Block MR, et al: Treating depressed primary care patients improves their physical, mental, and social functioning. Arch Intern Med 157:1113–1120, 1997

Craddock N, Jones I: Genetics of bipolar disorder. J Med Genet 36:585–594, 1999

Craighead WE, Miklowitz DJ: Psychosocial interventions for bipolar disorder. J Clin Psychiatry 61:58–64, 2000

Cuijpers P, Smit F: Excess mortality in depression: a meta-analysis of community studies. J Affect Disord 72:227–236, 2002

Cullberg J: Mood changes and menstrual symptoms with different gestagen/estrogen combinations: a double blind comparison with placebo. Acta Psychiatr Scand Suppl 236:1–86, 1972

Cummings EM, Davies P, Campbell SB: Developmental Psychopathology and Family Process: Theory, Research, and Clinical Implications. New York, Guilford, 2000

Depression Guideline Panel: Depression in Primary Care, Vol 2: Treatment of Major Depression (AHCPR Publication No. 93-0551). Rockville, MD, U.S. Department of Health and Human Services, Public Health Service, Agency for Health Care Policy and Research, 1993

DiGuiseppi C, Atkins D, Woolf SH: Report of the U.S. Preventive Services Task Force, 2nd Edition. Alexandria, VA, International Medical Publishing, 1996

Durand VM, Barlow DH: Abnormal Psychology: An Introduction. Scarborough, ON, Canada, Wadsworth, 2000

Eaton WW, Kessler LG: Rates of symptoms of depression in a national sample. Am J Epidemiol 114:528–538, 1981

Eaton WW, Anthony JC, Mandel W, et al: Occupations and the prevalence of major depressive disorder. J Occup Environ Med 32:1079–1087, 1990

Ehlers CL, Frank E, Kupfer DJ: Social zeitgebers and biological rhythms: a unified approach to understanding the etiology of depression. Arch Gen Psychiatry 45:948–952, 1988

Ellicott A, Hammen C, Gitlin M, et al: Life events and the course of bipolar disorder. Am J Psychiatry 147:1194–1198, 2001

El-Mallakh RS, Karippot A: Use of antidepressants to treat depression in bipolar disorder. Psychiatr Serv 53:580–584, 2002

Evans DL, Staab JP, Petitto JM, et al: Depression in the medical setting: biopsychological interactions and treatment considerations. J Clin Psychiatry 60 (suppl 4):40–55, 1999

Fava GA, Rafanelli C, Grandi S, et al: Prevention of recurrent depression with cognitive behavioral therapy: preliminary findings. Arch Gen Psychiatry 55:816–820, 1998

Fendrich M, Warner V, Weissman MM: Family risk factors, parental depression and childhood psychopathology. Dev Psychol 26:40–50, 1990

Fishbein D: The importance of neurobiological research to the prevention of psychopathology. Prev Sci 1:89–106, 2000

Frank E, Rush AJ, Blehar M, et al: Skating to where the puck is going to be: a plan for clinical trials and translation research in mood disorders. Biol Psychiatry 52:631–654, 2002

Garber J, Hilsman R: Cognition, stress, and depression in children and adolescents. Child Adolesc Psychiatr Clin N Am 1:129–167, 1992

Gerrity MS, Cole SA, Dietrich AJ, et al: Improving the recognition and management of depression: is there a role for physician education? J Fam Pract 48:949–957, 1999

Gershon ES, Mark A, Cohen N, et al: Transmitted factors in the morbid risk of affective disorders: a controlled study. J Psychiatr Res 12:283–299, 1975

Gershon ES, Hamovit J, Guroff JJ, et al: A family study of schizoaffective, bipolar I, bipolar II, unipolar, and normal control probands. Arch Gen Psychiatry 39:1157–1167, 1982

Hammen C, Burge D, Burney E, et al: Longitudinal study of diagnoses in children of women with unipolar and bipolar affective disorder. Arch Gen Psychiatry 47:1112–1117, 1990

Hedrick SC, Chaney EF, Felker B, et al: Effectiveness of collaborative care depression treatment in Veterans' Affairs primary care. J Gen Intern Med 18:9–16, 2003

Herman-Stahl MA, Petersen AC: The protective role of coping and social resources for depressive symptoms among young adolescents. J Youth Adolesc 25:733–753, 1996

Herman-Stahl MA, Stemmler M, Petersen AC: Approach and avoidant coping: implications for adolescent mental health. J Youth Adolesc 24:649–665, 1995

Hilsman R, Garber J: A test of the cognitive diathesis-stress model of depression in children: academic stressors, attributional style, perceived competence, and control. J Pers Soc Psychol 69:370–380, 1995

Hirsch BJ, Mickus M, Boerger R: Ties to influential adults among black and white adolescents: culture, social class, and family networks. Am J Community Psychol 30:289–303, 2002

Hirschfeld RM, Klerman GL, Clayton PJ, et al: Personality and depression: empirical findings. Arch Gen Psychiatry 40:993–998, 1983

Hirschfeld RM, Klerman GL, Lavori P, et al: Premorbid personality assessments of first onset of major depression. Arch Gen Psychiatry 46:345–350, 1989

Hirschfeld RM, Shea MT, Holzer CE: Personality dysfunction and depression, in Depression: Neurobiological, Psychopathological and Therapeutic Advances. Edited by Honig A, Van Praag HM. New York, Wiley, 1997, pp 327–341

Holahan CJ, Holahan CK, Moos RH, et al: Social support, coping and depressive symptoms in a late-middle-aged sample of patients reporting cardiac illness. Health Psychol 14:152–163, 1995

Hollon SD, Shelton RC: Treatment guidelines for major depressive disorder. Behav Ther 32:235–258, 2001

Hollon SD, Muñoz RF, Barlow DH, et al: Psychosocial intervention development for the prevention and treatment of depression: promoting innovation and increasing access. Biol Psychiatry 52:610–630, 2002

Hollon SD, DeRubeis RJ, Shelton RC, et al: Prevention of relapse following cognitive therapy vs medications in moderate to severe depression. Arch Gen Psychiatry 62:417–422, 2005

Hunter M, Battersby R, Whitehead M: Relationships between psychological symptoms, somatic complaints and menopausal status. Maturitas 8:217–228, 1986

Hyman SE: Bridging Science and Service: A Report by the National Advisory Mental Health Council's Clinical Treatment and Services Research Workgroup. Darby, PA, Diane Publishing, 1999

Institute of Medicine: Reducing Risks for Mental Disorders: Frontiers for Preventive Intervention Research. Washington, DC, National Academy Press, 1994

Izzo CV, Eckenrode JJ, Smith EG, et al: Reducing the impact of uncontrollable stressful life events through a program of nurse home visitation for new parents. Prev Sci 6:269–274, 2005

Jenaway A, Paykel ES: Life events and depression, in Depression: Neurobiological, Psychopathological and Therapeutic Advances. Edited by Honig A, Van Praag HM. New York, Wiley, 1997, pp 279–295

Jindal RD, Thase ME: Integrating psychotherapy and pharmacotherapy to improve outcomes among patients with mood disorders. Psychiatr Serv 54:1484–1490, 2003

Katon W, Schulberg H: Epidemiology of depression in primary care. Gen Hosp Psychiatry 14:237–247, 1992

Katon W, Von Korff M, Lin E, et al: Collaborative management to achieve treatment guidelines. Impact on depression in primary care. JAMA 273:1026–1031, 1995

Katon W, Robinson P, Von Korff M, et al: A multifaceted intervention to improve treatment of depression in primary care. Arch Gen Psychiatry 53:924–932, 1996

Kaufman J, Yang BZ, Douglas-Palumberi H, et al: Brain-derived neurotrophic factor-5-HTTLPR gene interactions and environmental modifiers of depression in children. Biol Psychiatry 59:673–680, 2006

Kendler KS, Prescott CA: A population-based twin study of lifetime major depression in men and women. Arch Gen Psychiatry 56:39–44, 1999

Kendler KS, Kessler RC, Neale MC, et al: The prediction of major depression in women: toward an integrated etiologic model. Am J Psychiatry 150:1139–1148, 1993

Kendler KS, Kessler RC, Walters EE, et al: Stressful life events, genetic liability, and onset of an episode of major depression in women. Am J Psychiatry 152:833–842, 1995

Kendler KS, Gardner CO, Prescott CA: A population-based twin study of self-esteem and gender. Psychol Med 28:1403–1409, 1998

Kendler KS, Thornton LM, Gardner CO: Genetic risk, number of previous depressive episodes, and stressful life events in predicting onset of major depression. Am J Psychiatry 158:582–586, 2001

Kessler RC, Rubinow DR, Holmes C, et al: The epidemiology of DSM-III-R bipolar I disorder in a general population survey. Psychol Med 27:1079–1089, 1997

Kessler RC, Berglund P, Demler O, et al: The epidemiology of major depressive disorder: results from the National Comorbidity Survey Replication (NCS-R). JAMA 289:3095–3105, 2003

Kessler RC, Chiu WT, Demler O, et al: Prevalence, severity, and comorbidity of twelve-month DSM-IV disorders in the National Comorbidity Survey Replication (NCS-R). Arch Gen Psychiatry 62:617–627, 2005

Kieseppa T, Partonen T, Haukka J, et al: High concordance of bipolar I disorder in a nationwide sample of twins. Am J Psychiatry 161:1814–1821, 2004

Kühner C, Angermeyer MC, Veiel HOF: Cognitive-behavioral group intervention as a means of tertiary prevention in depressed patients: acceptance and short-term efficacy. Cognit Ther Res 20:391–409, 1996

Leaf PJ, Bruce ML, Tischler GL: The differential effect of attitudes on the use of mental health services. Soc Psychiatry 21:187–192, 1986

Leverich GS, Post RM: Life charting of affective disorders. CNS Spectr 3:21–37, 1998

Lewinsohn PM, Clarke GN, Hoberman HM: The coping with depression course: review and future directions. Can J Behav Sci 21:470–493, 1989

Malkoff-Schwartz S, Frank E, Anderson B, et al: Stressful life events and social rhythm disruption in the onset of manic and depressive bipolar episodes: a preliminary investigation. Arch Gen Psychiatry 55:702–707, 1998

Marino S, Gallo JJ, Ford D, et al: Filters on the pathway to mental health care, I: incident mental disorders. Psychol Med 25:1135–1148, 1995

McCauley J, Kern DE, Kolodner K, et al: Clinical characteristics of women with a history of childhood abuse: unhealed wounds. JAMA 277:1362–1368, 1997

McPherson H, Herbison P, Romans S: Life events and relapse in established bipolar affective disorder. Br J Psychiatry 163:381–385, 1993

Miklowitz DJ: The Bipolar Disorder Survival Guide: What You and Your Family Need to Know. New York, Guilford, 2002

Mintz J, Mintz LI, Arruda MJ, et al: Treatments of depression and the functional capacity to work. Arch Gen Psychiatry 49:761–768, 1992

Muñoz RF, Ying YW, Bernal G, et al: Prevention of depression with primary care patients: a randomized controlled trial. Am J Community Psychol 23:199–222, 1995

Muñoz RF, Le HN, Clarke G, et al: Preventing the onset of major depression, in Handbook of Depression. Edited by Gotlib IH, Hammen CL. New York, Guilford, 2002, pp 383–403

Musselman DL, Evans DL, Nemeroff CB: The relationship of depression to cardiovascular disease: epidemiology, biology, and treatment. Arch Gen Psychiatry 55:580–592, 1998

National Institute of Mental Health: Bipolar Disorder (NIH Publication No. 08-3679). Rockville, MD, National Institute of Mental Health, U.S. Department of Health and Human Services, National Institute of Health, 2001

National Institute of Mental Health: Depression (NIH Publication No. 07-3561). Rockville, MD, National Institute of Mental Health, U.S. Department of Health and Human Services, National Institute of Health, 2007

Olds DL, Henderson Jr CR, Tatelbaum R, et al: Improving the life-course development of socially disadvantaged mothers: a randomized trial of nurse home visitation. Am J Public Health 78:1436–1445, 1988

Ormel J, Von Korff M, Usun TB, et al: Common mental disorders and disabilities across cultures: results from the WHO Collaborative Study on Psychological Problems in General Health Care. JAMA 272:1741–1748, 1994

Petersen AC, Compas BE, Brooks-Gunn J, et al: Depression in adolescence. Am Psychol 48:155–168, 1993

Post RM, Leverich GS: The role of psychosocial stress in the onset and progression of bipolar disorder and its comorbidities: the need for earlier and alternative modes of therapeutic intervention. Dev Psychopathol 18:1181–1211, 2006

Regier DA, Boyd JH, Burke Jr JD, et al: One-month prevalence of mental disorders in the United States: based on five Epidemiologic Catchment Area sites. Arch Gen Psychiatry 45:977–986, 1988

Regier DA, Narrow WE, Rae DS: The epidemiology of anxiety disorders: the Epidemiologic Catchment Area (ECA) experience. J Psychiatr Res 24 (suppl 2):3–14, 1990

Regier DA, Narrow WE, Rae DS, et al: The de facto US mental and addictive disorders service system: Epidemiologic Catchment Area prospective 1-year prevalence rates of disorders and services. Arch Gen Psychiatry 50:85–94, 1993

Resick PA: Clinical Psychology: A Modular Course. Philadelphia, PA, Taylor & Francis, 2001

Rhodes JE, Ebert L, Fischer K: Natural mentors: an overlooked resource in the social networks of young African American mothers. Am J Community Psychol 20:445–462, 1992

Rice J, Reich T, Andreasen NC, et al: The familial transmission of bipolar illness. Arch Gen Psychiatry 44:441–447, 1987

Rolf J, Masten AS, Cicchetti D, et al (eds): Risk and Protective Factors in the Development of Psychopathology. New York, Cambridge University Press, 1990

Rutter M, Chadwick O, Shaffer D: Head injury, in Developmental Neuropsychiatry. Edited by Rutter M. New York, Guilford, 1983, pp 83–111

Sachs GS, Thase ME: Bipolar disorder therapeutics: maintenance treatment. Biol Psychiatry 15:573–581, 2000

Sandler IN, West SG, Baca L, et al: Linking empirically based theory and evaluation: the Family Bereavement Program. Am J Community Psychol 20:491–521, 1992

Scott J, Colom F: Psychosocial treatments for bipolar disorders. Psychiatr Clin North Am 28:371–384, 2005

Simon GE, Ludman EJ, Unutzer J, et al: Randomized trial of a population-based care program for people with bipolar disorder. Psychol Med 35:13–24, 2005

Simon GE, Ludman EJ, Bauer MS, et al: Long-term effectiveness and cost of a systematic care program for bipolar disorder. Arch Gen Psychiatry 63:500–508, 2006

Southwick SM, Vythilingam M, Charney DS: The psychobiology of depression and resilience to stress: implications for prevention and treatment. Annu Rev Clin Psychol 1:255–291, 2005

Stice E, Ragan J, Randall P: Prospective relations between social support and depression: differential direction of effects for parent and peer support? J Abnorm Psychol 113:155–159, 2004

Stoner SC, Marken PA, Sommi RW: Psychiatric comorbidity and medical illness. Medical Update for Psychiatrists 3:64–70, 1998

Teicher MH, Andersen SL, Polcari A, et al: The neurobiological consequences of early stress and childhood maltreatment. Neurosci Biobehav Rev 27:33–44, 2003

Thomsen AF, Kvist TK, Andersen PK, et al: Increased risk of developing affective disorder in patients with hypothyroidism: a register-based study. Thyroid 15:700–707, 2005

Travis LA, Lyness JM, Shields CG, et al: Social support, depression, and functional disability in older adult primary-care patients. Am J Geriatr Psychiatry 12:265–271, 2004

Tsuang MT, Faraone SV: Summary and conclusions, in The Genetics of Mood Disorders. Edited by Tsuang MT, Faraone SV. Baltimore, MD, Johns Hopkins University Press, 1990

Turner RA, King PR, Tremblay PF: Coping styles and depression among psychiatric outpatients. Pers Individ Dif 13:1145–1147, 1992

Ustun TB, Ayuso-Mateos JL, Chatterji S, et al: Global burden of depressive disorders in the year 2000. Br J Psychiatry 184:386–392, 2004

Valle J, Ayuso-Gutierrez JL, Abril A, et al: Evaluation of thyroid function in lithium-naive bipolar patients. Eur Psychiatry 14:341–345, 1999

Vieta E, Colom F: Psychological interventions in bipolar disorder: from wishful thinking to an evidence-based approach. Acta Psychiatr Scand Suppl 422:34–38, 2004

Von Korff M, Katon W, Bush T, et al: Treatment costs, cost offset, and cost-effectiveness of collaborative management of depression. Psychosom Med 60:143–149, 1998

Warner V, Weissman MM, Mufson L, et al: Grandparents, parents, and grandchildren at high risk for depression: a three-generation study. J Am Acad Child Adolesc Psychiatry 38:289–296, 1999

Wehr TA, Sack DA, Rosenthal NE: Sleep reduction as a final common pathway in the genesis of mania. Am J Psychiatry 144:201–204, 1987

Weissman MM, Myers JK: Affective disorders in a US urban community: the use of research diagnostic criteria in an epidemiological survey. Arch Gen Psychiatry 35:1304–1311, 1978

Weissman MM, Kidd KK, Prusoff BA: Variability in rates of affective disorders in relatives of depressed and normal probands. Arch Gen Psychiatry 39:1397–1403, 1982

Weissman MM, Gershon ES, Kidd KK, et al: Psychiatric disorders in the relatives of probands with affective disorders: the Yale University—National Institute of Mental Health Collaborative Study. Arch Gen Psychiatry 41:13–21, 1984

Weissman MM, Leaf PJ, Tischler GL, et al: Affective disorders in five United States communities. Psychol Med 18:141–153, 1988

Weissman MM, Bland RC, Canino GJ, et al: Cross-national epidemiology of major depression and bipolar disorder. JAMA 276:293–299, 1996

Weissman MM, Warner V, Wickramaratne P, et al: Offspring of depressed parents: 10 years later. Arch Gen Psychiatry 54:932–940, 1997

Wells KB, Stewart A, Hays RD, et al: The functioning and wellbeing of depressed patients: results from the Medical Outcomes Study. JAMA 262:914–919, 1989

Zubin J, Spring B: Vulnerability: a new view of schizophrenia. J Abnorm Psychol 86:103–126, 1977

Zweifel JE, O'Brien WH: A meta-analysis of the effect of hormone replacement therapy upon depressed mood. Psychoneuroendocrinology 22:189–212, 1997

4

Prevention of Anxiety Disorders

O. Joseph Bienvenu, M.D., Ph.D.

Daniel J. Siegel

Golda S. Ginsburg, Ph.D.

This chapter is an expansion of a previous review on the prevention of anxiety disorders (Bienvenu and Ginsburg 2007). Specifically, in this chapter we discuss why one should consider prevention (i.e., the scope of the problem), risk factors for anxiety disorders, results of early prevention trials, and implications for clinical practice. This is not a systematic review of the prevention literature; rather, we focus on studies and concepts that illustrate trends in this field. This chapter does not address studies of the prevention of specific types

This work was supported by National Institute of Mental Health Grants K23 MH064543 and K23 MH063427.

of anxiety disorders or the prevention of anxiety disorders in specific contexts (e.g., after trauma) (for review, see Feldner et al. 2004).

Epidemiology of Anxiety Disorders

Anxiety disorders are the most common mental illnesses worldwide (Andrews et al. 2001; Demyttenaere et al. 2004; Wittchen and Jacobi 2005). In the U.S. National Comorbidity Survey Replication (NCS-R; Kessler et al. 2005a, 2005b), 18% of participants from the general population (ages 18 years and older) met DSM-IV criteria (American Psychiatric Association 1994) for an anxiety disorder in the last year, and 29% met the criteria at some point in their lifetime (for comparison, the lifetime prevalence of a mood disorder was 21%, and that of a substance use disorder was 16%). Anxiety disorders are also among the most common psychiatric disorders in school-age children and adolescents, with lifetime prevalences ranging between 8% and 27% (Costello et al. 2005). Partly because of their prevalence, early onset, and chronicity, anxiety disorders impose a substantial burden on society (Greenberg et al. 1999; Lepine 2002). Though anxiety disorders as a group tend to be less severe and costly than mood disorders on an individual basis, anxiety disorders may produce an even greater cost burden to populations than mood disorders because of their high prevalence (Smit et al. 2006). In addition, some anxiety disorders, such as panic disorder and obsessive-compulsive disorder, tend to be particularly severe and disabling conditions (Kessler et al. 2005b; Murray and Lopez 1996).

Adding to the burden associated with anxiety disorders is the fact that these conditions are highly comorbid with each other and with other *internalizing* conditions (e.g., depressive illnesses), and, to a lesser extent, with substance use disorders and other *externalizing* disorders (Costello et al. 2006; Kessler et al. 2005b; Krueger 1999). Importantly, anxiety disorders typically precede comorbid depressive and substance use disorders temporally; thus, it is possible that prevention or early treatment of anxiety could prevent the development of comorbid conditions in some people (Wittchen et al. 2003).

An additional reason to consider some form of prevention effort (especially a universal approach) is that, despite available effective treatments for anxiety disorders, many people do not receive treatment. For example, in the

NCS-R, only 37% of adults who recently had a DSM-IV anxiety disorder were treated in a health care setting, and only 42% used any type of services (Wang et al. 2005b). In the NCS-R, only 34% of persons with recent anxiety disorders received minimally adequate treatment. Similarly, a study in a pediatric primary care setting found that only 31% of children with anxiety disorders had received counseling or medication treatment during their lifetime (Chavira et al. 2004). Notably, although these studies were conducted in the United States, lack of treatment for mental disorders is certainly not specific to the United States (Andrews et al. 2001; Demyttenaere et al. 2004). That is, it is likely that this unmet treatment need exists worldwide. (However, diagnosis and treatment need are not necessarily identical, and controversy exists regarding priority of treatment in persons with less severe illnesses [Kessler et al. 2003; Narrow et al. 2002; Wakefield and Spitzer 2002].)

Onset of anxiety disorders tends to be early. For example, in the NCS-R, the median age at onset of anxiety disorders was 11 years (compared with 20 years for substance use disorders, and 30 years for mood disorders) (Kessler et al. 2005a). The distribution of onset ages is not completely uniform, of course, across the anxiety disorders. In the NCS-R, the median ages at onset of different anxiety disorders were as follows: specific phobia and separation anxiety disorder, 7 years; social phobia, 13 years; obsessive-compulsive disorder, 19 years; agoraphobia without panic, 20 years; posttraumatic stress disorder, 23 years; panic disorder, 24 years; and generalized anxiety disorder (GAD), 31 years. These findings are broadly consistent with prior epidemiological and clinic-based reports, although the median age at onset for GAD was a bit greater than in previous studies (GAD onset usually occurs between the late teens and late twenties; Kessler et al. 2001). Taken together, research suggests that in order to reduce the overall burden of anxiety disorders, prevention and early intervention should occur early in the life course.

Risk Factors for Anxiety Disorders

Demographic Factors

One fairly consistent demographic risk factor for anxiety disorders is female sex. Notably, obsessive-compulsive disorder and social phobia may have more equal sex distributions than other anxiety disorders (Bekker and van Mens-

Verhulst 2007; Merikangas 2005). As noted in the previous section ("Epidemiology of Anxiety Disorders"), anxiety disorders tend to have early onsets; thus, younger age is also a risk factor (e.g., Grant et al. 2008). Some longitudinal studies have also found that low income (or other aspects of socioeconomic status) elevates the risk of anxiety disorders (Grant et al. 2008; Moffitt et al. 2007; Phillips et al. 2005; Wittchen et al. 2000).

Genetics/Family History

Individuals with family histories of anxiety or depressive disorders are at greater risk of anxiety disorders than those without such family history (Hettema 2008; Hirshfeld-Becker et al. 2008). For example, Beidel and Turner (1997) found that offspring of anxious and/or anxious and depressed parents, compared with offspring of parents who did not have anxiety or depression, were more than four times as likely to have an anxiety disorder. This familiality appears to be mainly due to genetic factors, as opposed to shared environmental factors (Hettema 2008; Hettema et al. 2001).

Personality/Temperament

Personality/temperament traits like high neuroticism, low extraversion, or behavioral inhibition appear to be risk factors, or at least markers of risk, for most anxiety disorders (Brandes and Bienvenu 2006; Hirshfeld-Becker et al. 2008). Notably, these traits also appear to index genetic vulnerability to anxiety (and depressive) disorders (Bienvenu et al. 2007; Hettema et al. 2006); that is, personality traits and genetic vulnerabilities may not be independent risk factors.

Environmental Factors

Having overprotective and/or critical parents has been consistently associated with anxiety disorders in offspring (McLeod et al. 2007), although associations are modest and causal mechanisms remain incompletely understood (Hirshfeld-Becker et al. 2008). It is unclear whether the relationship between parental overprotection/criticism and childhood anxiety disorder reflects 1) a causal effect of parenting style, 2) anxious children eliciting overprotection, 3) anxiety in the parents (which could be genetically transmitted to the children), 4) reciprocal mechanisms, or 5) interactions of the above (e.g., Ginsburg et al. 2004). Researchers are just beginning to address these issues (Hirshfeld-Becker et al. 2008).

Studies of Anxiety Disorders Prevention

One of the issues that prevention scientists grapple with is "prevention in whom?" That is, based on the language suggested by the Institute of Medicine (1994), prevention efforts could be *indicated* (targeting persons with symptoms but not a disorder), *selective* (targeting persons at risk for a disorder), or *universal* (targeting an entire population). To date, few preventive interventions have been evaluated systematically at each of these levels of risk. With respect to how to prevent anxiety disorders, most interventions have been based on cognitive-behavioral principles. In the next sections we describe studies of preventive interventions targeting each of these three levels of risk and report their efficacy. These studies are largely examples of primary or secondary prevention, using the older prevention terminology (see Chapter 1, "Prevention in Mental Health").

Indicated Preventive Interventions

One of the first examples of an indicated preventive intervention focusing on childhood anxiety disorders was conducted by Dadds and colleagues (1997). These investigators targeted schoolchildren between ages 7 and 14 who did not have an anxiety disorder but who exhibited symptoms of anxiety, as well as children who met criteria for an anxiety disorder but were in the less severe range (the most common anxiety disorders were specific and social phobias, GAD, and separation anxiety disorder). After screening, 128 children were randomly assigned to the intervention group or a control condition (i.e., monitoring only). The intervention was based on Kendall's FEAR plan (F = feeling good by learning to relax; E = expecting good things to happen through positive self-talk; A = actions to take in facing up to fear stimuli; and R = rewarding oneself for efforts to overcome fear or worry; Kendall 1994) and involved a group cognitive-behavioral therapy (CBT) program in which children developed their own plans for graduated exposure to fear stimuli using physiological, cognitive, and behavioral coping strategies. Group sessions were held weekly for 10 weeks in school settings and involved 5–12 children per group. Three parental sessions were held during the 10-week period, to introduce parents to child management skills, to illustrate how parents could model and encourage use of the child intervention strategies, and to teach parents to use the intervention strategies to cope with their own anxiety.

The results of this study were encouraging (Dadds et al. 1997). Immediately postintervention, improvements in anxiety symptoms were noted in both groups, and there were equal rates of children having an anxiety disorder in each group (10%). At the 6-month follow-up, anxiety disorder prevalence was lower in the intervention group (16% vs. 54%), but at the 1-year follow-up there was no difference between the two groups in anxiety disorder prevalence. At the final assessment (at 24 months), children in the CBT group were less likely to have an anxiety disorder (20% vs. 39%). Thus, while the intervention may have had effects that varied over time, overall the CBT group had a lower burden of anxiety disorders.

Selective Preventive Interventions

Selective preventive interventions are aimed at persons who are at elevated risk based on specific known risk factors. Here, we discuss examples of selective interventions that have been evaluated in studies that target persons considered at high risk on three, likely related, bases: inhibited temperament, parental history of an anxiety disorder, and pessimistic attitudes.

Inhibited Temperament

Rapee and colleagues reasoned that a number of putative risk factors for anxiety disorders may be indexed or moderated/mediated by an inhibited temperament (Rapee 2002; Rapee et al. 2005). These investigators designed an intervention for parents of inhibited children to reduce parental anxiety, environmental support of avoidant coping, and vicarious and instructional learning of avoidance. They recruited 146 children, ages 3–5 years, who appeared behaviorally inhibited based on questionnaire and laboratory measures and randomly assigned half of them to an intervention group (parental education) and half to a control group (monitoring). Components of the intervention included the following:

- Education regarding the nature of withdrawal and anxiety
- Information about the importance of modeling competence and promoting independence

- Development of exposure hierarchies for the child and practice of gradual exposure
- Cognitive restructuring for the parent(s)
- Discussion of high-risk periods, such as the commencement of school

Parents in the intervention group attended six 90-minute, small-group sessions over the course of 2½ months. Diagnostic assessments were carried out at baseline (before the intervention or monitoring period began) and 1 year later.

In a preliminary report (Rapee 2002), the intervention seemed to have a significant effect on inhibited temperament (per mothers' ratings but not per laboratory assessments), with a greater reduction in the intervention group. There was also a greater reduction in the number of anxiety disorder diagnoses in the intervention group (the most common anxiety disorder diagnoses were specific and social phobias and separation anxiety disorder). In a subsequent report (Rapee et al. 2005) that included 26 more participants but used a different analytical method (with anxiety disorders and temperament apparently included simultaneously in a more complex statistical model), temperament did not appear to be independently affected by the intervention, although the number of anxiety disorders was. Specifically, the prevalence of anxiety disorders at the 1-year follow-up was significantly lower in children whose parents received the intervention, compared with children in the control group (50% vs. 63%).

Parental History of an Anxiety Disorder

Ginsburg (2009) has recently completed a prevention trial in children at high risk for anxiety disorders because of parental anxiety disorder. In contrast to the other studies reviewed in this chapter, an exclusionary criterion for this study was baseline anxiety disorder in the enrolled children. The means employed to potentially decrease the risk of anxiety disorders included a family-based intervention using the following:

- Psychoeducation (regarding the cognitive-behavioral conceptualization of anxiety)
- Contingency management (rewarding "brave" behaviors and using extinction techniques to reduce avoidant behaviors)

- Parental instruction in modeling coping behaviors
- Strategies to recognize and reduce parental anxiety levels
- Enhancement of specific problem-solving and communication skills in the family

The study included 40 children (mean age, 9 years) whose parents met DSM-IV criteria for a broad range of anxiety disorders. The children and their families were randomly assigned to the 8-week cognitive-behavioral intervention described above, the *Coping and Promoting Strength* program (CAPS; $n=20$), or a monitoring-only control condition ($n=20$). Independent evaluators conducted diagnostic interviews, and children and parents completed questionnaires regarding the children's anxiety symptoms before and after the intervention, as well as at 6 and 12 months following the postintervention assessment. In the intent-to-treat analyses, 30% of the children in the control group developed an anxiety disorder by the 12-month follow-up, compared with 0% in the CAPS group (Ginsburg 2009).

Pessimistic Attitudes

Seligman and colleagues (1999) assessed the efficacy of an 8-week CBT workshop (eight 2-hour meetings with 10–12 students) designed to prevent depression and anxiety in university students at risk because of a consistently pessimistic attributional style (established via questionnaire). Prior unpublished studies suggested that such students are at high risk for developing depression over the next few years. Students ($N=231$) were randomly assigned to either the intervention group or a control (monitoring) group. Topics in the intervention workshop included

- The cognitive theory of change
- Identification of automatic negative thoughts and underlying beliefs
- Marshaling of evidence to question and dispute automatic negative thoughts and irrational beliefs
- Replacement of automatic negative thoughts with more constructive interpretations, beliefs, and behaviors
- Behavioral activation strategies
- Interpersonal skills
- Stress management
- Generalizing coping skills to new situations

Students were given homework between workshop meetings, and they met with a trainer individually on six occasions over the next 1–2 years, to review skills and to have their questions addressed. The students were followed over a 3-year period, with repeated assessments of mental disorders and symptoms.

Results indicated that students in the intervention group had significantly fewer episodes of GAD and significantly fewer moderate (but not severe) episodes of depression (Seligman et al. 1999). In addition, the students in the intervention group reported significantly fewer anxiety and depressive symptoms, as well as changes in explanatory style, hope, and attitudes (cognitive measures). As might be expected, the cognitive changes appeared to mediate differences between groups on measures of anxiety and depression. Though effect sizes were moderate, most of these differences persisted during 3 years of follow-up.

Universal Preventive Interventions

Universal preventive interventions target an entire population without regard to risk status. Barrett and colleagues have conducted several universal prevention studies in children and adolescents in primary and secondary school settings, employing cognitive-behavioral techniques (e.g., Barrett and Turner 2001; Barrett et al. 2006; Lock and Barrett 2003, 2006). Arguments put forth for school-based universal interventions include less interventionist burden (i.e., no need to screen or recruit, as well as easier retention of participants), as well as potentially less stigma for the participants (Barrett et al. 2006). An argument against universal interventions is that resources are often limited and resources should therefore target those at highest risk. The interventions evaluated by Barrett and colleagues involved 10–12 classroom sessions for students, with four psychoeducational sessions for parents. The mnemonic FRIENDS is an acronym for the different skills taught in the sessions (F = feeling worried; R = relax and feel good; I = inner helpful thoughts; E = explore plans; N = nice work, reward yourself; D = don't forget to practice; and S = stay calm for life).

In one of the FRIENDS evaluation studies (Barrett and Turner 2001), 489 children ages 10–12 years were randomly assigned to one of three conditions: a psychologist-led intervention, a teacher-led intervention, or a usual care condition. At postintervention, children in both teacher-led and psychologist-led groups self-reported fewer anxiety symptoms compared with children in the usual care group. No differences were found in diagnoses (assessed in a subsample). Youths with high levels of anxiety symptoms at the preintervention assessment were more likely to move into the "normal" range if they had an intervention than if they received usual care. Positive outcomes for the prevention program were reported in replication studies, in which younger children, females, and those with greater anxiety severity at baseline benefited most from intervention (Lock and Barrett 2003). Although the majority of children in these Australian studies were white, Barrett and colleagues (2003) also reported positive findings in a similar study including a sample of non-English-speaking migrant youths with Yugoslavian, Chinese, and mixed-race backgrounds.

Public and Provider Education as a Prevention Tool

Publicity regarding the nature of, and effective treatments for, anxiety disorders is a potential prevention tool that unfortunately remains unstudied. In the United States, the public gets some education regarding anxiety disorders via news outlets (television, radio, print, and Internet media) and direct-to-consumer advertising via pharmaceutical companies. We know of no empirical studies explicitly addressing how such publicity affects persons' behaviors with regard to getting early treatment, or reducing the burden of anxiety disorders (secondary or tertiary prevention in the older terminology), but our anecdotal clinical experience suggests that publicity can facilitate persons' initiating psychiatric care.

In the United States, public health campaigns have attempted to educate the populace regarding mood disorders, and this may be facilitating treatment seeking to some extent (Insel and Fenton 2005). For example, in the 11 years between the original NCS (1990–1992) and the NCS-R (2001–2003), the proportion of persons with recent mood disorders who were in treatment in the health care sector increased from 28% to 51% (Kessler et al. 1999; Wang et al. 2005b). This increase may relate, at least in part, to increased public awareness. In the same period, the proportion of persons with recent anxiety disorders who were in treatment in the health care sector also increased, from

19% to 37%; unfortunately, the lag time between illness onset and receipt of treatment was long (i.e., 9–23 years) (Wang et al. 2005a). In the NCS-R, the majority of persons with mood disorders, panic disorder, or GAD eventually received some treatment; however, the cumulative lifetime probability of treatment was substantially lower for posttraumatic stress disorder and agoraphobia, and still lower for social and specific phobias (Wang et al. 2005a). An important goal for future research is to determine the effect of education on the outcomes of persons with, or at risk for, anxiety disorders.

It is worth noting that further education directed at primary care physicians (including pediatricians) about anxiety disorders seems vital. This is underscored by a recent study comparing U.S. service sectors used for mental health care (Wang et al. 2006). The researchers noted that, in comparing the NCS and NCS-R, a large increase was seen in the number of persons who sought psychiatric care exclusively in the general medical setting. In Australia, a national survey showed that most persons with recent mental disorders sought care, if any, from general practitioners (Andrews et al. 2001). Educational programs for primary care physicians regarding the prevention and treatment of anxiety disorders and their effects on patient outcomes also deserve study.

Mental health providers have an important role in prevention, in properly educating patients about the chronic/recurrent nature of anxiety problems, and in working with patients to develop plans for early intervention in the event of symptom recurrence. In addition, mental health providers can educate patients about anxiety disorders as risk factors for comorbid depressive and substance use disorders.

Important Considerations Pertaining to Prevention of Anxiety Disorders

As previously outlined in this chapter, anxiety disorders are common and burdensome conditions with early onset. Noted risk factors include demographic characteristics, family history, temperament/personality, and parenting styles. We have also presented evidence regarding the promise of cognitive-behavioral preventive interventions in groups characterized by varying levels of risk of anxiety disorders, and we have argued that simple education merits further study. Now we consider several limitations of this emerging field and suggest avenues for future research and public health policy.

The most glaring limitation of the prevention research literature is the dearth of studies. On the positive side, this means that the field is ripe for researchers who wish to make significant contributions. On the negative side, it means that we are limited in our ability to draw firm conclusions about whether, how, and in whom anxiety disorders can be prevented. Most studies have had small sample sizes, which limit their power to detect prevention effects. Also, most have used a narrow range of assessments (e.g., only self-reports or only anxiety disorder diagnoses) and have had limited follow-up periods (i.e., ≤3 years). The latter is a particular disadvantage, given that the impact of preventive interventions is hoped to be long-term, rather than short-term.

Many additional questions remain about the prevention of anxiety disorders, including the following:

- Exactly when in the life course should we consider prevention of anxiety disorders?
- Whom should prevention efforts target, and why?
- What intervention strategies, delivery formats, and settings would be most helpful?
- How much does prevention cost, and who will pay for it?

Below we attempt to address these issues as considerations for future research.

Exactly When in the Life Course Should We Consider Prevention of Anxiety Disorders?

Although most prevention scientists would agree that offering preventive interventions early in the life course makes good sense, *how* early has yet to be determined. For example, interventions to prevent childhood anxiety disorders aimed at anxious and expectant parents may have the most impact (i.e., intervening with parents prior to or shortly after the child's birth). Alternatively, delivering preventive interventions when children are very young (e.g., ages 3–5 years), perhaps to those with early signs of anxiety or behavioral inhibition, may have the greatest impact (Rapee et al. 2005). Finally, prevention efforts may be most useful when they are delivered during high-risk life transitions, such as when one is entering elementary school, middle school, high school, college, the workforce, marriage, or parenthood. There is still much to learn about when in the life course prevention may have its biggest effect.

Whom Should Prevention Efforts Target, and Why?

In order to determine whom to target, a critical need for the field is further empirical identification of risk and protective factors for the development of anxiety disorders. Theoretical models that specify how prevention might work (i.e., the mechanisms through which proximal and distal outcomes are expected to occur) must be articulated and tested. The study conducted by Seligman and colleagues (1999), discussed previously (see "Pessimistic Attitudes" in the "Selective Preventive Interventions" section), provides an example of this. Figure 4–1 (Bienvenu and Ginsburg 2007) displays a schematic of the CAPS program, a preventive intervention model for offspring of anxious parents that was developed by G. S. Ginsburg, one of the authors of this chapter. The CAPS program is a theoretically derived preventive intervention designed to change a set of modifiable risk and protective factors that, based on prior research and theory, are believed to mediate the development of anxiety disorders in children. The underlying theory of the intervention is that program-induced change in these mediators (e.g., parenting behaviors and maladaptive cognitions) will account for the effects of the program on reducing anxiety disorders. The first column of Figure 4–1 lists the modifiable risk factors (in children and parents); the second column lists the intervention strategies that target those risk factors; and the third and fourth columns list the hypothesized short-term (proximal) and long-term (distal) impacts of the intervention. Although the development of this model was informed by existing research (Ginsburg 2004), it awaits empirical validation. It is presented here as a heuristic of a theoretical model of intervention effects, but it is fully expected that the model and intervention components will be refined over time.

Related to the identification of risk and protective factors is an appreciation that these factors may not be stable over time and/or may be unique to specific developmental stages or life transitions (e.g., entry into elementary school or parenthood). Thus, identifying what to target might depend on when across the life span these risks occur. Donovan and Spence (2000) have detailed specific risk factors for anxiety disorders across the life span, and Kellam

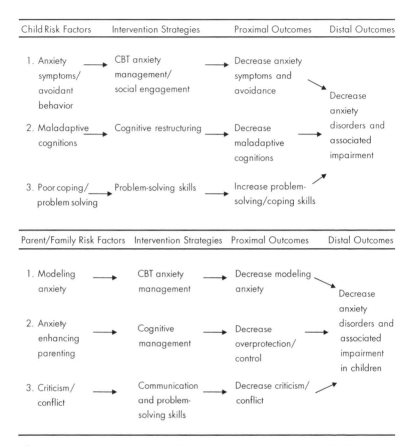

Figure 4–1.   The Coping and Promoting Strength program (CAPS) intervention model.

Note.   The top portion represents child risk factors and interventions. The bottom portion represents parental risk factors and interventions.
CBT = cognitive-behavioral therapy.
Source.   Adapted with permission from Informa Healthcare: *International Review of Psychiatry* (Bienvenu OJ, Ginsburg GS: "Prevention of Anxiety Disorders." *International Review of Psychiatry [Abingdon, England]* 19:647–654, 2007).

and Van Horn (1997) have presented a prevention model that highlights how the timing of interventions should account for the prevalence of risk factors at different ages, the timing of disorder onset, and the specific life task demands at different developmental stages.

What Intervention Strategies, Delivery Formats, and Settings Would Be Most Helpful?

Another goal for future research should be to clarify which specific preventive intervention strategies are most effective. Currently, most interventions combine a number of cognitive-behavioral ingredients; thus, it is difficult to determine which ones may have the greatest short-term and long-term impact. Studies examining theory-based mechanisms of interventions will help to answer these questions.

Also unclear is whether preventive intervention strategies are most effective when delivered on a community-wide basis, as in public service announcements or public education campaigns, or whether work with smaller groups or individual families is needed. The recent success of bibliotherapy (Rapee et al. 2006) and Web-based formats for the treatment of anxiety disorders suggests that additional options may be viable for preventive interventions.

Currently, most preventive interventions for children are delivered in schools. Although there are many advantages to this (e.g., increased access) there are also disadvantages (e.g., time diverted from academics) that need to be weighed. In addition, involving family members or adults is often not practical in this milieu. Alternative settings, such as places of worship, community settings, the workplace, and hospital clinics should also be examined as potential venues for interventions to prevent anxiety disorders.

How Much Does Prevention Cost, and Who Will Pay for It?

Few studies have examined the cost-effectiveness of anxiety disorder prevention programs. Indeed, a top priority for the field is to conduct a cost-benefit analysis for potential payers of such interventions. Currently, routine preventive interventions for anxiety disorders are not, to the authors' knowledge, subsidized by governments or insurance companies. Data on the cost savings of such interventions would be useful leverage for soliciting third-party payers. Evidence will be needed about which strategies might be the most cost-effective in the long term. For instance, would indicated and selective interventions be more cost-effective than universal interventions? Whether or not preventive cognitive-behavioral interventions are adopted by governments or insurers in the near future, based on the apparent efficacy of prevention programs, some persons may elect to seek these interventions and pay for them themselves. Importantly, the potential benefits for individuals and their families are compelling enough to warrant further financial support of research.

Conclusion

Clinicians should recognize that anxiety disorders are very common illnesses with early onsets, and have substantial lifetime comorbidity with other anxiety disorders, depressive disorders, and, to a lesser extent, substance use disorders. Thus, prevention and early treatment of anxiety disorders may substantially reduce the psychiatric burden for individuals over their lifetime.

Knowledge of risk factors can help clinicians recognize which of their patients (and their patients' family members) are at greatest risk (see "Key Points" below). Such information can be used in determining whom to educate regarding anxiety disorders and whom to target for prevention, monitoring, and early intervention.

The most commonly studied interventions in the growing prevention literature involve cognitive-behavioral techniques. Though it is hoped that such interventions will have long-lasting effects (e.g., from childhood to early adulthood), this remains to be determined. Nevertheless, shorter-term results are encouraging.

Key Points

- Anxiety disorders are the most common mental illnesses worldwide, affecting almost one-third of the U.S. population at some point. These disorders place a significant burden on individuals and society, yet many people do not receive treatment.

- Risk factors for anxiety disorders include female sex; young age; low socioeconomic status; family history of anxiety or depressive disorders; personality traits such as neuroticism, behavioral inhibition, and a low level of extraversion; and having overprotective and/or critical parents.

- Prevention efforts could be indicated (targeting persons with symptoms but not a disorder), selective (targeting persons at elevated risk for a disorder), or universal (targeting an entire population). Cognitive-behavioral interventions have shown promise in studies focusing on each of these levels of risk: indicated prevention for anxious children; selective prevention for young persons at risk due to inhibited temperament, parental history of an anxiety disorder, or pessimistic attitudes; and universal prevention strategies in school settings.

• Publicity regarding the nature of and effective treatments for anxiety disorders may help facilitate anxious persons' initiating psychiatric care (secondary and tertiary prevention), although this remains unstudied. Education of primary care physicians regarding prevention and treatment of anxiety disorders, and patient education by mental health providers, are essential.

• Additional research is necessary to address the following questions: Exactly when in the life course might preventive interventions have the greatest impact? Whom should prevention efforts target, and why? What intervention strategies, delivery formats, and settings would be most helpful? Finally, how much does prevention cost, and who will pay for it?

References

American Psychiatric Association: Diagnostic and Statistical Manual of Mental Disorders, 4th Edition. Washington, DC, American Psychiatric Association, 1994

Andrews G, Henderson S, Hall W: Prevalence, comorbidity, disability and service utilization: overview of the Australian National Mental Health Survey. Br J Psychiatry 178:145–153, 2001

Barrett PM, Turner C: Prevention of anxiety symptoms in primary school children: preliminary results from a universal school-based trial. Br J Clin Psychol 40:399–410, 2001

Barrett P, Sonderegger R, Xenos S: Using FRIENDS to combat anxiety and adjustment problems among young migrants to Australia: a national trial. Clin Child Psychol Psychiatry 8:241–260, 2003

Barrett PM, Farrell LJ, Ollendick TH, et al: Long-term outcomes of an Australian universal prevention trial of anxiety and depression symptoms in children and youth: an evaluation of the FRIENDS program. J Clin Child Adolesc Psychol 35:403–411, 2006

Beidel DC, Turner SM: At risk for anxiety: I: psychopathology in the offspring of anxious parents. J Am Acad Child Adolesc Psychiatry 36:918–924, 1997

Bekker MH, van Mens-Verhulst J: Anxiety disorders: sex differences in prevalence, degree, and background, but gender-neutral treatment. Gend Med 4 (suppl B): S178–S193, 2007

Bienvenu OJ, Ginsburg GS: Prevention of anxiety disorders. Int Rev Psychiatry 19:647–654, 2007

Bienvenu OJ, Hettema JM, Neale MC, et al: Low extraversion and high neuroticism as indices of genetic and environmental risk for social phobia, agoraphobia, and animal phobia. Am J Psychiatry 164:1714–1721, 2007

Brandes M, Bienvenu OJ: Personality and anxiety disorders. Curr Psychiatry Rep 8:263–269, 2006

Chavira DA, Stein MB, Bailey K, et al: Child anxiety in primary care: prevalent but untreated. Depress Anxiety 20:155–164, 2004

Costello EJ, Egger H, Angold A: The developmental epidemiology of anxiety disorders: phenomenology, prevalence, and comorbidity. Child Adolesc Psychiatr Clin N Am 14:631–648, 2005

Costello EJ, Foley DL, Angold A: 10-year research update review: the epidemiology of child and adolescent psychiatric disorders: II: developmental epidemiology. J Am Acad Child Adolesc Psychiatry 45:8–25, 2006

Dadds MR, Spence SH, Holland DE, et al: Prevention and early intervention for anxiety disorders: a controlled trial. J Consult Clin Psychol 65:627–635, 1997

Demyttenaere K, Bruffaerts R, Posada-Villa J, et al: Prevalence, severity, and unmet need for treatment of mental disorders in the World Health Organization World Mental Health Surveys. JAMA 291:2581–2590, 2004

Donovan CL, Spence SH: Prevention of childhood anxiety disorders. Clin Psychol Rev 20:509–531, 2000

Feldner MT, Zvolensky MJ, Schmidt NB: Prevention of anxiety psychopathology: a critical review of the empirical literature. Clinical Psychology: Science and Practice 11:405–424, 2004

Ginsburg GS: Anxiety prevention programs for youth: practical and theoretical considerations. Clinical Psychology: Science and Practice 11:430–434, 2004

Ginsburg GS: The Child Anxiety Prevention Study: intervention model and primary outcomes. J Consult Clin Psychol 77:580–587, 2009

Ginsburg GS, Grover R, Ialongo N: Parenting behaviors among anxious and non-anxious mothers: relation with concurrent and long-term child outcomes. Child Fam Behav Ther 26:23–41, 2004

Grant BF, Goldstein RB, Chou SP, et al: Sociodemographic and psychopathologic predictors of first incidence of DSM-IV substance use, mood and anxiety disorders: results from the Wave 2 National Epidemiologic Survey on Alcohol and Related Conditions. Mol Psychiatry 2008 Apr 22 [Epub ahead of print]

Greenberg PE, Sisitsky T, Kessler RC, et al: The economic burden of anxiety disorders in the 1990s. J Clin Psychiatry 60:427–435, 1999

Hettema JM: What is the genetic relationship between anxiety and depression? Am J Med Genet C Semin Med Genet 148:140–146, 2008

Hettema JM, Neale MC, Kendler KS: A review and meta-analysis of the genetic epidemiology of anxiety disorders. Am J Psychiatry 158:1568–1578, 2001

Hettema JM, Neale MC, Myers JM, et al: A population-based twin study of the relationship between neuroticism and internalizing disorders. Am J Psychiatry 163:857–864, 2006

Hirshfeld-Becker DR, Micco JA, Simoes NA, et al: High risk studies and developmental antecedents of anxiety disorders. Am J Med Genet C Semin Med Genet 148:99–117, 2008

Insel T, Fenton W: Psychiatric epidemiology: it's not just about counting anymore. Arch Gen Psychiatry 62:590–592, 2005

Institute of Medicine: Reducing Risks for Mental Disorders: Frontiers for Preventive Intervention Research. Washington, DC, National Academy Press, 1994

Kellam SG, Van Horn YV: Life course development, community epidemiology, and preventive trials: a scientific structure for prevention research. Am J Community Psychol 25:177–188, 1997

Kendall PC: Treatment of anxiety disorders in children: a randomized controlled trial. J Consul Clin Psychol 62:100–110, 1994

Kessler RC, Zhao S, Katz SJ, et al: Past-year use of outpatient services for psychiatric problems in the National Comorbidity Survey. Am J Psychiatry 156:115–123, 1999

Kessler RC, Keller MB, Wittchen HU: The epidemiology of generalized anxiety disorder. Psychiatr Clin North Am 24:19–39, 2001

Kessler RC, Merikangas KR, Berglund P, et al: Mild disorders should not be eliminated from the DSM-V. Arch Gen Psychiatry 60:1117–1122, 2003

Kessler RC, Berglund P, Demler O, et al: Lifetime prevalence and age-of-onset distributions of DSM-IV disorders in the National Comorbidity Survey Replication. Arch Gen Psychiatry 62:593–602, 2005a

Kessler RC, Chiu WT, Merikangas KR, et al: Prevalence, severity, and comorbidity of 12-month DSM-IV disorders in the National Comorbidity Survey Replication. Arch Gen Psychiatry 62:617–627, 2005b

Krueger RF: The structure of common mental disorders. Arch Gen Psychiatry 56:921–926, 1999

Lepine JP: The epidemiology of anxiety disorders: prevalence and societal costs. J Clin Psychiatry 63:4–8, 2002

Lock S, Barrett PM: A longitudinal study of developmental differences in universal preventive intervention for child anxiety. Behav Change 20:183–199, 2003

McLeod BD, Wood JJ, Weisz JR: Examining the association between parenting and childhood anxiety: a meta-analysis. Clin Psychol Rev 27:155–172, 2007

Merikangas KR: Vulnerability factors for anxiety disorders in children and adolescents. Child Adolesc Psychiatr Clin N Am 14:649–679, 2005

Moffitt TE, Caspi A, Harrington H, et al: Generalized anxiety disorder and depression: childhood risk factors in a birth cohort followed to age 32. Psychol Med 37:441–452, 2007

Murray CL, Lopez AD: The Global Burden of Disease. Cambridge, MA, Harvard University Press, 1996

Narrow WE, Rae DS, Robins LN, et al: Revised prevalence estimates of mental disorders in the United States: using a clinical significance criterion to reconcile 2 surveys' estimates. Arch Gen Psychiatry 59:115–123, 2002

Phillips NK, Hammen CL, Brennan PA, et al: Early adversity and the prospective prediction of depressive and anxiety disorders in adolescents. J Abnorm Child Psychol 33:13–24, 2005

Rapee RM: The development and modification of temperamental risk for anxiety disorders: prevention of a lifetime of anxiety? Biol Psychiatry 52:947–957, 2002

Rapee RM, Kennedy S, Ingram M, et al: Prevention and early intervention of anxiety disorders in inhibited preschool children. J Consult Clin Psychol 73:488–497, 2005

Rapee RM, Abbott MJ, Lyneham HJ: Bibliotherapy for children with anxiety disorders using written materials for parents: a randomized controlled trial. J Consult Clin Psychol 74:436–444, 2006

Seligman MEP, Schulman P, DeRubeis RJ, et al: The prevention of depression and anxiety. Prevention and Treatment 2: article 8, 1999

Smit F, Cuijpers P, Oostenbrink J, et al: Costs of nine common mental disorders: implications for curative and preventive psychiatry. J Ment Health Policy Econ 9:193–200, 2006

Wakefield JC, Spitzer RL: Lowered estimates—but of what? Arch Gen Psychiatry 59:129–130, 2002

Wang PS, Berglund P, Olfson M, et al: Failure and delay in initial treatment contact after first onset of mental disorders in the National Comorbidity Survey Replication. Arch Gen Psychiatry 62:603–613, 2005a

Wang PS, Lane M, Olfson M, et al: Twelve-month use of mental health services in the United States. Arch Gen Psychiatry 62:629–640, 2005b

Wang PS, Demler O, Olfson M, et al: Changing profiles of service sectors used for mental health care in the United States. Am J Psychiatry 163:1187–1198, 2006

Wittchen HU, Jacobi F: Size and burden of mental disorders in Europe—a critical review and appraisal of 27 studies. Eur Neuropsychopharmacol 15:357–376, 2005

Wittchen HU, Kessler RC, Pfister H, et al: Why do people with anxiety disorders become depressed?: a prospective-longitudinal community study. Acta Psychiatr Scand 102 (suppl 406):14–23, 2000

Wittchen HU, Beesdo K, Bittner A, et al: Depressive episodes—evidence for a causal role of primary anxiety disorders? Eur Psychiatry 18:384–393, 2003

5

Complementary and Alternative Medicine in the Prevention of Depression and Anxiety

Ashli A. Owen-Smith, Ph.D.

Charles L. Raison, M.D.

The use of complementary and alternative medicine (CAM) is becoming increasingly widespread, particularly among individuals with depression and anxiety. In this chapter we review research on the efficacy of various CAM modalities for both treating and preventing depression and anxiety, discuss the implications of patients' CAM use for mental health practitioners, and provide directions for future research.

Definition of Complementary and Alternative Medicine

The National Center for Complementary and Alternative Medicine (NCCAM) defines *complementary and alternative medicine* as a group of medical and health care systems, therapies, and products that are not currently considered part of mainstream, conventional (biomedical) medicine (Lake and Spiegel 2007; National Center for Complementary and Alternative Medicine 2008). *Integrative medicine*, a term often used in conjunction with CAM in the scientific literature, is the combining of biomedical, complementary, and alternative therapies such that the treatment regimen is tailored to each individual's unique symptoms and specific circumstances (Lake 2007).

The NCCAM has grouped these practices into five main categories:

1. Mind-body medicine
2. Biologically based practices
3. Manipulative and body-based practices
4. Energy medicine
5. Whole medical systems

Mind-body medicine focuses primarily on the interactions between the mind and body and the ways in which these interactions can impact health. Examples of mind-body therapies include prayer/spiritual healing, meditation, yoga, tai chi, and hypnosis. Biologically based practices are those that utilize dietary supplements (e.g., herbs, vitamins, fatty acids, probiotics). Manipulative and body-based practices include chiropractic and osteopathic manipulation, massage, rolfing (deep tissue massage), and reflexology. Energy medicine is based on the idea that human beings possess subtle forms of energy that can be manipulated for both physical and mental health. Practices considered forms of energy medicine include reiki, qi gong, and acupuncture. Whole medical systems are systems that have been developed independently from conventional medicine and are typically practiced by specific cultures. Examples include traditional Chinese medicine and ayurvedic medicine (National Center for Complementary and Alternative Medicine 2008).

It is important to note that which particular therapies are considered outside of mainstream, conventional medicine depends on a specific culture's dominant medical system. For example, the use of herbs to treat various psychological disturbances is a common practice by some Indian health care providers and is considered part of conventional medicine in certain parts of India. The most common herbs used to treat and prevent psychological disturbances are brahmi, vacha, and kapikacchu (Lake and Spiegel 2007). The use of those same herbs in the United States would be labeled as CAM because, in contrast to India, herbal supplements are not typically included in Western medical school curricula or in best-practice protocols. Additionally, therapies labeled as CAM are constantly fluctuating based on myriad factors including 1) the emergence of efficacy research about the therapy, 2) insurance coverage of the therapy, and 3) the availability of the therapy. For example, although chiropractic care was once considered belonging solely to the genre of CAM, research suggests that many physicians may be more frequently referring patients for chiropractic care and believe in its efficacy (Astin et al. 1998), suggesting that this particular modality may be transitioning from the category of CAM to that of conventional, or at least integrative, medicine.

Distinction Between "Complementary" and "Alternative" Medicine

Though the terms *complementary* and *alternative* are often used interchangeably, they have different meanings (and this distinction can have important clinical implications, which is discussed further at the end of the chapter; see "Implications for Mental Health Practitioners"). A *complementary* medicine is one that is used *in conjunction with* another therapy. Typically the other therapy is conventional in nature—for example, the use of St. John's wort (*Hypericum perforatum*) to treat depression in addition to psychotherapy (Lake and Spiegel 2007). An *alternative* therapy, by contrast, is one that is used *instead of* a conventional therapy—for example, the use of kava (*Piper methysticum*) for anxiety in place of benzodiazepines (Pittler and Ernst 2000).

Complementary and Alternative Medicine Use in the United States

Estimates from the National Health Interview Survey suggest that approximately 35% of Americans use at least one CAM modality (Tindle et al. 2005). Individuals report using myriad therapies and practices (one study assessed 1,600 different CAM modalities); the most commonly used therapies include spiritual healing/prayer, herbal medicine, chiropractic care, massage, and relaxation techniques (e.g., meditation, yoga, breathing exercises) (Barnes et al. 2004; Bausell et al. 2001; Ni et al. 2002; Standish et al. 2001). Interestingly, the use of herbal therapies and yoga has increased in recent years while the use of chiropractic care and massage therapy has decreased. These shifts in utilization rates may be due to the fact that access to and insurance coverage of the latter therapies have become more limited under managed care (Tindle et al. 2005).

Not all individuals are equally likely to use CAM. Users are typically more likely to be younger than age 65, be female, reside in the western United States, live in urban areas, have at least a high school education, and have a higher annual household income than individuals who do not use CAM (Barnes et al. 2004; Bausell et al. 2001; Ni et al. 2002; Tindle et al. 2005). White Americans are more likely to use manipulative and body-based practices whereas African Americans are more likely to use mind-body therapies including prayer (Barnes et al. 2004). CAM users are also more likely to report experiencing a greater number of health conditions compared with nonusers, suggesting that CAM users may be in poorer health (Ni et al. 2002; Paramore 1997). The fact that individuals most often seek CAM therapies for the treatment of certain health conditions, as opposed to using CAM for prevention purposes, further supports this hypothesis. The most common medical conditions treated with CAM are chronic pain (specifically neck, back, and joint-related pain), colds, headaches, anxiety, and depression (Barnes et al. 2004; Eisenberg et al. 1998; Paramore 1997). The most frequently reported reasons for using CAM include dissatisfaction with conventional medicine (Ritchie et al. 2005), that the user believes current medications are ineffective and/or that alternative therapies would help (Cauffield 2000), that a conventional health care provider suggested it, and that access to conventional health care is complicated by certain barriers (Ritchie et al. 2005).

Complementary and Alternative Medicine and Mental Illness Treatment

Overview

Given that most individuals seek CAM for the treatment of health problems, it is not surprising that individuals with mental illnesses are among the most frequent users of CAM (Grzywacz et al. 2006; Lake and Spiegel 2007). Unützer and colleagues (2000) reported that individuals who meet criteria for major depression, panic disorder, generalized anxiety disorder, mania, or psychosis, assessed by structured interviews based on the World Health Organization Composite International Diagnostic Interview, are significantly more likely than individuals not meeting criteria for a mental illness to use CAM. Another study reported that the types of CAM most frequently used by individuals with a mental illness are spiritual healing/prayer, meditation, massage, yoga, guided imagery, herbs, chiropractic care, and nutritional supplements (Russinova et al. 2002).

Among those with a mental illness, individuals with depression or anxiety are particularly likely to use CAM: 41% of depressed patients and 43% of individuals with panic attacks report using CAM compared with 35% of the general population (Eisenberg et al. 1998; Tindle et al. 2005). The most common CAM therapies used by people with depression or anxiety are relaxation techniques, spiritual practices, herbs, and multivitamins (Kessler et al. 2001; Knaudt et al. 1999).

Efficacy of CAM in the Treatment of Anxiety and Depression

Not only is CAM frequently used among individuals with symptoms of anxiety and depression, several CAM therapies have been demonstrated to be efficacious in the treatment of these disorders. For example, mindfulness meditation—a form of meditation in which individuals are encouraged to intentionally and nonjudgmentally pay attention to the present moment—is one CAM therapy that has been used in the treatment of individuals with anxiety disorders. In one seminal study conducted by Kabat-Zinn and colleagues (1992), participants with DSM-III-R–defined anxiety disorders (American Psychiatric Association 1987) showed significant reductions in Hamilton Rating Scale for Depression (Ham-D) and Beck Depression Inventory scores following participation in an 8-week mindfulness meditation program. These reductions were also maintained at 3-month and 3-year follow-ups (Miller et al. 1995). In another study, individuals participating in a mindfulness-based cognitive therapy program who had experienced three or more depressive episodes in their lifetime had significantly fewer relapses at 1-year follow-up compared with those receiving standard (conventional) treatment (Teasdale et al. 2000).

Yoga, a form of meditation that incorporates physical postures, stretching, deep relaxation, and mindful breathing, has also been investigated as a treatment strategy for anxiety and depressive disorders (Gerbarg and Brown 2007). Several studies suggest that as few as ten 1-hour yoga classes can significantly improve anxiety, reduce panic attacks, and reduce fatigue (Miller et al. 1995; Woolery et al. 2004) and can be as effective as antidepressants in reducing depressive symptoms (Janakiramaiah et al. 2000).

Although routine exercise is not included in the NCCAM's categorization of CAM described above (see "Definition of Complementary and Alternative Medicine"), it is briefly mentioned here because many people use exercise as a complementary treatment for both medical and psychiatric disorders. Research clearly demonstrates the importance of regular physical exercise in the prevention of diverse chronic illnesses such as diabetes, cardiovascular disease, and osteoporosis; physical activity/exercise may also be an effective therapy for depressed individuals. For example, one study found that depressed women who engaged in 10 weeks of moderate aerobic exercise had significantly lower Beck Depression Inventory scores than women who were in the relaxation comparison group or control (no treatment) group (McCann and Holmes 1984). A more recent study examined the impact of exercise on Ham-D scores for adults with moderate major depressive disorder (Dunn et al. 2005). Results showed that the mean Ham-D score at 12 weeks was reduced by 47% from baseline among participants who engaged in the most vigorous exercise compared with control participants, suggesting that physical activity alleviates symptoms of depression and may be a useful treatment for major depressive disorder.

Research has also investigated the efficacy of several herbal products as possible treatments for depression and anxiety. For example, St. John's wort—a plant common in the United States, Europe, and Asia—has been investigated as an herbal treatment for depression. In fact, research suggests that the herb may be as effective as antidepressants and superior to placebo in the treatment of mild to moderate depression (Lee et al. 2007). Additionally, kava, a plant that originated in the Pacific Islands, has been demonstrated to have moderate efficacy in the treatment of anxiety (Pittler and Ernst 2000). This study reported that participants who received kava had significantly greater reductions in scores on the Hamilton Anxiety Scale compared with those who received placebo.

Complementary and Alternative Medicine and the Prevention of Depressive and Anxiety Disorders

Background

The primary prevention of depressive and anxiety disorders is of great importance, particularly given that individuals with such disorders are also prone to substance abuse, high-risk sexual behavior, physical health problems, impaired social relationships, and a 30-fold increased risk of suicide (Birmaher et al. 1996; Brent et al. 1988; Rohde et al. 1994). Further, though secondary and tertiary approaches are undoubtedly imperative for improving the health and quality of life for those afflicted, they may not be the most effective or efficient method for managing such disorders (Kazdin 1987).

Unfortunately, there has been very little research examining the efficacy of CAM in the prevention of mental illnesses in general, and in the prevention of depression and anxiety specifically. There are several possible reasons for the absence of research on the efficacy of CAM in the prevention of mental illnesses:

1. Prevention research in general is often methodologically difficult to conduct. In order to examine whether a certain treatment or behavior reduces one's risk of subsequently developing a mental illness, the research approach must be longitudinal in design with a relatively long follow-up period. These studies are time consuming, expensive, and subject to substantial participant attrition. Therefore, researchers may be less likely to undertake such investigations because of time- and budget-related constraints.
2. The prevention of mental illnesses is often more challenging than the prevention of purely physical illnesses. The etiology and pathogenesis of malaria, for example, is relatively clear: malarial parasites are transmitted during the feeding of a female mosquito on a human. Thus, prevention efforts have focused primarily on strengthening human resistance to infection through prophylactic medication and preventing transmission of malaria from mosquitoes to humans through the use of topical repellants and bed nets. By contrast, most mental illnesses develop from an interaction between genetic, biological, psychological, and social influences, making prevention efforts complicated at best.

3. Other challenges to conducting CAM-related research include the disparities in funding that unfortunately still exist for CAM research compared with conventional biomedical research. This limits the number of rigorous studies that can be conducted on the efficacy of CAM in treating and preventing mental illnesses.

4. Furthermore, it is often difficult to identify appropriate control/comparison conditions in many CAM efficacy studies. For example, when examining the efficacy of mindfulness meditation for reducing depression there is some debate about whether control participants should receive no treatment, treatment as usual, or some other relaxation program that does not include a mindfulness component. This lack of consistent comparison conditions often makes interpretation and generalizability of CAM efficacy research challenging.

5. Finally, many CAM therapies are highly individualized. For example, the efficacy of yoga for reducing anxiety may be partly dependent on the expertise of the yoga instructor. What type of yoga and how the yoga is taught can further contribute to the variability in yoga practice. These inconsistencies make it difficult to draw conclusions across multiple studies about the efficacy of certain CAM therapies in the treatment and prevention of mental illnesses.

In the absence of rigorous research on CAM use for the prevention of mental illnesses, it may be useful to examine the ways in which CAM use can impact various psychological precursors to mental illnesses. For example, although no evidence exists demonstrating that yoga decreases an individual's likelihood of developing a subsequent anxiety *disorder* there is evidence that yoga may reduce stress and minimize anxiety. Therefore, given that symptoms of anxiety and depression are risks factors for the development of subsequent anxiety and depressive disorders, respectively (Horowitz et al. 2007; Schmidt et al. 2006; van Lang et al. 2007), it is reasonable to hypothesize that a CAM therapy that ameliorates subclinical depressive or anxiety symptoms could reduce the likelihood that an individual will develop a future depressive or anxiety disorder. Given this, the subsequent section discusses the ways in which various CAM therapies have been successful in improving mental health by reducing symptoms of depression and anxiety in nonclinical populations.

Efficacy of CAM for Enhancing Mental Health

Meditation

Several studies examining the impact of meditation on depression and anxiety symptoms in healthy individuals (i.e., without a diagnosed disorder) have reported promising findings. One study that implemented a 7-week mindfulness-based meditation program among medical students found significant decreases in anxiety, psychological distress, and depression symptoms at follow-up for the program participants compared with the wait-list control subjects (Shapiro et al. 1998). Other studies similarly have indicated that participants report significantly lower stress levels, experience reduced anxiety, feel less depressed, and even have decreases in stress-related cortisol levels following meditation interventions (Lane et al. 2007; Tang et al. 2007).

Depressed individuals recovering from major depressive episodes may also benefit from mindfulness-based meditation. As noted earlier, one study found that for patients who had experienced three or more previous depressive episodes, the risk of relapse and recurrence in those who received mindfulness-based cognitive therapy was half that in those who received treatment as usual (Teasdale et al. 2000). This finding suggests that meditation and/or mindfulness-based therapy can also be effective for tertiary prevention of mental illnesses.

The pathways by which meditation reduces symptoms of depression and anxiety are unclear, although some have speculated that the practice of focusing on the breath and present moment can interrupt anxiogenic or depressogenic thought patterns, thereby affording the individual an opportunity to engage in more effective coping methods (Toneatto and Nguyen 2007). Others have examined possible physiological mechanisms. For example, evidence suggests that stress-related conditions such as major depression are frequently associated with increased inflammatory activity in the nervous system. Interestingly, recent research indicates that frequent meditators may, when faced with a stressful experience, have reduced inflammatory responses compared with infrequent meditators or nonmeditators, suggesting that meditation may affect the body's response to stressful stimuli (Pace et al. 2008).

In addition to evidence investigating the impact of meditation on symptoms of anxiety and depression, research also suggests that meditation can reduce one's risk of cognitive decline. Lazar and colleagues (2005) reported that brain regions associated with attention, interoception, and sensory process-ing—specifically, the prefrontal cortex and right anterior insula—were thicker in frequent meditators compared with matched control subjects. Further, this finding was most profound in older participants, suggesting that meditation might offset cortical thinning related to neural degeneration.

Yoga

Promising evidence also exists for the efficacy of yoga in reducing depression and anxiety in healthy populations. One recent study (Kjellgren et al. 2007) implemented a *sudarshan kriya* program (a form of yoga that emphasizes breathing exercises) with a group of Swedish university students. The authors reported that program participants had significantly lower anxiety, depres-sion, and stress compared with control participants. Similar findings were re-ported among American university students who engaged in an Iyengar yoga-based program, which emphasizes certain postures that are hypothesized to specifically target depression (including back bends, standing poses, and inver-sions [poses in which the head is positioned lower than the heart, e.g., head-stands or handstands]). Results indicate that program recipients experienced significant decreases in symptoms of depression and anxiety traits following only two 1-hour sessions per week for 5 weeks (Woolery et al. 2004). In addi-tion to the research suggesting that yoga practice can have a profound impact on the self-reported depression and anxiety of study participants, there is also evidence that yoga can have important physiological consequences. For exam-ple, yoga practice has been demonstrated to cause decreases in salivary cortisol levels and lower sympathetic nervous system activity, both of which may be markers of anxiety and depression (Michalsen et al. 2005; Ray et al. 2001). Other research has found that brain γ-aminobutyric acid (GABA) levels increase fol-lowing a yoga session, which may be particularly important given that low GABA states are associated with depression and anxiety disorders (Streeter et al. 2007).

Exercise

There is some evidence that exercise may be another method of preventing depression and anxiety in healthy individuals. In one recent prospective study conducted in the Netherlands (Bernaards et al. 2006) involving 1,747 indi-viduals, researchers investigated the impact of physical activity on subsequent psychological complaints. Study participants who engaged in physical activity more frequently (at least one to two times per week) were significantly less likely to report experiencing depression, emotional exhaustion, and general poor health than those who exercised less than once a month. Results also suggested that a dose-response relationship exists between amount of physical activity and depression: the higher the frequency of exercise the lower the risk of depression. Other similar prospective studies have found that higher amounts of physical activity are associated with a greater reduction in depressive symptoms (Camacho et al. 1991; Cooper-Patrick et al. 1997; Morgan and Bath 1998; Paffenbarger et al. 1994). It is hypothesized that physical activity and depression may be associated through several pathways. Physiologically, exercise may reduce depression by affecting serotonin, noradrenalin, and dopamine transmission; by lowering the hypothalamic-pituitary-adrenal axis response to stress; and/or by stimulating the production of endorphins (Brosse et al. 2002). Psychologically, physical activity may increase self-efficacy, interrupt unpleasant emotions, and/or facilitate social support (Bernaards et al. 2006). Most likely, these physiological and psychological pathways interact synergistically to reduce the risk of depression among those individuals who frequently exercise.

Implications for Mental Health Practitioners

Anxiety disorders, affecting almost 20% of the population, and mood disorders, affecting approximately 10% of the population, are by far the most common mental disorders in the United States (Center for Mental Health Services 2006). Given that these illnesses are so widespread and disabling, and that conventional anxiolytic and antidepressant medications can cause myriad unpleasant side effects, it is not surprising that patients and mental health care practitioners alike often explore alternative approaches to prevention and treatment.

Many CAM modalities offer several advantages over conventional psychiatric approaches:

1. After some recommended initial instruction, meditation, yoga, and exercise generally can be practiced on one's own, making these approaches cost-effective. This is particularly important for economically disadvan-

taged individuals and/or for those who lack sufficient health insurance coverage.

2. Some individuals may feel there is stigma associated with seeking mental health care services; more independent treatment approaches such as relaxation techniques and physical activity can minimize this feeling.

3. Individuals often report that CAM use yields a greater sense of agency in their own health care, resulting in a sense of control over their lives and increased self-confidence (Astin 1998; Cauffield 2000).

Therefore, the benefits of CAM use may extend beyond any immediate effects on depressive/anxiety symptomatology to facilitate more general well-being.

CAM use is not without its risks, however. Meditation should be supervised by a trained instructor, at least for those participants who are beginners. Participants always should be counseled to discontinue any meditative practice that produces discomfort or distress, physically or emotionally. Practitioners should also be wary of organizations that have commercialized various meditation techniques (in fact, some have even been accused of unethical and cult-like practices). Patients should be able to learn and practice meditation at low cost and without any pressure, judgment, or coercion (Arias et al. 2006).

Although yoga is one of the safest forms of physical activity, it is also not risk free. As with other forms of physical activity, there is risk of muscle strain, inflamed joints, bruises, and other musculoskeletal damage, especially if the postures are not executed correctly. Therefore, patients who express interest in beginning a yoga program should practice under a trained yoga instructor before attempting any poses independently. Further, people have occasionally reported that they need their medication less frequently when they practice yoga regularly. Practitioners should caution patients against discontinuing any prescribed medications without consulting their health care providers, and should encourage patients to disclose all physical and mental health problems to their yoga instructor before beginning a yoga regimen (McCall 2007).

In this same vein, practitioner-patient communication is of critical importance when patients are contemplating or currently using any CAM modality. Research suggests that patients typically underreport their CAM use, in part because health care practitioners often fail to ask their patients about it. Health care providers may not ask patients about their CAM use because, as is often reported, they do not feel knowledgeable about these modalities or they feel uncomfortable talking with patients about them (Giveon et al. 2003; Milden and Stokols 2004; Winslow and Shapiro 2002). For example, 61% of physicians in one study reported that they did not feel sufficiently informed about CAM safety or efficacy (Milden and Stokols 2004); more than 70% of providers in another study claimed that they had little or no knowledge about herbal remedies (Giveon et al. 2003). Although many medical schools in the United States now offer CAM courses and CAM rotations for residents, these findings underscore the need for additional training in CAM for conventional health care providers.

Regardless of their own education about and comfort with CAM, practitioners should recognize that some patients may be using a nonconventional modality concurrently with a prescribed medication (as a *complementary* medicine), which could cause potentially harmful drug interactions. For example, research suggests that there may be potentially harmful interactions between hypericin, one of the active ingredients in St. John's wort, and benzodiazepines and selective serotonin reuptake inhibitors (Fugh-Berman 2000; Lantz et al. 1999) as well as between ginseng (*Panax spp.*) and some antidepressants (Fugh-Berman 2000). Other patients may be using a nonconventional modality instead of a prescribed medication (as an *alternative* medicine), which will undoubtedly impact the efficacy of treatment of the condition for which the medication was prescribed. Practitioners need to initiate conversations with patients about:

1. Whether they are using any nonprescribed therapies
2. If so, what they are using
3. How often they are using the therapies
4. How much they are using (the doses, if applicable)
5. How long they have been using and intend to use the therapies

Patients' quality of care, and the therapeutic alliance, can only be enhanced by such dialogues.

Conclusion

About one-third of Americans use at least one type of CAM and report seeking complementary and alternative therapies/practices most commonly for the treatment of chronic pain, the common cold, headaches, depression, and anxiety. Individuals with depression and anxiety—the most frequent users of CAM among those who have been diagnosed with a mental illness—are most likely to use relaxation techniques (meditation and yoga), spiritual practices, herbs, and multivitamins.

There is some evidence that meditation, yoga, exercise, St. John's wort, and kava can be efficacious in treating the symptoms of depression and anxiety among individuals who have been diagnosed with related mental illnesses. Less research has investigated the efficacy of these modalities in the prevention of these conditions. However, results from studies that have examined reductions in depressive and anxiety-related symptoms among healthy, nonclinical populations are promising. The findings indicate that mindfulness-based meditation, yoga, and exercise may be successful methods of preventing the onset of or reducing the severity of depressive and anxiety disorders. Longitudinal research is needed to further evaluate whether such practices reduce individuals' risk of developing mental illnesses.

Key Points

- Although a limited amount of literature does exist on the efficacy of a number of complementary and alternative medicine (CAM) modalities for the *treatment* of some mental illnesses, there is a paucity of research on CAM modalities for the *prevention* of such illnesses. Specifically, future longitudinal research is needed to investigate the efficacy of meditation, yoga, exercise, and herbal supplements for the prevention of depression and anxiety.

- The available research with nonclinical populations suggests that meditation, yoga, and exercise may be effective methods for reducing depressive and anxiety symptomatology.

- Although the research on the efficacy of these modalities is promising, they are not without risks. Both physical and psychological harm is possible. Individuals wanting to explore such approaches should be monitored by trained instructors.

- In order to avoid possible drug interactions and treatment inefficacy, practitioners should initiate conversations with patients about their CAM use.

References

American Psychiatric Association: Diagnostic and Statistical Manual of Mental Disorders, 3rd Edition, Revised. Washington, DC, American Psychiatric Association, 1987

Arias AJ, Steinberg K, Banga A, et al: Systematic review of the efficacy of meditation techniques as treatments for medical illness. J Altern Complement Med 12:817–832, 2006

Astin JA: Why patients use alternative medicine: results of a national study. JAMA 279:1548–1553, 1998

Astin JA, Marie A, Pelletier KR, et al: A review of the incorporation of complementary and alternative medicine by mainstream physicians. Arch Intern Med 158:2303–2310, 1998

Barnes PM, Powell-Griner E, McFann K, et al: Complementary and alternative medicine use among adults: United States, 2002. Adv Data 343:1–19, 2004

Bausell RB, Lee WL, Berman BM: Demographic and health-related correlates to visits to complementary and alternative medical providers. Med Care 39:190–196, 2001

Bernaards CM, Jans MP, van den Heuvel SG, et al: Can strenuous leisure time physical activity prevent psychological complaints in a working population? Occup Environ Med 63:10–16, 2006

Birmaher B, Ryan ND, Williamson DE, et al: Childhood and adolescent depression: a review of the past 10 years: part I. J Am Acad Child Adolesc Psychiatry 35:1427–1439, 1996

Brent DA, Perper JA, Goldstein CE, et al: Risk factors for adolescent suicide: a comparison of adolescent suicide victims with suicidal inpatients. Arch Gen Psychiatry 45:581–588, 1988

Brosse AL, Sheets ES, Lett HS, et al: Exercise and the treatment of clinical depression in adults: recent findings and future directions. Sports Med 32:741–760, 2002

Camacho TC, Roberts RE, Lazarus NB, et al: Physical activity and depression: evidence from the Alameda County Study. Am J Epidemiol 134:220–231, 1991

Cauffield JS: The psychosocial aspects of complementary and alternative medicine. Pharmacotherapy 20:1289–1294, 2000

Center for Mental Health Services: Mental Health, United States, 2004 (DHHS Publ No SMA-06-4195). Edited by Manderscheid RW, Berry JT. Rockville, MD, Substance Abuse and Mental Health Services Administration, 2006

Cooper-Patrick L, Ford DE, Mead LA, et al: Exercise and depression in midlife: a prospective study. Am J Public Health 87:670–673, 1997

Dunn AL, Trivedi MH, Kampert JB, et al: Exercise treatment for depression: efficacy and dose response. Am J Prev Med 28:1–8, 2005

Eisenberg DM, Davis RB, Ettner SL, et al: Trends in alternative medicine use in the United States, 1990-1997: results of a follow-up national survey. JAMA 280:1569–1575, 1998

Fugh-Berman A: Herb-drug interactions. Lancet 355:134–138, 2000

Gerbarg PL, Brown RP: Yoga, in Complementary and Alternative Treatments in Mental Health Care. Edited by Lake J, Spiegel D. Washington, DC, American Psychiatric Publishing, 2007, pp 381–400

Giveon SM, Liberman N, Klang S, et al: A survey of primary care physicians' perceptions of their patients' use of complementary medicine. Complement Ther Med 11:254–260, 2003

Grzywacz JG, Suerken CK, Quandt SA, et al: Older adults' use of complementary and alternative medicine for mental health: findings from the 2002 National Health Interview Survey. J Altern Complement Med 12:467–473, 2006

Horowitz JL, Garber J, Ciesla JA, et al: Prevention of depressive symptoms in adolescents: a randomized trial of cognitive-behavioral and interpersonal prevention programs. J Consult Clin Psychol 75:693–706, 2007

Janakiramaiah N, Gangadhar BN, Naga Venkatesha Murthy PJ, et al: Antidepressant efficacy of Sudarshan Kriya Yoga (SKY) in melancholia: a randomized comparison with electroconvulsive therapy (ECT) and imipramine. J Affect Disord 57:255–259, 2000

Kabat-Zinn J, Massion AO, Kristeller J, et al: Effectiveness of a meditation-based stress reduction program in the treatment of anxiety disorders. Am J Psychiatry 149:936–943, 1992

Kazdin AE: Child Psychotherapy. New York, Sage, 1987

Kessler RC, Soukup J, Davis RB, et al: The use of complementary and alternative therapies to treat anxiety and depression in the United States. Am J Psychiatry 158:289–294, 2001

Kjellgren A, Bood SA, Axelsson K, et al: Wellness through a comprehensive yogic breathing program: a controlled pilot trial. BMC Complement Altern Med 7:43, 2007. Available at: http://www.biomedcentral.com/content/pdf/1472-6882-7-43.pdf. Accessed July 27, 2009.

Knaudt PR, Connor KM, Weisler RH, et al: Alternative therapy use by psychiatric outpatients. J Nerv Ment Dis 187:692–695, 1999

Lake J: Integrative approaches, in Complementary and Alternative Treatments in Mental Health Care. Edited by Lake J, Spiegel D. Washington, DC, American Psychiatric Publishing, 2007, pp 63–82

Lake J, Spiegel D: Complementary and alternative treatments in mental health care: overview and significant trends, in Complementary and Alternative Treatments in Mental Health Care. Edited by Lake J, Spiegel D. Washington, DC, American Psychiatric Publishing, 2007, pp 3–20

Lane JD, Seskevich JE, Pieper CF: Brief meditation training can improve perceived stress and negative mood. Altern Ther Health Med 13:38–44, 2007

Lantz MS, Buchalter E, Giambanco V: St. John's wort and antidepressant drug interactions in the elderly. J Geriatr Psychiatry Neurol 12:7–10, 1999

Lazar SW, Kerr CE, Wasserman RH, et al.: Meditation experience is associated with increased cortical thickness. Neuroreport 16:1893–1897, 2005

Lee R, Yee PS, Naing G: Western herbal medicines, in Complementary and Alternative Treatments in Mental Health Care. Edited by Lake J, Spiegel D. Washington, DC, American Psychiatric Publishing, 2007, pp 87–114

McCall T: Yoga as Medicine: The Yogic Prescription for Health and Healing. New York, Bantam Dell, 2007

McCann IL, Holmes DS: Influence of aerobic exercise on depression. J Pers Soc Psychol 46:1142–1147, 1984

Michalsen A, Grossman P, Acil A, et al: Rapid stress reduction and anxiolysis among distressed women as a consequence of a three-month intensive yoga program. Med Sci Monit 11:CR555–CR561, 2005

Milden SP, Stokols D: Physicians' attitudes and practices regarding complementary and alternative medicine. Behav Med 30:73–82, 2004

Miller JJ, Fletcher K, Kabat-Zinn J: Three-year follow-up and clinical implications of a mindfulness meditation-based stress reduction intervention in the treatment of anxiety disorders. Gen Hosp Psychiatry 17:192–200, 1995

Morgan K, Bath PA: Customary physical activity and psychological wellbeing: a longitudinal study. Age Ageing 27 (suppl 3):35–40, 1998

National Center for Complementary and Alternative Medicine: What Is CAM? (NCCAM Publ No D347). February 2007. Available at: http://nccam.nih.gov/health/whatiscam/. Accessed November 4, 2008.

Ni H, Simile C, Hardy AM: Utilization of complementary and alternative medicine by United States adults: results from the 1999 national health interview survey. Med Care 40:353–358, 2002

Pace T, Negi LT, Adame D, et al: Effect of compassion meditation on autonomic, neuroendocrine and inflammatory pathway reactivity to psychosocial stress. Brain Behav Immun 22:29–35, 2008

Paffenbarger RS Jr, Lee IM, Leung R: Physical activity and personal characteristics associated with depression and suicide in American college men. Acta Psychiatr Scand Suppl 377:16–22, 1994

Paramore LC: Use of alternative therapies: estimates from the 1994 Robert Wood Johnson Foundation National Access to Care Survey. J Pain Symptom Manage 13:83–89, 1997

Pittler MH, Ernst E: Efficacy of kava extract for treating anxiety: systematic review and meta-analysis. J Clin Psychopharmacol 20:84–89, 2000

Ray US, Mukhopadhyaya S, Purkayastha SS, et al: Effect of yogic exercises on physical and mental health of young fellowship course trainees. Indian J Physiol Pharmacol 45:37–53, 2001

Ritchie CS, Gohmann SF, McKinney WP: Does use of CAM for specific health problems increase with reduced access to care? J Med Syst 29:143–153, 2005

Rohde P, Lewinsohn PM, Seeley JR: Are adolescents changed by an episode of major depression? J Am Acad Child Adolesc Psychiatry 33:1289–1298, 1994

Russinova Z, Wewiorski NJ, Cash D: Use of alternative health care practices by persons with serious mental illness: perceived benefits. Am J Public Health 92:1600–1603, 2002

Schmidt NB, Zvolensky MJ, Maner JK: Anxiety sensitivity: prospective prediction of panic attacks and Axis I pathology. J Psychiatr Res 40:691–699, 2006

Shapiro SL, Schwartz GE, Bonner G: Effects of mindfulness-based stress reduction on medical and premedical students. J Behav Med 21:581–599, 1998

Standish LJ, Greene KB, Bain S, et al: Alternative medicine use in HIV-positive men and women: demographics, utilization patterns and health status. AIDS Care 13:197–208, 2001

Streeter CC, Jensen JE, Perlmutter RM, et al: Yoga Asana sessions increase brain GABA levels: a pilot study. J Altern Complement Med 13:419–426, 2007

Tang YY, Ma Y, Wang J, et al: Short-term meditation training improves attention and self-regulation. Proc Natl Acad Sci U S A 104:17152–17156, 2007

Teasdale JD, Segal ZV, Williams JM, et al: Prevention of relapse/recurrence in major depression by mindfulness-based cognitive therapy. J Consult Clin Psychol 68:615–623, 2000

Tindle HA, Davis RB, Phillips RS, et al: Trends in use of complementary and alternative medicine by US adults: 1997–2002. Altern Ther Health Med 11:42–49, 2005

Toneatto T, Nguyen L: Does mindfulness meditation improve anxiety and mood symptoms?: a review of the controlled research. Can J Psychiatry 52:260–266, 2007

Unützer J, Klap R, Sturm R, et al.: Mental disorders and the use of alternative medicine: results from a national survey. Am J Psychiatry 157:1851–1857, 2000

van Lang ND, Ferdinand RF, Verhulst FC: Predictors of future depression in early and late adolescence. J Affect Disord 97:137–144, 2007

Winslow LC, Shapiro H: Physicians want education about complementary and alternative medicine to enhance communication with their patients. Arch Intern Med 162:1176–1181, 2002

Woolery A, Myers H, Sternlieb B, et al: A yoga intervention for young adults with elevated symptoms of depression. Altern Ther Health Med 10:60–63, 2004

6

Applying Prevention Principles to Schizophrenia and Other Psychotic Disorders

Michael T. Compton, M.D., M.P.H.

Serious mental illnesses, exemplified by schizophrenia and other psychotic disorders, are important causes of disability that lead to major losses in overall health and productivity throughout the world (Murray and Lopez 1996; U.S. Department of Health and Human Services 2000). Schizophrenia is one of the most severe mental disorders. It is commonly associated with academic, interpersonal, occupational, and social dysfunction, as well as reduced quality

This work was supported by National Institute of Mental Health Grants K23 MH067589 and R01 MH081011, as well as research funding from the American Psychiatric Institute for Research and Education, the Emory Medical Care Foundation, and the Emory University Research Committee.

of life and socioeconomic decline. Schizophrenia and other psychotic disorders—though relatively rare conditions compared to other more highly prevalent psychiatric and substance use disorders like major depressive disorder, anxiety disorders, and alcohol use disorders—exact a tremendous toll in terms of direct medical costs and diverse indirect costs to society (Knapp et al. 2004; Wu et al. 2005). Compounding these problems, schizophrenia is one of the most highly stigmatized of all medical and psychiatric conditions. Stigmatization is one of a multitude of factors leading to delays in seeking help, poor treatment engagement, poor access to care, and lack of treatment or undertreatment among individuals affected by the disorder. Clearly, like other chronic and serious health conditions, schizophrenia is worthy of focused attention pertaining to prevention in addition to treatment, rehabilitation, and recovery. Thus, besides crucial efforts to ameliorate the ongoing inadequate treatment of serious mental illnesses, which is an enormous public health problem itself (P.S. Wang et al. 2002), considerations of prevention approaches are crucial.

This chapter presents some ways in which prevention principles can be applied to schizophrenia and other primary psychotic disorders (i.e., schizophreniform disorder, schizoaffective disorder, delusional disorder, brief psychotic disorder, shared psychotic disorder, and psychotic disorder not otherwise specified). Psychotic disorders due to general medical conditions and substance-induced psychotic disorders are not discussed given the obvious prevention principles for those conditions. After a brief introduction to the epidemiology of schizophrenia, the early course (i.e., the premorbid period, the prodrome, and the onset of psychotic symptoms) is described, as are the phenomenology, course, and DSM-IV-TR-defined criteria and course specifiers. Risk factors and risk markers are then outlined. Prevention paradigms are considered vis-à-vis these serious mental illnesses, and three examples of the application of prevention principles to schizophrenia are presented.

Epidemiology of Schizophrenia

Schizophrenia occurs in all populations, with a prevalence in the range of 1.4–4.6 per 1,000 (Jablensky 2000). Others estimate the point prevalence of schizophrenia to be roughly 3–8 per 1,000 (Eaton and Chen 2006), or around 0.5%

(Yung et al. 2007). The lifetime prevalence of schizophrenia is commonly cited to be approximately 1%. Prevalence estimates and symptomatic presentation appear to be relatively consistent across different countries (World Health Organization 1973), though the prevalence has been reported to be slightly higher in some geographically isolated areas (Kendler et al. 1993).

Given the chronic nature of schizophrenia, the incidence of the disorder is much lower than the point prevalence. Incidence rates are generally cited as being about 0.1–0.7 per 1,000 per year (Eaton and Chen 2006; Goldner et al. 2002). Incidence rates peak in late adolescence and young adulthood, and women tend to have a later age at onset. Some recent studies suggest that incidence rates may be higher for males than females (Kirkbride et al. 2006; Thorup et al. 2007). Ethnic minority groups may have a higher incidence, a finding that is thought to be mediated by risk factors such as discrimination and social adversity (Fearon et al. 2006; Kirkbride et al. 2006).

Sequential Onset, Symptoms, Phenomenology, and Course of Schizophrenia

As discussed elsewhere (Compton and Harvey, in press), schizophrenia and other psychotic disorders are commonly characterized by a gradual accumulation of symptoms and psychosocial dysfunction—a sequential onset—prior to the first initiation of treatment. That is, the early course is often described in terms of the premorbid period, the prodrome, the onset of psychosis, the duration of untreated psychosis, and the first treatment. Numerous studies have shown deficits in premorbid functioning (in the elementary, middle, and high school years) prior to the onset of any psychiatric symptoms among those who later develop schizophrenia. Then, the gradual and cumulative development of prodromal symptoms (i.e., nonspecific psychiatric symptoms, early negative symptoms, and subthreshold or attenuated positive symptoms and disorganization) marks the end of the premorbid phase.

The prodrome of schizophrenia has been viewed traditionally as a prepsychotic state (an attenuated form of psychosis) identifiable only retrospectively after the onset of psychosis. However, ongoing efforts aim to prospectively identify individuals meeting criteria for one or more prodromal syndromes that confer an increased, though not absolute, vulnerability to developing psychosis (Yung et al. 1996, 2007). Such conceptualizations of the retrospective *prodrome* concept as a current/prospective *at-risk mental state* form the basis of currently studied indicated preventive interventions, described in the section "Delaying or Averting Conversion From the Prodrome to Psychosis (Indicated Preventive Interventions)."

The emergence of psychotic symptoms, marking the end of the prodrome, is characterized by a heterogeneous mode of onset, with an acute onset conferring a better prognosis than a gradual or insidious mode of onset of psychotic symptoms. Once psychotic symptoms emerge, there is commonly an extended delay before seeking treatment, the so-called *duration of untreated psychosis* (DUP); this is the target of secondary prevention efforts, which are discussed in the section "Detecting the Illness Early and Providing Comprehensive First-Episode Treatment (Secondary Prevention)."

No single sign or symptom is pathognomonic for schizophrenia, and at present no biological, electrophysiological, or neuroimaging tests are diagnostic. Characteristic domains of symptoms include positive symptoms (e.g., hallucinations, delusions, ideas of reference, grandiosity, excitement, and suspiciousness/paranoia); negative symptoms (e.g., alogia, anhedonia, avolition, blunted or flat affect, emotional withdrawal, and passive social isolation); disorganization of thoughts, speech, and behavior; and cognitive impairments. The latter, increasingly recognized as important causes of functional disability though not part of the formal diagnostic criteria, occur in domains such as abstraction, attention, executive function, processing speed, reasoning and problem solving, social cognition, verbal learning and memory, visual learning and memory, and verbal and spatial working memory (Friis et al. 2002; Jaeger et al. 2003; Nuechterlein et al. 2004).

Hostility and aggression are sometimes present, typically driven by paranoia or other positive symptoms. Affective and motor symptoms may be observed as well. Importantly, many individuals with schizophrenia have substantial impairments in insight that seriously complicate treatment adherence. Also of particular importance, given the related adverse health consequences, is the fact that individuals with schizophrenia have very high rates of substance use disorder comorbidities and markedly high rates of cigarette smoking/nicotine dependence.

Schizophrenia is currently conceptualized based on neurodevelopmental and diathesis-stress models (Keshavan et al. 2006; Mueser and McGurk 2004;

Walker 1994; Walker and Diforio 1997). Schizophrenia is a disorder with a polythetic structure; that is, signs of the illness are variable across individuals and some combination of these signs is required to meet criteria for the disorder, though as noted above there is no single pathognomonic sign or symptom. In addition to this heterogeneity in symptoms, the course and outcomes of schizophrenia are highly heterogeneous (Carpenter and Kirkpatrick 1988; L. Davidson and McGlashan 1997). The majority of patients have a relapsing and remitting course of acute, positive symptoms, while negative symptoms and cognitive impairments are more persistent. The deficit syndrome, which represents a subtype characterized by asociality, relatively poor functioning, and a prominence of stable, primary negative symptoms (Kirkpatrick and Buchanan 1990; Kirkpatrick et al. 1993), may be present in a minority of patients.

A relatively small proportion of patients have a chronic, unremitting (and in some cases, treatment-refractory) course with poor outcome and severe dysfunction in self-care, sometimes referred to as *Kraepelinian schizophrenia* (Keefe et al. 1996). Another small proportion has a course characterized by complete recovery after an initial episode of nonaffective psychosis (Mojtabai et al. 2003). For most patients, however, the long-term course of schizophrenia is marked by substantial psychosocial disability, largely due to the usual age at onset of the disorder being in late adolescence and early adulthood—educational progress is often disrupted, more than 70% of people with the disorder remain unemployed, approximately 70% never marry, and most people with schizophrenia have limited social contacts and supports.

Diagnostic Criteria and Course Specifiers

Current diagnostic criteria for schizophrenia, provided in DSM-IV-TR (American Psychiatric Association 2000), are shown in Table 6–1. The current descriptive diagnostic system, which is not based on etiology, pathophysiology, or biological markers, may not represent the true underlying pathophysiology of schizophrenia (Tsuang and Faraone 2002).

The criteria are designed to be reliable, though their validity is highly questionable (Allardyce et al. 2007; Dutta et al. 2007; Jablensky 2006) and they do not take into account the dimensional nature of psychotic experiences

Table 6–1.   DSM-IV-TR diagnostic criteria for schizophrenia

A. *Characteristic symptoms:*   Two (or more) of the following, each present for a significant portion of time during a 1-month period (or less if successfully treated):

(1)   delusions

(2)   hallucinations

(3)   disorganized speech (e.g., frequent derailment or incoherence)

(4)   grossly disorganized or catatonic behavior

(5)   negative symptoms, i.e., affective flattening, alogia, or avolition

Note: Only one Criterion A symptom is required if delusions are bizarre or hallucinations consist of a voice keeping up a running commentary on the person's behavior or thoughts, or two or more voices conversing with each other.

B. *Social/occupational dysfunction:*   For a significant portion of the time since the onset of the disturbance, one or more major areas of functioning such as work, interpersonal relations, or self-care are markedly below the level achieved prior to the onset (or when the onset is in childhood or adolescence, failure to achieve expected level of interpersonal, academic, or occupational achievement).

C. *Duration:*   Continuous signs of the disturbance persist for at least 6 months. This 6-month period must include at least 1 month of symptoms (or less if successfully treated) that meet Criterion A (i.e., active-phase symptoms) and may include periods of prodromal or residual symptoms. During these prodromal or residual periods, the signs of the disturbance may be manifested by only negative symptoms or two or more symptoms listed in Criterion A present in an attenuated form (e.g., odd beliefs, unusual perceptual experiences).

D. *Schizoaffective and mood disorder exclusion:*   Schizoaffective disorder and mood disorder with psychotic features have been ruled out because either (1) no major depressive, manic, or mixed episodes have occurred concurrently with the active-phase symptoms; or (2) if mood episodes have occurred during active-phase symptoms, their total duration has been brief relative to the duration of the active and residual periods.

E. *Substance/general medical condition exclusion:*   The disturbance is not due to the direct physiological effects of a substance (e.g., a drug of abuse, a medication) or a general medical condition.

F. *Relationship to a pervasive developmental disorder:*   If there is a history of autistic disorder or another pervasive developmental disorder, the additional diagnosis of schizophrenia is made only if prominent delusions or hallucinations are also present for at least a month (or less if successfully treated).

Table 6–1.   DSM-IV-TR diagnostic criteria for schizophrenia *(continued)*

Classification of longitudinal course (can be applied only after at least 1 year has elapsed since the initial onset of active-phase symptoms):

Episodic With Interepisode Residual Symptoms (episodes are defined by the reemergence of prominent psychotic symptoms); *also specify if:* **With Prominent Negative Symptoms**

Episodic With No Interepisode Residual Symptoms

Continuous (prominent psychotic symptoms are present throughout the period of observation); *also specify if:* **With Prominent Negative Symptoms**

Single Episode In Partial Remission; *also specify if:* **With Prominent Negative Symptoms**

Single Episode In Full Remission

Other or Unspecified Pattern

Source.   Reprinted from American Psychiatric Association: *Diagnostic and Statistical Manual of Mental Disorders,* 4th Edition, Text Revision. Washington, DC, American Psychiatric Association, 2000. Copyright 2000, American Psychiatric Association. Used with permission.

in the general population (Allardyce et al. 2007; van Os and Delespaul 2005). Phenotypic and genetic heterogeneity confounds the search for causes of schizophrenia-spectrum disorders (Dutta et al. 2007; Jablensky 2006). That is, "lumping" very different disorders into an artificial diagnostic category creates difficulties in interpreting the vast and accumulating research literature, some of which may be very relevant to prevention efforts. For example, prevention of pellagra and syphilis, facilitated by knowledge of their risk factors and etiologies, has been an effective strategy for preventing mental illnesses including psychosis (C. H. Brown and Faraone 2004), but such prevention is facilitated by "splitting" the diagnosis based on etiological entities (rather than using an artificial category that is reliable but doubtfully valid).

In addition to the current diagnostic criteria, DSM-IV-TR provides five course specifiers that clinicians can use to further describe the course of the disorder. These specifiers, listed below, can be applied when at least 1 year has passed since the initial onset of active-phase symptoms:

- Episodic with interepisode residual symptoms, with or without prominent negative symptoms
- Episodic with no interepisode residual symptoms

- Continuous, with or without prominent negative symptoms
- Single episode in partial remission, with or without prominent negative symptoms
- Single episode in full remission

These course specifiers reflect the heterogeneity in course and outcomes commonly observed by mental health professionals who treat individuals with schizophrenia.

Risk Factors and Risk Markers for Schizophrenia

Future prospects for prevention efforts for schizophrenia and related psychotic disorders are based in part on the identification of risk factors and risk markers for these disorders. As described in Chapter 2 ("Identifying and Understanding Risk Factors and Protective Factors in Clinical Practice") and discussed by C. H. Brown and Faraone (2004), the term *risk factors* refers to antecedents of a problem or disorder that are statistically, but not necessarily causally, related to the development of the disorder. In this chapter, *risk markers* are also discussed. Risk markers are biological or neuropsychological markers of the disorder or the genetic liability for the disorder. Thus, because they are thought to be trait markers present before symptom onset, risk markers can be considered risk factors that are not necessarily causal. The notion of risk markers is closely related to *endophenotypes*, which are biological or psychological abnormalities thought to be more closely related to the genotype than are the outward clinical phenotypes of the disorder. Both risk factors and risk markers for schizophrenia and related psychotic disorders are briefly reviewed below.

Risk Factors

A prevention-oriented goal of schizophrenia research is to identify and influence malleable causal risk factors to delay or prevent the disorder (McGorry 1998; Silverman 1989). Many potential risk factors for the development of schizophrenia have been proposed and studied, some of which are shown in Table 6–2. However, it is not always clear which risk factors are causally related to the development of the disorder. The most widely replicated factor that clearly increases the risk of schizophrenia is a family history of the disorder in a first-degree relative (Hallmayer 2000; Sobell et al. 2002; Tsuang 2000). A comparatively strong risk factor is the presence of velocardiofacial syndrome (VCFS), caused by microdeletions involving chromosome *22q11* (Murphy and Owen 2001). VCFS, which is characterized by variable phenotypes such as cleft palate, congenital heart anomalies, and immune disorders (Shprintzen et al. 2005), is associated with a lifetime prevalence of psychosis of approximately 25 times that in the general population (Hodgkinson et al. 2001). Several studies suggest that advanced paternal age is a risk factor for schizophrenia (A.S. Brown et al. 2002; Dalman and Allebeck 2002; Malaspina et al. 2001; Zammit et al. 2003). This could be explained by de novo mutations arising in paternal germ cells, which may be compatible with recent evidence of significantly more microdeletions and microduplications in patients with schizophrenia compared with healthy control subjects and biological relatives of patients (Walsh et al. 2008).

Table 6–2.   Select risk factors for schizophrenia

Family history of schizophrenia

Microdeletions of chromosome 22q11 (velocardiofacial syndrome)

Advanced paternal age

Maternal infection during pregnancy, including first-trimester rubella, influenza, and other viral infections

Famine during pregnancy

Low maternal vitamin D intake or other prenatal nutritional deficiencies

Obstetric (pregnancy and delivery) complications

    Rh factor incompatibility and other pregnancy complications

    Abnormal fetal growth and low birth weight

    Delivery complications such as uterine atony

Birth during winter or spring months

Greater urbanization of place of birth/upbringing

Early central nervous system infection

Immigrant status

Cannabis use during adolescence

Several of the established risk factors pertain to prenatal exposures (Susser et al. 1999). Prenatal exposures to viruses, famine, or malnutrition are risk factors for schizophrenia. Obstetric complications are known risk factors for schizophrenia (M. Cannon et al. 2002; Dalman et al. 2001; Hollister et al. 1996; Hultman et al. 1997; McNeil 1995; McNeil and Cantor-Graae 2000; Palmer et al. 2002), although like most other risk factors for the disorder, effect sizes are generally small. A meta-analysis of eight prospective, population-based studies revealed that three groups of pregnancy and delivery complications were associated with schizophrenia (M. Cannon et al. 2002):

1. Pregnancy complications including bleeding, diabetes, Rh factor incompatibility, and preeclampsia
2. Abnormal fetal growth and development, such as low birth weight, congenital malformations, and small head circumference
3. Delivery complications including uterine atony, asphyxia, and emergency cesarean section

It is relatively well established that being born in winter or spring months and having a more urban place of birth and upbringing are associated with an elevated risk of schizophrenia, and both of these likely represent proxy risk factors in which the actual mediating causal factors remain unknown or unproven (Kraemer et al. 2001).

Other potential risk factors for primary psychotic disorders include perinatal or childhood exposure to infections such as central nervous system viral infections, and being a first- or second-generation immigrant (this may be mediated by social adversity and discrimination). Researchers have become interested particularly in evidence that cannabis use in adolescence is an independent risk factor for, or component cause of, psychosis and schizophrenia (Compton et al. 2007a; DiForti and Murray 2005; Henquet et al. 2005; Smit et al. 2004).

Among the various proposed risk factors for schizophrenia, some have been thoroughly established by epidemiological studies (e.g., family history), some require additional investigation (e.g., immigration), and the biological significance of others requires clarification (e.g., urbanization of place of birth/upbringing) (Compton 2004). Additionally, whereas some risk factors, such as a family history of schizophrenia, may be more strongly associated with the development of schizophrenia, other more commonly occurring factors, like obstetric complications, may be more important in terms of population-attributable risk (Warner 2001). Thus, as discussed by C.H. Brown and Faraone (2004), both the prevalence of the risk factor and the strength of the risk factor (generally assessed using relative risks and odds ratios) in terms of later outcomes must be considered in evaluating the potential usefulness of any given prevention approach. Moreover, environmental risk factors may interact with genetic factors (Tienari et al. 2004). For example, specific gene-environment interactions have be demonstrated between fetal and/or early postnatal malnutrition and ε4 genotypes of the apolipoprotein E gene (APOE; Liu et al. 2003) and between adolescent cannabis use and a functional polymorphism of the catechol-*O*-methyltransferase (COMT) gene (Caspi et al. 2005).

Some "risk factors" may represent early manifestations of the emerging disorder that occur during the premorbid or prodromal periods. These include the following:

- Delayed childhood motor, cognitive, or social development
- Social adjustment difficulties in childhood and adolescence
- Lower intelligence or declining scholastic performance
- Being unmarried
- Being unemployed
- Psychopathological conditions in adolescence and early adulthood, including obsessive-compulsive disorder, social phobia, panic attacks, and certain personality disorders

Regarding the latter, schizotypal personality disorder is thought to be closely related, both genetically and phenotypically, to schizophrenia and other Axis I primary psychotic disorders. Schizotypal personality traits, which may be indistinguishable from prodromal features, are often determined to have been present prior to the onset of psychotic symptoms. However, it should be noted that the prevalence of such traits, as well as the prevalence of self-reported, clinically inconsequential, intermittent psychotic symptoms, is much higher in the general population than the prevalence of a psychotic illness (van Os and Delespaul 2005). Nonetheless, schizotypy, symptoms that appear in the prodromal period, and self-reported psychotic symptoms in the general population may help in targeting future preventive interventions. *Schizotaxia*, a constellation of negative symptoms, neuropsychological impairment, and psychosocial dysfunction present in some of the nonpsychotic and nonschizotypal relatives of patients with schizophrenia, is also of interest for the potential targeting of prevention efforts (Faraone et al. 2004).

Further elucidation of risk factors for schizophrenia is crucial to advancing a prevention paradigm. Understanding risk factors will clarify the etiology and pathophysiology of schizophrenia and ultimately inform primary prevention efforts that aim to reduce malleable risk factors (e.g., adolescent cannabis use, prenatal nutritional deficiencies). Clarification even of nonmodifiable risk factors is beneficial because they may be useful in risk stratification efforts and the targeting of preventive interventions to those at highest risk. An understanding of risk markers, discussed briefly in the following section, may also be productive in achieving prevention goals.

Risk Markers

A risk marker for schizophrenia (also called a *vulnerability indicator* or a *trait marker*) is any biological or neuropsychological trait that reflects an elevated underlying liability toward developing the disorder (Jones and Tarrant 2000; Kremen et al. 1992; Pardes et al. 1989). If one had to choose a limited population to target for a prevention program, one would choose a population high in risk markers or endophenotypes (also called *elementary phenotypes* or *intermediate phenotypes*), which, as mentioned earlier, represent an intermediate expression between causative mechanisms such as genes, and overt symptoms (Flint and Munafò 2007; Gottesman and Gould 2003; Michie et al. 2000; Moldin and Erlenmeyer-Kimling 1994). Some of the most widely studied risk markers or endophenotypes for schizophrenia are shown in Table 6–3.

Table 6–3.   Select risk markers for schizophrenia

Minor physical anomalies

Neurological soft signs

Neurocognitive deficits in abstraction, perceptual-motor speed, sustained attention, executive functioning, verbal learning/memory, and working memory

Eye tracking dysfunction involving smooth-pursuit eye movements and the antisaccade task

Electrophysiological findings such as increased latency and reduced P300 amplitude

Physical and neurological risk markers include minor physical anomalies (Compton and Walker 2009) and neurological soft signs (Bombin et al. 2005). Neuropsychological endophenotypes include deficits in concept formation and abstraction, perceptual-motor speed, sustained attention, executive functioning, verbal learning/memory, and working memory (Egan et al. 2000; Gur et al. 2007; Kremen et al. 1992, 1994; Michie et al. 2000; Snitz et al. 2006; Tsuang et al. 2002; Q. Wang et al. 2007).

Many studies indicate that laboratory-measured eye tracking dysfunction is a risk marker for schizophrenia, and the high prevalence of smooth-pursuit eye tracking dysfunction in patients and their relatives suggests that this deficit may be a genetically transmitted trait marker (Hong et al. 2006; K.H. Lee and Williams 2000; Levy et al. 1994). The antisaccade task, in which research participants must move their eyes in the direction opposite of a visual target, has also been studied as a risk marker (Curtis et al. 2001; McDowell et al. 1999, 2002).

Electrophysiological endophenotypes include specific features of event-related potentials, deficiencies in sensory gating and prepulse inhibition of the startle reflex, and the mismatch negativity component of event-related potentials (Blackwood 2000; Friedman and Squires-Wheeler 1994; Light and Braff 2001; O'Donnell et al. 1999; Price et al. 2006).

These and other proven and putative risk markers may be useful in future attempts at risk prediction or risk stratification, which would inform the targeting of preventive interventions. Currently, none of the measures of elevated risk has satisfactory predictive performance, noninvasiveness, ease of testing, and low cost to enable widespread clinical use (Copolov and Crook 2000). However, as measures are refined, it may become possible to develop tools to identify high-risk individuals who could then be included in indicated intervention strategies (M. Davidson and Weiser 2000). Such risk identification and risk stratification (as is done using the Framingham risk score to predict 10-year cardiovascular disease outcomes based on risk factors; Eichler et al. 2007) could rely on several risk markers or endophenotypes in order to improve predictive accuracy (John et al. 2008; Price et al. 2006). Risk prediction in another area of mental health is exemplified by a recent report in which King and colleagues (2008) studied a risk algorithm for the prediction of the onset of major depression based on a combination of risk factors, which performed as well as similar risk algorithms for cardiovascular events. However, regarding the prediction of schizophrenia, it has been pointed out that although combining multiple factors improves the prediction that transition to a psychotic disorder is going to take place (i.e., it enhances predictive value), a relatively small proportion of cases is predictable using such combinations (van Os and Delespaul 2005).

Schizophrenia and the Prevention Paradigm

Schizophrenia and other serious mental illnesses traditionally have not been widely considered from the prevention perspective (C.H. Brown and Faraone 2004; Compton 2004; Sartorius and Henderson 1992). This is thought by some to partly reflect an entrenched, pessimistic, and fundamentally inaccurate, Kraepelinian notion of schizophrenia being progressive and inevitably debilitating (McGorry 1991; Yung et al. 2007). However, similar to other chronic diseases with variable courses, schizophrenia can be considered from the perspectives of the traditional public health classifications of primary, secondary, and tertiary prevention, as well as the newer Institute of Medicine categories of universal, selective, and indicated preventive interventions (Institute of Medicine 1994).

Primary, Secondary, and Tertiary Prevention

The primary prevention of schizophrenia—reducing actual incidence through health promotion or specific protective interventions that modify risk factors—is a prospect that is likely to be realized only in the future. Secondary prevention is a more proximal goal for contemporary schizophrenia research and clinical programs. Such efforts, exemplified by work aiming to reduce treatment delays and promote early detection and phase-specific treatment of the early illness, are discussed below (see subsection "Detecting the Illness Early and Providing Comprehensive First-Episode Treatment [Secondary Prevention]"). A stricter definition of secondary prevention would refer to the detection of latent disease *before* symptoms become apparent; however, community screening for early stages of the illness may not be feasible due to the low incidence of schizophrenia and other psychotic disorders (C.H. Brown and Faraone 2004). Rather, screening measures may someday be appropriate for those at established elevated risk. Despite variations in the definition of secondary prevention, many view early detection and treatment to be a facet of secondary prevention.

Important aspects of tertiary prevention include minimizing morbidity, disability, and mortality by preventing relapse, treatment nonadherence, substance abuse comorbidity, physical illness comorbidity, and suicide, as briefly discussed below. Tertiary prevention should also aim to reduce psychosocial decline, family alienation, unemployment, homelessness, and incarceration (the latter being particularly relevant given the problem of criminalization; Wood and Kotwicki 2007). *Healthy People 2010*, an extensive report of the U.S. Department of Health and Human Services (2000) that documents the most significant preventable threats to health and establishes national goals to reduce these threats, has addressed several tertiary prevention concerns pertaining to serious mental illnesses like schizophrenia. These include reducing the suicide rate, reducing the proportion of homeless adults who have a serious mental illness, and increasing the proportion of persons with a serious mental illness who are employed.

Universal, Selective, and Indicated Preventive Interventions

Schizophrenia can also be considered using the newer classification of prevention, which is based not on the stage of disease during which the intervention is applied, but on the level of risk of the target population to which the intervention is directed (Compton 2008; Institute of Medicine 1994). In relation to schizophrenia, a universal preventive intervention would be one applied to the population in general, such as enhanced accessibility of prenatal care for all women to reduce prenatal and obstetric risk factors for development of the disorder among offspring (Faraone et al. 2002). Population-based efforts to decrease cannabis use during adolescence have also been postulated as a way to contribute to the prevention of some incident cases of psychosis (Ferdinand et al. 2005a; Verdoux et al. 2005). However, it should be noted that many universal interventions such as these would likely have broad effects on health in many domains, and detecting a specific effect on reducing the incidence of schizophrenia may be difficult (Raphael 1980). Nonetheless, it has been argued that some risk factors for mental illnesses in general (including schizophrenia) are so widespread that targeting them through universal preventive interventions could provide broad benefits (Yung et al. 2007). Such risk factors include low levels of social capital (poor social cohesion, exclusion, social marginalization, and discrimination), poverty and low socioeconomic status, and childhood trauma (Yung et al. 2007).

A selective intervention targets a specific subgroup at elevated risk, such as a subset of the population experiencing a specific risk factor. Examples of selective preventive interventions for schizophrenia may include prophylaxis for Rh factor incompatibility (Wyatt 1996), minimizing the risk of obstetric complications in women with schizophrenia (Warner 2001), and efforts to reduce cannabis exposure among young people with an elevated vulnerability to schizophrenia (i.e., with a genetic predisposition evidenced by family history) (Ferdinand et al. 2005b). Thus, selective interventions could be directed toward those at genetic risk (i.e., the biological offspring of individuals with schizophrenia) (C. Lee et al. 2005). However, Yung and colleagues (2007) point out that because individuals receiving a selective preventive intervention would be asymptomatic, the type of intervention that would be used is not clear; thus, at present, indicated preventive interventions primarily are being studied.

An indicated intervention is given only to a small group of individuals who are at particularly high risk for a psychotic disorder, such as those with clinical features and psychosocial decline consistent with the prodrome of schizophrenia. Several research groups are studying indicated preventive interventions using atypical antipsychotic agents or cognitive-behavioral therapy in putatively prodromal adolescents and young adults (Compton et al. 2007b; Yung et al. 1998); this research is described in the "Delaying or Averting Conversion From the Prodrome to Psychosis (Indicated Preventive Interventions)" section below. Another suggested indicated preventive intervention is reducing or eliminating cannabis use among young people at *ultra-high* risk for psychosis (Compton and Ramsay 2009; Compton et al. 2007a). Three examples of applying prevention principles to schizophrenia and other psychotic disorders are reviewed in more detail below:

1. Indicated preventive interventions that target putatively prodromal adolescents and young adults
2. Secondary prevention efforts aimed at early detection and intervention for new-onset psychosis

3. Tertiary prevention strategies that are routinely employed by mental health professionals treating patients with schizophrenia

Three Applications of Prevention Principles to Schizophrenia

Delaying or Averting Conversion From the Prodrome to Psychosis (Indicated Preventive Interventions)

Indicated preventive interventions target individuals who are at particularly high risk, such as adolescents who are at high genetic risk or who exhibit clinical features consistent with the prodrome of schizophrenia. To facilitate such prospective research on the prodrome, several prodromal syndromes have been defined. For example, Yung and colleagues in Melbourne, Australia, outlined criteria for *ultra-high risk* clinical states, including 1) an attenuated positive symptom syndrome; 2) brief, limited, intermittent psychotic symptoms; and 3) a genetic risk and recent deterioration syndrome (Yung et al. 1998, 2007). The syndromal criteria used by McGlashan and colleagues at Yale University are based closely on these categories (Hawkins et al. 2004; Tully and McGlashan 2006). Similarly, individuals meeting criteria for clinical high risk (CHR) status, developed by Cornblatt and colleagues at Zucker Hillside Hospital in Glen Oaks, New York, have been categorized as CHR– (attenuated negative/disorganized symptoms) or CHR+ (attenuated positive symptoms in addition to attenuated negative/disorganized symptoms) (Auther et al. 2008; Cornblatt and Auther 2005; Cornblatt et al. 2002). Across a number of studies, an average annual transition rate (from the putatively prodromal state to psychosis) of about 30%–40% has been observed (Yung et al. 2007). van Os and Delespaul (2005) have described such methods that rely on consecutive referral processes and clinical criteria as "sample enrichment strategies" that lead to this relatively high predictive value.

An example of an indicated preventive intervention approach is the Personal Assistance and Crisis Evaluation (PACE) clinic developed by McGorry and colleagues in Melbourne, Australia (McGorry 2000; Phillips et al. 2002), to monitor and study interventions for young people who are at putatively high risk of impending psychosis (Phillips et al. 1999; Yung et al. 1996) based on three *ultra-high risk* syndromal definitions. Studies at the PACE clinic are based on sequential screening using a combination of markers to define individuals at increased risk, and research is being done to investigate the predictive power of a number of risk markers (Yung et al. 1996). The clinic provides phase-specific psychosocial treatments aimed at reducing stress and enhancing coping abilities with an emphasis on individualized case management, problem solving, and stress management. Thus, even if the young person's condition does not progress to psychosis, he or she is not actually receiving unnecessary treatment, because treatment is provided for the particular presenting problems (Yung and McGorry 1996, 1997, 2002).

In 2002, researchers at the PACE clinic published results of a randomized, controlled trial of low-dose risperidone and cognitive-behavioral therapy versus a needs-based (control) intervention for 6 months in 59 patients at ultra-high risk (in a putatively prodromal state) of progression to psychosis (McGorry et al. 2002). After 6 months, 10 of 28 individuals receiving the control intervention progressed to psychosis, compared with only 3 of 31 in the preventive intervention group. This was the first study to demonstrate the promising approach of identifying and treating adolescents and young adults who are prodromal or at incipient risk of progression to psychosis. Further research is needed, however, given that the study was not blinded and the differential effects of risperidone and cognitive-behavioral therapy could not be separated. Thus, it remains unclear whether the low-dose antipsychotic or the cognitive-behavioral therapy provided the preventive effect.

Several other groups have studied interventions among putatively prodromal adolescents and young adults. Morrison and colleagues (2004) in the United Kingdom conducted a randomized, controlled trial comparing cognitive therapy with treatment as usual (i.e., monitoring only) in 58 patients at ultra-high risk of psychosis. Results suggested that cognitive therapy significantly reduced the likelihood of progressing to psychosis, having antipsychotic medication prescribed, or meeting diagnostic criteria for a psychotic disorder over the course of 12 months. For example, 2 of 35 (6%) of participants receiving cognitive therapy met the a priori criteria for transition to psychosis, compared with 5 of 23 (22%) in the group receiving monitoring only. This study was noteworthy because a purely psychological treatment with few side effects was tested. Although promising, this study, like the others, had several methodological limitations that warrant caution in interpretation (Auther et al. 2008).

In 2006, results from the PRIME study (Prevention Through Risk Identification Management and Education), conducted at four sites—Yale University, the University of North Carolina at Chapel Hill, the University of Toronto, and Foothills Hospital, Calgary, Alberta, Canada—were published (McGlashan et al. 2006). This study was a double-blind, randomized, parallel-group, placebo-controlled trial of olanzapine in 60 patients meeting criteria for the prodrome of schizophrenia. During the year of treatment, 16% of olanzapine-treated patients and 38% of placebo-administered patients experienced a conversion to psychosis. Results from a Cox proportional hazards model showed that the treatment groups differed to a nearly significant degree ($P=0.09$) in terms of conversion to psychosis after adjustment for the baseline severity of positive prodromal symptoms. These results are consistent with the findings from Australia (McGorry et al. 2002) but require replication in larger samples. In addition to a possible reduction in rates of conversion from the prodrome to psychosis, after 8 weeks of treatment olanzapine was significantly more efficacious at improving prodromal symptoms than placebo. However, the drop-out rate was very high (27 of 60; 45%) and the antipsychotic agent was associated with dramatic weight gain, which averaged 9.9 kg, compared with 0.7 kg in the placebo group.

In Germany, both psychosocial and pharmacological interventions are being studied in putatively prodromal individuals (Bechdolf et al. 2005a, 2005b; Ruhrmann et al. 2005, 2006), using the "basic symptoms" concept studied by Klosterkötter and colleagues (1996, 1997, 2001) as a basis for classifying adolescents and young adults who appear to be in a prodromal state. Preliminary data suggest that treatment of prodromal adolescents with a low dose of atypical antipsychotic medication may result in improvements in behavioral and neurocognitive functioning (T.D. Cannon et al. 2002). These findings suggest that treatment during the prodrome may provide symptomatic relief in addition to possibly delaying the onset of psychosis. However, when medications are used, side effects must be monitored closely. Ongoing assessment of the risk-benefit ratio, along with several other important ethical concerns including the problem of false-positive cases (C. Lee et al. 2005), are being considered by early psychosis researchers. Experimental neuroprotective drug strategies are also being considered by investigators of early psychosis (Berger et al. 2007; Yung et al. 2007), though such research is in its infancy.

In the United States and Canada, prodromal researchers are collaborating in an effort called the North American Prodrome Longitudinal Study (NAPLS) in order to maximize the sample size and thus enhance the statistical power for detecting predictors of conversion to psychosis (Addington et al. 2007). The NAPLS dataset constitutes the largest currently available longitudinal set of data on potentially prodromal patients and is currently being utilized to address a series of scientific questions about the nature of the currently defined prodromal syndromes (T. D. Cannon et al. 2008).

Detecting the Illness Early and Providing Comprehensive First-Episode Treatment (Secondary Prevention)

Early detection and intervention for schizophrenia have been of increasing interest (Falloon 1992; Johannessen et al. 2001; Linzsen et al. 1998; McGlashan 1996; McGorry et al. 1996; Wyatt and Henter 2001). The prodromal (ultra-high risk) phase is considered to end when frank psychotic symptoms develop. However, even after the onset of psychosis, many patients remain psychotic in the community for weeks, months, or even years before seeking treatment. This delay in treatment is termed the *DUP* (duration of untreated psychosis), which is typically defined as the period from the onset of positive psychotic symptoms to the initiation of adequate treatment (Compton et al. 2007b, 2008; McGlashan 1999; Norman and Malla 2001).

Like delays in treatment of other chronic health conditions, DUP is recognized as a critical variable in light of evidence associating longer DUP with poorer outcomes, despite large methodological variation between studies (Bottlender et al. 2002). Two independent meta-analyses have strongly suggested that treatment delay, or DUP, adversely affects short-term outcomes in first-episode psychosis. Marshall and colleagues (2005) examined data from 26 studies involving prospective cohorts (4,490 participants) recruited during the first episode of psychosis. They found a significant association, not attributable solely to premorbid adjustment, between DUP and several outcomes in symptomatic and functional domains at 6 and 12 months. Perkins and colleagues (2005) summarized data from 44 studies involving 5,491 participants. Shorter DUP was associated with greater response to antipsychotic treatment (as measured by severity of global psychopathology, positive symptoms, negative symptoms, and functional outcomes), and again the effect persisted even in studies that controlled for premorbid functioning. These conclusions support the potential of secondary prevention efforts.

The promise of secondary prevention also is evidenced by findings suggesting that community-level interventions may lead to a reduction in median DUP. Researchers in the Treatment and Intervention in Psychosis Study study in Norway assessed DUP in 281 first-episode patients from four Scandinavian health care sectors with specialized first-episode services, two of which were involved in an extensive early detection program (Melle et al. 2004). This community-based program consisted of educational campaigns (through newspaper, radio, and cinema advertisements) directed at the general population, as well as targeted information to general practitioners, social workers, and high school health professionals (Joa et al. 2008). DUP was significantly shorter for the patients from the early detection areas (median, 5 weeks) compared with patients from the other two health care sectors (median, 16 weeks; $P=0.003$). Results from this study suggest that it may be possible to reduce DUP through community-based and health system–based early detection efforts, leading to better outcomes (Larsen et al. 2006; Melle et al. 2006; Simonsen et al. 2006).

Such findings have prompted early psychosis experts to suggest that community-wide education should be encouraged to ensure that the public has a better understanding of psychosis and how to obtain effective and timely treatment (International Early Psychosis Association Writing Group 2005). Research on causes or determinants of DUP at the patient, family, and health system levels (Compton and Broussard, in press) may inform the development of interventions to reduce DUP, thus leading to earlier detection and treatment, and ultimately to improved outcomes. A number of early detection and intervention programs have been developed, primarily in Australia, Europe, and North America as described in several books (Edwards and McGorry 2002; Ehmann et al. 2004; Miller et al. 2001).

Preventing Relapse, Nonadherence, Substance Abuse, Physical Morbidity, and Suicide (Tertiary Prevention)

Given the prominent burden of untreated or undertreated schizophrenia and related psychotic disorders, ongoing attention must be given to enhancing treatment and encouraging tertiary prevention. Though beyond the scope of this review, some of the many tertiary prevention goals in schizophrenia are:

- Prevention of relapse of psychotic symptoms after stabilization and remission of active-phase symptoms (Herz et al. 2000; Pecenak 2007; Taylor et al. 2005)
- Prevention of nonadherence to medication regimens (Dolder et al. 2003; Lacro et al. 2002; Weiden 2007)
- Prevention of substance abuse, physical morbidity, and suicide in schizophrenia (Brunette et al. 2006; Compton et al. 2006; Dixon et al. 2006; Meltzer 2002; Montross et al. 2005)

Conclusion: Advice for Clinicians

As prevention sciences develop within psychiatry and the neurosciences, there will be a need to design and evaluate effective prevention efforts and translate results into appropriate, cost-effective changes at the clinical, community, and public policy levels. When considering schizophrenia from a prevention perspective, a number of potential preventive interventions are apparent, some of which may already be feasible for mental health professionals to incorporate into their clinical interactions with patients and their families.

Given our knowledge of modifiable risk factors for schizophrenia and related psychotic disorders, it is particularly important that patients with a psychotic disorder who are pregnant or plan to become pregnant be advised to engage in comprehensive prenatal care. This should emphasize attention to nutrition, prevention of influenza and other infections, and guarding against pregnancy/delivery complications and low birth weight to the extent possible. The importance of prenatal care as an intervention to prevent mental illness may extend to women with a family history of schizophrenia or a family history in their sexual partner (indicating a potentially heritable diathesis) as well, even if the disorder is not present in that particular woman herself.

Given the emerging and convincing (though not entirely conclusive) evidence that cannabis use in adolescence is a risk factor for the later development of psychotic disorders (perhaps especially among those with a genetic tendency or schizotypal traits), adolescents with a family history of a psychotic disorder should be advised against the use of marijuana, as well as other drugs. More generally, all adolescents seen by mental health professionals should be advised against the use of cannabis and other addictive substances.

Several research groups are currently working on indicated interventions involving adolescents and young adults who have a syndrome consistent with the schizophrenia prodrome. Such researchers also work with adolescents and young adults who have a family history of a psychotic disorder along with schizotypal traits or a recent decline in psychosocial functioning. Because those interventions, both pharmacological (e.g., low-dose atypical antipsychotics or other agents targeted at specific symptoms, such as antidepressants for prominent dysphoria) and psychosocial (e.g., cognitive-behavioral therapy and phase-specific case management and other psychosocial treatments) are currently under investigation, they cannot yet be generally recommended for routine clinical practice. However, Addington and colleagues (2006) have provided a detailed review of such interventions for help-seeking individuals who are clearly at high risk for developing psychosis. Mental health professionals should also consider referring such adolescents to specialized clinical and research programs (Auther et al. 2008).

Clinicians have an important role in reducing the duration of untreated psychosis. Mental health professionals evaluating and treating individuals with new-onset or first-episode psychosis should aim to provide comprehensive and timely care, using both pharmacological (Bradford et al. 2003; Tandon et al. 2006; Zipursky 2002) and psychosocial and rehabilitative approaches (Bustillo et al. 2001; Jackson et al. 2002; Penn et al. 2005; Torrey et al. 2005) based on expert guidelines (International Early Psychosis Association Writing Group 2005; Lehman et al. 2004; Sheitman et al. 1997). First-episode patients, and their families (Collins 2002; Gleeson et al. 1999), should be engaged intensively in terms of psychoeducation, optimizing insight, and enhancing motivation for treatment with a goal of symptom remission and illness recovery. The latter outcome is based on contemporary conceptualizations of the recovery approach to serious mental illnesses (Buckley et al. 2007; Liberman and Kopelowicz 2005). The first few years of a psychotic disorder have been argued to represent a *critical period* in the long-term trajectory of psychosis, which has major implications for secondary prevention (Birchwood 1999). Age-appropriate, community- or home-based, phase-specific treatment that is based on a clinical staging model (which postulates that patients in the early stages have a better response to treatment and better prognosis than those in later stages, and that treatments offered in the earlier stages should be more benign as well as more effective; Yung et al. 2007), is currently recommended (International Early Psychosis Association Writing Group 2005).

Promoting access to care in the early course of psychosis is crucially important (Yung et al. 2002). This may include community-based efforts to enhance mental health literacy (Jorm 2000), multimedia campaigns (Wright et al. 2006), and "mental health first aid" training for the public (Kitchener and Jorm 2002, 2006; Jorm et al. 2005).

Key Points

- Schizophrenia and other psychotic disorders—often characterized by positive, negative, and disorganized symptoms in addition to diverse cognitive impairments—are commonly associated with major psychosocial dysfunction in academic, interpersonal, occupational, and social domains, as well as reduced quality of life and socioeconomic decline.

- Fairly well-established risk factors for schizophrenia include: a family history of the disorder in a first-degree relative, VCFS (velocardiofacial syndrome) associated with microdeletions involving chromosome 22q11, advanced paternal age at birth, prenatal exposure to viruses, prenatal nutritional deficiencies, obstetric complications, perinatal or childhood central nervous system viral infections, being a first- or second-generation immigrant, and cannabis use in adolescence. Environmental risk factors likely interact with genetic factors in elevating risk.

- Risk markers or endophenotypes, such as minor physical anomalies, neurological soft signs, diverse neurocognitive deficits, eye tracking dysfunction, and specific electrophysiological markers, may be useful in future attempts at risk prediction or risk stratification. This would inform the targeting of preventive interventions, as is done with the Framingham risk score to estimate the 10-year risk of developing myocardial infarction or coronary death.

- True primary prevention of schizophrenia—reducing its actual incidence through health promotion or specific protective interventions that modify risk factors—is a prospect that is likely to be realized only in the future.

- Many individuals with new-onset, first-episode psychosis remain psychotic for weeks, months, or even years before seeking treatment. Research suggests that initiating treatment as early as possible is associated with improved outcomes. Thus secondary prevention, through reducing treatment delays and promoting early detection and comprehensive, phase-specific treatment of the early illness, should be a key clinical goal. Programs focusing on early detection and intervention have been established in numerous developed countries.

- Some research programs are working to intervene even earlier, during the prodromal stage, in an effort to improve prodromal symptoms and potentially delay or even avert conversion from the prodrome to psychosis. These research efforts can be considered indicated preventive interventions.

- Important aspects of tertiary prevention include minimizing morbidity, disability, and mortality by preventing relapse, medication nonadherence, substance abuse comorbidity, physical illness comorbidity, and suicide as well as psychosocial decline, family alienation, unemployment, homelessness, and incarceration.

References

Addington J, Francey SM, Morrison AP (eds): Working with People at High Risk of Developing Psychosis: A Treatment Handbook. West Sussex, UK, Wiley, 2006

Addington J, Cadenhead KS, Cannon TD, et al: North American Prodrome Longitudinal Study: a collaborative multisite approach to prodromal schizophrenia research. Schizophr Bull 33:665–672, 2007

Allardyce J, Gaebel W, Zielasek J, et al: Deconstructing Psychosis conference February 2006: the validity of schizophrenia and alternative approaches to the classification of psychosis. Schizophr Bull 33:863–867, 2007

American Psychiatric Association: Diagnostic and Statistical Manual of Mental Disorders, 4th Edition, Text Revision. Washington, DC, American Psychiatric Association, 2000

Auther AM, Gillett DA, Cornblatt BA: Expanding the boundaries of early intervention for psychosis: intervening during the prodrome. Psychiatr Ann 38:528–537, 2008

Bechdolf A, Ruhrmann S, Wagner M, et al: Interventions in the initial prodromal states of psychosis in Germany: concept and recruitment. Br J Psychiatry Suppl 48:s45–s48, 2005a

Bechdolf A, Veith V, Schwarzer D, et al: Cognitive-behavioral therapy in the pre-psychotic phase: an exploratory study. Psychiatry Res 136:251–255, 2005b

Berger G, Dell'Olio M, Amminger P, et al: Neuroprotection in emerging psychotic disorders. Early Interv Psychiatry 1:114–127, 2007

Birchwood M: Early intervention in psychosis: the critical period, in The Recognition and Management of Early Psychosis: A Preventive Approach. Edited by McGorry PD, Jackson HJ. Cambridge, UK, Cambridge University Press, 1999, pp 226–264

Blackwood D: P300, a state and a trait marker in schizophrenia. Lancet 355:771–772, 2000

Bombin I, Arango C, Buchanan RW: Significance and meaning of neurological signs in schizophrenia: two decades later. Schizophr Bull 31:962–977, 2005

Bottlender R, Sato T, Jäger M, et al: The impact of duration of untreated psychosis and premorbid functioning on outcome of first inpatient treatment in schizophrenic and schizoaffective patients. Eur Arch Psychiatry Clin Neurosci 252:226–231, 2002

Bradford DW, Perkins DO, Lieberman JA: Pharmacological management of first-episode schizophrenia and related psychoses. Drugs 63:2265–2282, 2003

Brown AS, Schaefer CA, Wyatt RJ, et al: Paternal age and risk of schizophrenia in adult offspring. Am J Psychiatry 159:1528–1533, 2002

Brown CH, Faraone SV: Prevention of schizophrenia and psychotic behavior: definitions and methodological issues, in Early Clinical Intervention and Prevention in Schizophrenia. Edited by Stone WS, Faraone SV, Tsuang MT. Totowa, NJ, Humana Press, 2004, pp 255–283

Brunette MF, Noordsy DL, Green AI: Co-occurring substance use and other psychiatric disorders, in The American Psychiatric Publishing Textbook of Schizophrenia. Edited by Lieberman JA, Stroup TS, Perkins DO. Washington, DC, American Psychiatric Publishing, 2006, pp 223–244

Buckley PF, Fenley G, Mabe A, et al: Recovery and schizophrenia. Clin Schizophrenia and Related Psychoses 1:96–100, 2007

Bustillo JR, Lauriello J, Horan W, et al: The psychosocial treatment of schizophrenia: an update. Am J Psychiatry 158:163–175, 2001

Cannon M, Jones PB, Murray RM: Obstetric complications and schizophrenia: historical and meta-analytic review. Am J Psychiatry 159:1080–1092, 2002

Cannon TD, Huttunen MO, Dahlström M, et al: Antipsychotic drug treatment in the prodromal phase of schizophrenia. Am J Psychiatry 159:1230–1232, 2002

Cannon TD, Cadenhead K, Cornblatt B, et al: Prediction of psychosis in youth at high clinical risk: a multisite longitudinal study in North America. Arch Gen Psychiatry 65:28–37, 2008

Carpenter WT, Kirkpatrick B: The heterogeneity of the long-term course of schizophrenia. Schizophr Bull 14:645–652, 1988

Caspi A, Moffitt TE, Cannon M, et al: Moderation of the effect of adolescent-onset cannabis use on adult psychosis by a functional polymorphism in the catechol-O-methyltransferase gene: longitudinal evidence of a gene X environment interaction. Biol Psychiatry 57:1117–1127, 2005

Collins AA: Family intervention in the early stages of schizophrenia, in The Early Stages of Schizophrenia. Edited by Zipursky RB, Schulz SC. Washington, DC, American Psychiatric Publishing, 2002, pp 129–157

Compton MT: Considering schizophrenia from a prevention perspective. Am J Prev Med 26:178–185, 2004

Compton MT: Incorporating the prevention paradigm into administrative psychiatry. Psychiatr Clin N Am 31:73–84, 2008

Compton MT, Broussard B: Conceptualizing the multi-faceted determinants of the duration of untreated psychosis. Early Interv Psychiatry (in press)

Compton MT, Harvey PD: Schizophrenia: elucidating vulnerability and moving toward prevention, in Vulnerability to Psychopathology: Risk Across the Lifespan, 2nd Edition. Edited by Ingram RE, Price JM. New York, Guilford (in press)

Compton MT, Ramsay CE: The impact of pre-onset cannabis use on age at onset of prodromal and psychotic symptoms. Prim Psychiatry 16:35–43, 2009

Compton MT, Walker EF: Physical manifestations of neurodevelopmental disruption: are minor physical anomalies part of the syndrome of schizophrenia? Schizophr Bull 35:425–436, 2009

Compton MT, Daumit GL, Druss BG: Cigarette smoking and overweight/obesity among individuals with serious mental illnesses: a preventive perspective. Harv Rev Psychiatry 14:212–222, 2006

Compton MT, Goulding SM, Walker EF: Cannabis use, first-episode psychosis, and schizotypy: a summary and synthesis of recent literature. Curr Psychiatry Rev 3:161–171, 2007a

Compton MT, McGlashan TH, McGorry PD: Toward prevention approaches for schizophrenia: an overview of prodromal states, the duration of untreated psychosis, and early intervention paradigms. Psychiatr Ann 37:340–348, 2007b

Compton MT, Goulding SM, Broussard B, et al: Treatment delay in the early course of schizophrenia and the duration of untreated psychosis. Psychiatr Ann 38:504–511, 2008

Copolov D, Crook J: Biological markers and schizophrenia. Aust N Z J Psychiatry 34 (suppl 1):S108–S112, 2000

Cornblatt BA, Auther AM: Treating early psychosis: who, what, and when? Dialogues Clin Neurosci 7:39–49, 2005

Cornblatt B, Lencz T, Obuchowski M: The schizophrenia prodrome: treatment and high-risk perspectives. Schizophr Res 54:177–186, 2002

Curtis CE, Calkins ME, Grove WM, et al: Saccadic disinhibition in patients with acute and remitted schizophrenia and their first-degree biological relatives. Am J Psychiatry 158:100–106, 2001

Dalman C, Allebeck P: Paternal age and schizophrenia: further support for an association. Am J Psychiatry 159:1591–1592, 2002

Dalman C, Thomas HV, David AS, et al: Signs of asphyxia at birth and risk of schizophrenia: population-based case-control study. Br J Psychiatry 179:403–408, 2001

Davidson L, McGlashan TH: The varied outcomes of schizophrenia. Can J Psychiatry 42:34–43, 1997

Davidson M, Weiser M: Early diagnosis of schizophrenia—the first step towards secondary prevention. Acta Psychiatr Scand Suppl 400:7–10, 2000

DiForti M, Murray RM: Cannabis consumption and risk of developing schizophrenia: myth or reality. Epidemiol Psichiatr Soc 14:184–187, 2005

Dixon L, Messias E, Wohlheiter K: Nonpsychiatric comorbid disorders, in The American Psychiatric Publishing Textbook of Schizophrenia. Edited by Lieberman JA, Stroup TS, Perkins DO. Washington, DC, American Psychiatric Publishing, 2006, pp 383–393

Dolder CR, Lacro JP, Leckband S, et al: Interventions to improve antipsychotic medication adherence: review of recent literature. J Clin Psychopharmacol 23:389–399, 2003

Dutta R, Greene T, Addington J, et al: Biological, life course, and cross-cultural studies all point toward the value of dimensional and developmental ratings in the classification of psychosis. Schizophr Bull 33:868–876, 2007

Eaton WW, Chen CY: Epidemiology, in The American Psychiatric Publishing Textbook of Schizophrenia. Edited by Lieberman JA, Stroup TS, Perkins DO. Washington, DC, American Psychiatric Publishing, 2006, pp 17–37

Edwards J, McGorry PD: Implementing Early Intervention in Psychosis: A Guide to Establishing Early Psychosis Services. London, UK, Martin Dunitz, 2002

Egan MF, Goldberg TE, Gscheidle T, et al: Relative risk of attention deficits in siblings of patients with schizophrenia. Am J Psychiatry 157:1309–1316, 2000

Ehmann T, MacEwan GW, Honer WG (eds): Best Care in Early Psychosis Intervention: Global Perspectives. Abingdon, UK, Taylor & Francis, 2004

Eichler K, Puhan MA, Steurer J, et al: Prediction of first coronary events with the Framingham score: a systematic review. Am Heart J 153:722–731, 2007

Falloon IRH: Early intervention for first episodes of schizophrenia: a preliminary exploration. Psychiatry 55:4–15, 1992

Faraone SV, Brown CH, Glatt SJ, et al: Preventing schizophrenia and psychotic behavior: definitions and methodological issues. Can J Psychiatry 47:527–537, 2002

Faraone SV, Tsuang MT, Tarbox SI: The nature of schizotaxia, in Early Clinical Intervention and Prevention in Schizophrenia. Edited by Stone WS, Faraone SV, Tsuang MT. Totowa, NJ, Humana Press, 2004, pp 93–114

Fearon P, Kirkbride JB, Morgan C, et al: ÆSOP Study Group: Incidence of schizophrenia and other psychoses in ethnic minority groups: results from the MRC ÆSOP Study. Psychol Med 36:1541–1550, 2006

Ferdinand RF, Sondeijker F, van der Ende J, et al: Cannabis use predicts future psychotic symptoms, and vice versa. Addiction 100:612–618, 2005a

Ferdinand RF, Van der Ende J, Bongers I, et al: Cannabis—psychosis pathway independent of other types of psychopathology. Schizophr Res 79:289–295, 2005b

Flint J, Munafò MR: The endophenotype concept in psychiatric genetics. Psychol Med 37:163–180, 2007

Friedman D, Squires-Wheeler E: Event-related potentials (ERPs) as indicators of risk for schizophrenia. Schizophr Bull 20:63–74, 1994

Friis S, Sundet K, Rund BR, et al: Neurocognitive dimensions characterising patients with first-episode psychosis. Br J Psychiatry 181 (suppl 43):s85–s90, 2002

Gleeson J, Jackson HJ, Stavely H, et al: Family intervention in early psychosis, in The Recognition and Management of Early Psychosis: A Preventive Approach. Edited by McGorry PD, Jackson HJ. Cambridge, UK, Cambridge University Press, 1999, pp 376–406

Goldner EM, Hsu L, Waraich P, et al: Prevalence and incidence studies of schizophrenic disorders: a systematic review of the literature. Can J Psychiatry 47:833–843, 2002

Gottesman II, Gould TD: The endophenotype concept in psychiatry: etymology and strategic intentions. Am J Psychiatry 160:636–645, 2003

Gur RE, Nimgaonkar VL, Almasy L, et al: Neurocognitive endophenotypes in a multiplex multigenerational family study of schizophrenia. Am J Psychiatry 164:813–819, 2007

Hallmayer J: The epidemiology of the genetic liability for schizophrenia. Aust N Z J Psychiatry 34(suppl):S47–S55, 2000

Hawkins KA, McGlashan TH, Quinlan D, et al: Factorial structure of the Scale of Prodromal Symptoms. Schizophr Res 68:339–347, 2004

Henquet C, Murray R, Linszen D, et al: The environment and schizophrenia: the role of cannabis use. Schizophr Bull 31:608–612, 2005

Herz MI, Lamberti JS, Mintz J, et al: A program for relapse prevention in schizophrenia: a controlled study. Arch Gen Psychiatry 57:277–283, 2000

Hodgkinson KA, Murphy J, O'Neill S, et al: Genetic counselling for schizophrenia in the era of molecular genetics. Can J Psychiatry 46:123–130, 2001

Hollister JM, Laing P, Mednick SA: Rhesus incompatibility as a risk factor for schizophrenia in male adults. Arch Gen Psychiatry 53:19–24, 1996

Hong LE, Mitchell BD, Avila MT, et al: Familial aggregation of eye-tracking endophenotypes in families of schizophrenic patients. Arch Gen Psychiatry 63:259–264, 2006

Hultman CM, Ohman A, Cnattingius S, et al: Prenatal and neonatal risk factors for schizophrenia. Br J Psychiatry 170:128–133, 1997

Institute of Medicine: Reducing Risks for Mental Disorders: Frontiers for Preventive Intervention Research. Edited by Mrazek PJ, Haggerty RJ. Washington, DC, National Academy Press, 1994

International Early Psychosis Association Writing Group: International clinical practice guidelines for early psychosis. Br J Psychiatry 187:s120–s124, 2005

Jablensky A: Epidemiology of schizophrenia: the global burden of disease and disability. Eur Arch Psychiatry Clin Neurosci 250:274–285, 2000

Jablensky A: Subtyping schizophrenia: implications for genetic research. Mol Psychiatry 11:815–836, 2006

Jackson HJ, Edwards J, Hulbert C, et al: Recovery from psychosis: psychosocial interventions, in The Recognition and Management of Early Psychosis: A Preventive Approach. Edited by McGorry PD, Jackson HJ. Cambridge, UK, Cambridge University Press, 1999, pp 265–307

Jaeger J, Czobor P, Berns SM: Basic neuropsychological dimensions in schizophrenia. Schizophr Res 65:105–116, 2003

Joa I, Johannessen JO, Larsen TK, et al: Information campaigns: 10 years of experience in the Early Treatment and Intervention in Psychosis (TIPS) study. Psychiatr Ann 38:512–520, 2008

Johannessen JO, McGlashan TH, Larsen TK, et al: Early detection strategies for untreated first-episode psychosis. Schizophr Res 51:39–46, 2001

John JP, Arunachalam V, Ratnam B, et al: Expanding the schizophrenia phenotype: a composite evaluation of neurodevelopmental markers. Compr Psychiatry 48:78–86, 2008

Jones PB, Tarrant CJ: Developmental precursors and biological markers for schizophrenia and affective disorders: specificity and public health implications. Eur Arch Psychiatry Clin Neurosci 250:286–291, 2000

Jorm AF: Mental health literacy: public knowledge and beliefs about mental disorders. Br J Psychiatry 177:396–401, 2000

Jorm AF, Blewitt KA, Griffiths KM, et al: Mental health first aid responses of the public: results from an Australian national survey. BMC Psychiatry 5:9, 2005. Available at: http://www.biomedcentral.com/1471-244X/5/9. Accessed July 15, 2009.

Keefe RS, Frescka E, Apter SH, et al: Clinical characteristics of Kraepelinian schizophrenia: replication and extension of previous findings. Am J Psychiatry 153:806–811, 1996

Kendler KS, McGuire M, Gruenberg AM, et al: The Roscommon Family Study: I: methods, diagnosis of probands, and risk of schizophrenia in relatives. Arch Gen Psychiatry 50:527–540, 1993

Keshavan MS, Gilbert AR, Diwadkar VA: Neurodevelopmental theories, in The American Psychiatric Publishing Textbook of Schizophrenia. Edited by Lieberman JA, Stroup TS, Perkins DO. Washington, DC, American Psychiatric Publishing, 2006, pp 69–83

King M, Walker C, Levy G, et al: Development and validation of an international risk prediction algorithm for episodes of major depression in general practice attendees: the PredictD Study. Arch Gen Psychiatry 65:1368–1376, 2008

Kirkbride JB, Fearon P, Morgan C, et al: Heterogeneity in incidence rates of schizophrenia and other psychotic syndromes: findings from the 3-center ÆSOP study. Arch Gen Psychiatry 63:250–258, 2006

Kirkpatrick B, Buchanan RW: Anhedonia and the deficit syndrome of schizophrenia. Psychiatry Res 31:25–30, 1990

Kirkpatrick B, Buchanan RW, Breier A, et al: Case identification and stability of the deficit syndrome of schizophrenia. Psychiatry Res 47:47–56, 1993

Kitchener BA, Jorm AF: Mental health first aid training for the public: evaluation of effects on knowledge, attitudes and helping behavior. BMC Psychiatry 2:10, 2002. Available at: http://www.biomedcentral.com/1471-244X/2/10. Accessed July 15, 2009.

Kitchener BA, Jorm AF: Mental health first aid training: a review of evaluation studies. Aust N Z J Psychiatry 40:6–8, 2006

Klosterkötter J, Ebel H, Schultze-Lutter F, et al: Diagnostic validity of basic symptoms. Eur Arch Psychiatry Clin Neurosci 246:147–154, 1996

Klosterkötter J, Gross G, Huber G, et al: Evaluation of the 'Bonn Scale for the Assessment of Basic Symptoms – BSABS' as an instrument for the assessment of schizophrenia proneness: a review of recent findings. Neurology, Psychiatry and Brain Research 5:137–150, 1997

Klosterkötter J, Hellmich MI, Steinmeyer EM, et al: Diagnosing schizophrenia in the initial prodromal phase. Arch Gen Psychiatry 58:158–164, 2001

Knapp M, Mangalore R, Simon J: The global costs of schizophrenia. Schizophr Bull 30:279–293, 2004

Kraemer HC, Stice E, Kazdin A, et al: How do risk factors work together?: mediators, moderators, and independent, overlapping, and proxy risk factors. Am J Psychiatry 158:848–856, 2001

Kremen WS, Tsuang MT, Faraone SV, et al: Using risk markers to compare conceptual models of genetic heterogeneity in schizophrenia. J Nerv Ment Dis 180:141–152, 1992

Kremen WS, Seidman LJ, Pepple JR, et al: Neuropsychological risk indicators for schizophrenia: a review of family studies. Schizophr Bull 20:103–119, 1994

Lacro JP, Dunn LB, Dolder CR, et al: Prevalence of and risk factors for medication nonadherence in patients with schizophrenia: a comprehensive review of recent literature. J Clin Psychiatry 63:892–909, 2002

Larsen TK, Melle I, Auestad B, et al: Early detection of first-episode psychosis: the effect on 1-year outcome. Schizophr Bull 32:758–764, 2006

Lee C, McGlashan TH, Woods SW: Prevention of schizophrenia: can it be achieved? CNS Drugs 19:193–206, 2005

Lee KH, Williams LM: Eye movement dysfunction as a biological marker of risk for schizophrenia. Aust N Z J Psychiatry 34(suppl):S91–S100, 2000

Lehman AF, Lieberman JA, Dixon LB, et al: American Psychiatric Association; Steering Committee on Practice Guidelines: Practice guideline for the treatment of patients with schizophrenia, second edition. Am J Psychiatry 161 (2 suppl):1–56, 2004

Levy DL, Holzman PS, Matthysse S, et al: Eye tracking and schizophrenia: a selective review. Schizophr Bull 20:47–62, 1994

Liberman RP, Kopelowicz A: Recovery from schizophrenia: a concept in search of research. Psychiatr Serv 56:735–742, 2005

Light GA, Braff DL: Measuring P50 suppression and prepulse inhibition in a single recording session. Am J Psychiatry 158:2066–2068, 2001

Linszen DH, Dingemans PMAJ, Lenior ME, et al: Early detection and intervention in schizophrenia. Int Clin Psychopharmacol 13 (suppl 3):S31–S34, 1998

Liu W, Breen G, Zhang J, et al: Association of APOE gene with schizophrenia in Chinese: a possible risk factor in times of malnutrition. Schizophr Res 62:225–230, 2003

Malaspina D, Harlap S, Fennig S, et al: Advancing paternal age and the risk of schizophrenia. Arch Gen Psychiatry 58:361–367, 2001

Marshall M, Lewis S, Lockwood A, et al: Association between duration of untreated psychosis and outcome in cohorts of first-episode patients: a systemic review. Arch Gen Psychiatry 62:975–983, 2005

McDowell JE, Myles-Worsley M, Coon H, et al: Measuring liability for schizophrenia using optimized antisaccade stimulus parameters. Psychophysiology 36:138–141, 1999

McDowell JE, Brown GG, Paulus M, et al: Neural correlates of refixation saccades and antisaccades in normal and schizophrenia subjects. Biol Psychiatry 51:216–223, 2002

McGlashan TH: Early detection and intervention in schizophrenia: research. Schizophr Bull 22:327–345, 1996

McGlashan TH: Duration of untreated psychosis in first-episode schizophrenia: marker or determinant of course? Biol Psychiatry 46:899–907, 1999

McGlashan TH, Zipursky RB, Perkins D, et al: Randomized, double-blind trial of olanzapine versus placebo in patients prodromally symptomatic for psychosis. Am J Psychiatry 163:790–799, 2006

McGorry PD: Paradigm failure in functional psychosis: review and implications. Aust N Z J Psychiatry 25:43–55, 1991

McGorry PD: "A stitch in time"…the scope of preventive strategies in early psychosis. Eur Arch Psychiatry Clin Neurosci 248:22–31, 1998

McGorry PD: The nature of schizophrenia: signposts to prevention. Aust N Z J Psychiatry 34(suppl):S14–S21, 2000

McGorry PD, Edwards J, Mihalopoulos C, et al: EPPIC: an evolving system of early detection and optimal management. Schizophr Bull 22:305–326, 1996

McGorry PD, Yung AR, Phillips LJ, et al: Randomized controlled trial of interventions designed to reduce the risk of progression to first-episode psychosis in a clinical sample with subthreshold symptoms. Arch Gen Psychiatry 59:921–928, 2002

McNeil TF: Perinatal risk factors and schizophrenia: selective review and methodological concerns. Epidemiol Rev 17:107–112, 1995

McNeil TF, Cantor-Graae E: Minor physical anomalies and obstetric complications in schizophrenia. Aust N Z J Psychiatry 34(suppl):S65–S73, 2000

Melle I, Larsen TK, Haahr U, et al: Reducing the duration of untreated first-episode psychosis: effects on clinical presentation. Arch Gen Psychiatry 16:143–150, 2004

Melle I, Johannesen JO, Friis S, et al: Early detection of the first episode of schizophrenia and suicidal behavior. Am J Psychiatry 163:800–804, 2006

Meltzer HY: Suicidality in schizophrenia: a review of the evidence for risk factors and treatment options. Curr Psychiatry Rep 4:279–283, 2002

Michie PT, Kent A, Stienstra R, et al: Phenotypic markers as risk factors in schizophrenia: neurocognitive functions. Aust N Z J Psychiatry 34(suppl):S74–S85, 2000

Miller T, Mednick SA, McGlashan TH, et al: Early Intervention in Psychotic Disorders: Proceedings of the NATO Advanced Research Workshop on Early Intervention in Psychiatric Disorders, Prague, Czech Republic, October 22–27, 1998 (NATO Science Series D, Vol 91). New York, Springer, 2001

Mojtabai R, Susser ES, Bromet EJ: Clinical characteristics, 4-year course, and DSM-IV classification of patients with nonaffective acute remitting psychosis. Am J Psychiatry 160:2108–2115, 2003

Moldin SO, Erlenmeyer-Kimling L: Measuring liability to schizophrenia: progress report 1994: editors' introduction. Schizophr Bull 20:25–29, 1994

Montross LP, Zisook S, Kasckow J, et al: Suicide among patients with schizophrenia: a consideration of risk and protective factors. Ann Clin Psychiatry 17:173–182, 2005

Morrison AP, French P, Walford L, et al: Cognitive therapy for the prevention of psychosis in people at ultra-high risk: randomised controlled trial. Br J Psychiatry 185:291–297, 2004

Mueser KT, McGurk SR: Schizophrenia. Lancet 363:2063–2072, 2004

Murphy KC, Owen MJ: Velo-cardio-facial syndrome: a model for understanding the genetics and pathogenesis of schizophrenia. Br J Psychiatry 179:397–402, 2001

Murray CJL, Lopez AD: The Global Burden of Disease. Cambridge, MA, Harvard University Press, 1996

Norman RMG, Malla AK: Duration of untreated psychosis: a critical examination of the concept and its importance. Psychol Med 31:381–400, 2001

Nuechterlein KH, Barch DM, Gold JM, et al: Identification of separable cognitive factors in schizophrenia. Schizophr Res 72:29–39, 2004

O'Donnell BF, McCarley RW, Potts GF, et al: Identification of neural circuits underlying P300 abnormalities in schizophrenia. Psychophysiology 36:388–398, 1999

Palmer CGS, Turunen JA, Sinsheimer JS, et al: RHD maternal-fetal genotype incompatibility increases schizophrenia susceptibility. Am J Hum Genet 71:1312–1319, 2002

Pardes H, Silverman MM, West A: Prevention and the field of mental health: a psychiatric perspective. Annu Rev Pub Health 10:403–422, 1989

Pecenak J: Relapse prevention in schizophrenia: evidence from longterm, randomized, double-blind clinical trials. Neuro Endocrinol Lett 28 (suppl 1):49–70, 2007

Penn DL, Waldheter EJ, Perkins DO, et al: Psychosocial treatment for first-episode psychosis: a research update. Am J Psychiatry 162:2220–2232, 2005

Perkins DO, Gu H, Boteva K, et al: Relationship between duration of untreated psychosis and outcome in first-episode schizophrenia: a critical review and meta-analysis. Am J Psychiatry 162:1785–1804, 2005

Phillips LJ, Leicester SB, O'Dwyer LE, et al: The PACE Clinic: identification and management of young people at "ultra" high risk of psychosis. J Psychiatr Pract 8:255–269, 2002

Phillips LJ, Yung AR, Hearn N, et al: Preventative mental health care: accessing the target population. Aust N Z J Psychiatry 33:912–917, 1999

Price GW, Michie PT, Johnston J, et al: A multivariate electrophysiological endophenotype, from a unitary cohort, shows greater research utility than any single feature in the Western Australian Family Study of Schizophrenia. Biol Psychiatry 60:1–10, 2006

Raphael B: Primary prevention: fact or fiction. Aust N Z J Psychiatry 14:163–174, 1980

Ruhrmann S, Schultze-Lutter F, Maier W, et al: Pharmacological intervention in the initial prodromal phase of psychosis. Eur Psychiatry 20:1–6, 2005

Ruhrmann S, Hoppmann B, Theysohn S, et al: Acute symptomatic treatment effects in persons clinically at risk for psychosis. Schizophr Res 86(suppl):S8, 2006

Sartorius N, Henderson AS: The neglect of prevention in psychiatry. Aust N Z J Psychiatry 26:550–553, 1992

Sheitman BB, Lee H, Strauss R, et al: The evaluation and treatment of first-episode psychosis. Schizophr Bull 23:653–661, 1997

Shprintzen RJ, Higgins AM, Antshel K, et al: Velo-cardio-facial syndrome. Curr Opin Pediatr 17:725–730, 2005

Silverman MM: Children of psychiatrically ill parents: a prevention perspective. Hosp Community Psychiatry 40:1257–1265, 1989

Simonsen E, Friis S, Haahr U, et al: Two year outcome and predictors in first episode psychosis (abstract). Schizophr Res 86(suppl):S155–S156, 2006

Smit F, Boiler L, Cuijpers P: Cannabis use and the risk of later schizophrenia: a review. Addiction 99:425–430, 2004

Snitz BE, MacDonald AW 3rd, Carter CS: Cognitive deficits in unaffected first-degree relatives of schizophrenia patients: a meta-analytic review of putative endophenotypes. Schizophr Bull 32:179–194, 2006

Sobell JL, Mikesell MJ, McMurray CT: Genetics and etiopathophysiology of schizophrenia. Mayo Clin Proc 77:1068–1082, 2002

Susser ES, Brown AS, Gorman JM (eds): Prenatal Exposures in Schizophrenia. Washington, DC, American Psychiatric Press, 1999

Tandon R, Targum SD, Nasrallah HA, et al: Strategies for maximizing clinical effectiveness in the treatment of schizophrenia. J Psychiatr Pract 12:348–363, 2006

Taylor M, Chaudhry I, Cross M, et al: Relapse Prevention in Schizophrenia Consensus Group: towards consensus in the long-term management of relapse prevention in schizophrenia. Hum Psychopharmacol 20:175–181, 2005

Thorup A, Waltoft BL, Pedersen CB, et al: Young males have a higher risk of developing schizophrenia: a Danish register study. Psychol Med 37:479–484, 2007

Tienari PA, Wynne LC, Sorri A, et al: Genotype-environment interaction in schizo-phrenia-spectrum disorder: long-term follow-up study of Finnish adoptees. Br J Psychiatry 184:216–222, 2004

Torrey WC, Green RL, Drake RE: Psychiatrists and psychiatric rehabilitation. J Psy-chiatr Pract 11:155–160, 2005

Tsuang M: Schizophrenia: genes and environment. Biol Psychiatry 47:210–220, 2000

Tsuang MT, Faraone SV: Diagnostic concepts and the prevention of schizophrenia. Can J Psychiatry 47:515–517, 2002

Tsuang MT, Stone WS, Tarbox SI, et al: An integration of schizophrenia with schizo-typy: identification of schizotaxia and implications for research on treatment and prevention. Schizophr Res 54:169–175, 2002

Tully EM, McGlashan TH: The prodrome, in The American Psychiatric Publishing Textbook of Schizophrenia. Edited by Lieberman JA, Stroup TS, Perkins DO. Washington, DC, American Psychiatric Publishing, 2006, pp 341–352

U.S. Department of Health and Human Services: Healthy People 2010: Understanding and Improving Health, 2nd Edition. Rockville, MD, U.S. Department of Health and Human Services, Office of Disease Prevention and Health Promotion, 2000. Available at: http://www.healthypeople.gov/Document/pdf/uih/2010uih.pdf. Accessed July 15, 2008.

van Os J, Delespaul P: Toward a world consensus on prevention of schizophrenia. Dialogues Clin Neurosci 7:53–67, 2005

Verdoux H, Tournier M, Cougnard A: Impact of substance use on the onset and course of early psychosis. Schizophr Res 79:69–75, 2005

Walker EF: Developmentally moderated expressions of the neuropathology underlying schizophrenia. Schizophr Bull 20:453–480, 1994

Walker EF, Diforio D: Schizophrenia: a neural diathesis-stress model. Psychol Rev 104:667–685, 1997

Walsh T, McClellan JM, McCarthy SE, et al: Rare structural variants disrupt multiple genes in neurodevelopmental pathways in schizophrenia. Science 320:539–543, 2008

Wang PS, Demler O, Kessler RC: Adequacy of treatment for serious mental illness in the United States. Am J Publ Health 92:92–98, 2002

Wang Q, Chan R, Sun J, et al: Reaction time of the Continuous Performance Test is an endophenotypic marker for schizophrenia: a study of first-episode neuroleptic-naive schizophrenia, their non-psychotic first-degree relatives and healthy popu-lation controls. Schizophr Res 89:293–298, 2007

Warner R: The prevention of schizophrenia: what interventions are safe and effective? Schizophr Bull 27:551–562, 2001

Weiden PJ: Understanding and addressing adherence issues in schizophrenia: from theory to practice. J Clin Psychiatry 68 (suppl 14):14–19, 2007

Wood K, Kotwicki RJ: Criminalization of mental illnesses, in Responding to Individuals with Mental Illnesses. Edited by Compton MT, Kotwicki RJ. Sudbury, MA, Jones & Bartlett, 2007, pp 13–20

World Health Organization: Report of the International Pilot Study of Schizophrenia. Geneva, Switzerland, World Health Organization, 1973

Wright A, McGorry PD, Harris MG, et al: Development and evaluation of a youth mental health community awareness campaign—The Compass Strategy. BMC Public Health 6:215, 2006. Available at: http://www.biomedcentral.com/1471-2458/6/215. Accessed July 15, 2009.

Wu EQ, Birnbaum HG, Shi L, et al: The economic burden of schizophrenia in the United States in 2002. J Clin Psychiatry 66:1122–1129, 2005

Wyatt RJ: Neurodevelopmental abnormalities in schizophrenia: a family affair. Arch Gen Psychiatry 53:11–15, 1996

Wyatt RJ, Henter I: Rationale for the study of early intervention. Schizophr Res 51:69–76, 2001

Yung AR, McGorry PD: The prodromal phase of first-episode psychosis: past and current conceptualizations. Schizophr Bull 22:353–370, 1996

Yung AR, McGorry PD: Is pre-psychotic intervention realistic in schizophrenia and related disorders? Aust N Z J Psychiatry 31:799–805, 1997

Yung AR, McGorry PD, McFarlane CA, et al: Monitoring and care of young people at incipient risk of psychosis. Schizophr Bull 22:283–303, 1996

Yung AR, Phillips LJ, McGorry PD, et al: Prediction of psychosis: a step towards indicated prevention of schizophrenia. Br J Psychiatry 172(suppl):14–20, 1998

Yung AR, Phillips LJ, Drew LT: Promoting access to care in early psychosis, in The Recognition and Management of Early Psychosis: A Preventive Approach. Edited by McGorry PD, Jackson HJ. Cambridge, UK, Cambridge University Press, 1999, pp 80–114

Yung AR, Killackey E, Hetrick SE, et al: The prevention of schizophrenia. Int Rev Psychiatry 19:633–646, 2007

Zammit S, Allebeck P, Dalman C, et al: Paternal age and risk for schizophrenia. Br J Psychiatry 183:405–408, 2003

Zipursky RB: Optimal pharmacologic management of the first episode of schizophrenia, in The Early Stages of Schizophrenia. Edited by Zipursky RB, Schulz SC. Washington, DC, American Psychiatric Publishing, 2002, pp 81–106

7

Prevention of Alcohol and Drug Abuse

Rebecca A. Powers, M.D., M.P.H.

Substance use disorders (SUDs) and related problems cause several types of complications, consequences, and even disabilities for a large proportion of the U.S. population. We are aware of the immediate ill effects, the difficulties of treatment, and the high morbidity and mortality rates associated with substance abuse. Everyone agrees that prevention can benefit individuals, families, and the community. What may be in dispute is the type of prevention. No single intervention will have a dramatic or instantaneous effect given the complexity of the problem. The risk factors and etiologies are multifactorial and complex, as are the protective factors. The issue becomes even more convoluted when one considers legal issues and the potentially positive health benefits of low to moderate alcohol intake. The politics, control of their use, and drive for financial gain and power that underlie substances of abuse add to the problem.

The pain and suffering associated with alcohol and drug abuse and dependence are real but usually immeasurable. One may not even have a diagnosis associated with substances, but misuse of a substance just once could lead to poor judgment resulting in an accident. The effects are far reaching and involve the individual with the problem, his or her family and friends, other people involved with the individual, the medical community, the economy, the workforce, and so forth. Comorbidity diagnoses occur in 60%–90% of those affected with substance-related disorders, thereby magnifying and complicating the problem. Adolescents with a severe SUD have other psychiatric disorders more frequently than adults with an SUD (Powers 1998). Practicing mental health professionals are affected daily by the consequences of SUDs in their patients. For these reasons, a consideration of alcohol and drug abuse prevention is crucial.

Alcohol Use as a Problem and a Benefit: The Paradox

Alcohol use creates a paradox more than the use of any other substance, legal or not. It is used all over the world more than any other substance and probably more safely; yet, it can also be a powerful and hazardous drug. Only tobacco use causes more morbidity and mortality. The fact that it is legal, easy to obtain, and the product of a multibillion dollar industry makes it alluring to many.

Alcohol abuse is more common than any other SUD. The consequences of alcohol abuse and dependence can be all encompassing and insidious. Alcohol abuse presents a unique dilemma for the public health community, referred to as the *prevention paradox* (B. L. Cook and Abreu 1998). This means that the patterns associated with the formal diagnosis of alcohol use disorders have less health and economic consequences than hazardous drinking alone. This paradox is complicated by the suggestion that low to moderate alcohol use may be protective against cardiovascular disease. Therefore, the level of intake of alcohol, the risk factors for alcohol abuse, the protective factors in an individual to resist becoming a problem drinker, and the context of the individual in society all must be taken into account when understanding the overall dilemma. The effects of alcohol on the individual vary along a continuum of use from abstinence to dependence.

Physically, alcohol affects the brain reward pathway through its effects on dopamine, γ-aminobutyric acid, serotonin, opioid, and N-methyl-D-aspartate neurotransmitter systems (Grant 1994). Nicotinic receptors in the ventral tegmental area are partially responsible for the reinforcing properties, and likely account for why people who are alcohol dependent are more likely to smoke cigarettes as well (Tizabi et al. 2002; see also Chapter 13, "The Prevention of Cigarette Smoking: Principles for Psychiatric Practice"). Both the interactions of substances with and the genetic underpinnings of these pathways contribute to the possibility of abuse and dependence.

People drink alcohol for many different reasons, including pleasure, reduction of anxiety or tension, social ties (including peer relations), self-medication, peer relatedness, and addiction. Approximately 90% of adults in the United States have had some experience with alcohol in their lifetime. About half of individuals older than 12 years, or 121 million persons, are current consumers of alcohol according to the National Survey on Drug Use and Health (Substance Abuse and Mental Health Services Administration 2006). More than one in five (23%) had engaged in binge drinking once or more in the 30 days preceding the 2006 survey. It was estimated that 17 million, or almost 7%, of those age 12 or older are heavy drinkers, similar to the 2002–2003 estimates (Schuckit 2000). About 40% of those who drink experience an alcohol-related problem (Schuckit 2000).

Alcohol abuse and dependence are highly prevalent in the United States. About 10% of women and 20% of men have met DSM-IV-TR criteria for alcohol abuse in their lifetime (American Psychiatric Association 2000). This constitutes about 20%–30% of the psychiatric population. Full-time college students have higher rates of alcohol use, binge drinking, and heavy use compared with others in their age group (18–22 years) (Substance Abuse and Mental Health Services Administration 2006). About 31% of college students abuse alcohol and 6% more are alcohol dependent. Male students are at greater risk than females. For those younger than 24 years, alcohol dependence has been reported to occur in 10% of males and 5% of females (Knight et al. 2002). Dependence typically develops in the midtwenties through age 40, but can occur at any age. Schuckit (2000) found that repeated intoxication at an early age increases the risk of developing an alcohol use disorder.

Alcohol use disorders affect at least 20–30 million people in the United States at any given time (B. L. Cook and Abreu 1998). This number increases through complications that affect marriage, family, or work; motor vehicle crashes and other accidents; physical health conditions; and overall direct and indirect costs to society. The disorders associated with alcohol generally can be divided into three groups, as listed below. DSM-IV-TR criteria for the third group, substance (including alcohol) abuse and dependence, are given in Tables 7–1 and 7–2.

1. Disorders due to the direct effect of alcohol on the brain (intoxication, withdrawal, and withdrawal delirium; alcohol-induced mood, anxiety, sexual, and sleep disorders; and hallucinosis)
2. Disorders with persisting effects from alcohol (amnestic disorder, dementia, Wernicke encephalopathy, and Korsakoff syndrome)
3. Disorders associated with the behavioral effects of alcohol (alcohol abuse and alcohol dependence)

A lifelong syndrome affecting children with confirmed prenatal exposure to alcohol is fetal alcohol syndrome. The syndrome is associated with stunted growth, abnormal facial features, neurocognitive deficits, and problems with vision and hearing. The National Task Force on Fetal Alcohol Syndrome/Fetal Alcohol Effects recommends that a child be referred for full fetal alcohol syndrome evaluation when there is confirmed significant prenatal alcohol use (i.e., seven or more drinks per week and/or three or more drinks on multiple occasions) (Agency for Healthcare Research and Quality 2008a). The task force recommends that if prenatal alcohol exposure in the high-risk range is known in the absence of any other positive screening criteria, the primary health care provider should document this exposure and closely monitor the child's ongoing growth and development.

In addition to the personal and family-related costs of alcohol abuse and dependence, diverse groups such as the federal, state, and local governments; private insurance companies; employers; and society at large are affected. Up to 20% of patients (outpatients) of primary care physicians are problem drinkers, and 20%–40% of those admitted to the hospital have an alcohol use disorder, thereby costing society a great deal in terms of medical care. Industry must face large costs due to absenteeism, sick leave, decreased worker efficiency, health care expenditures, and employee replacement costs through people quitting, being fired, or dying prematurely. Other alcohol-related costs include property and administrative costs related to motor vehicle accidents, as well as alcohol-related crime. A person's life span is reduced by about 15 years

Table 7–1. DSM-IV-TR diagnostic criteria for substance abuse

A. A maladaptive pattern of substance use leading to clinically significant impairment or distress, as manifested by one (or more) of the following, occurring within a 12-month period:

    (1) recurrent substance use resulting in a failure to fulfill major role obligations at work, school, or home (e.g., repeated absences or poor work performance related to substance use; substance-related absences, suspensions, or expulsions from school; neglect of children or household)

    (2) recurrent substance use in situations in which it is physically hazardous (e.g., driving an automobile or operating a machine when impaired by substance use)

    (3) recurrent substance-related legal problems (e.g., arrests for substance-related disorderly conduct)

    (4) continued substance use despite having persistent or recurrent social or interpersonal problems caused or exacerbated by the effects of the substance (e.g., arguments with spouse about consequences of intoxication, physical fights)

B. The symptoms have never met the criteria for Substance Dependence for this class of substance.

Source. Reprinted from American Psychiatric Association: *Diagnostic and Statistical Manual of Mental Disorders,* 4th Edition, Revised. Washington, DC, American Psychiatric Association, 2000. Copyright 2000, American Psychiatric Association. Used with permission.

in the context of alcohol dependence (Schuckit 2000). Deaths associated with alcohol are not always coded accordingly on death certificates. The National Institute on Drug Abuse and the National Institute on Alcohol Abuse and Alcoholism estimate the economic burden on society to be about $246 billion for alcohol and drug abuse (Harwood 2000). Alcohol problems accounted for about 60% of the costs, whereas the remaining 40% were due to drug abuse and dependence (Harwood 2000).

In addition to the previously mentioned prevention paradox pertaining to alcohol use, the use of this substance presents another type of paradox, because alcohol consumed responsibly can be beneficial. Low to moderate alcohol intake from any source may decrease cardiovascular disease risk, which may lead to a reduction in all-cause mortality. Although low doses can be protective for coronary artery disease, higher doses increase the rate of deaths from all causes (World Health Organization 2002). The protective effects may be secondary to genetic variations in alcohol dehydrogenase (ADH) and other

Table 7–2.   DSM-IV-TR diagnostic criteria for substance dependence

A maladaptive pattern of substance use, leading to clinically significant impairment or distress, as manifested by three (or more) of the following, occurring at any time in the same 12-month period:

(1)   tolerance, as defined by either of the following:

    (a)   a need for markedly increased amounts of the substance to achieve intoxication or desired effect

    (b)   markedly diminished effect with continued use of the same amount of the substance

(2)   withdrawal, as manifested by either of the following:

    (a)   the characteristic withdrawal syndrome for the substance (refer to Criteria A and B of the criteria sets for Withdrawal from the specific substances)

    (b)   the same (or a closely related) substance is taken to relieve or avoid withdrawal symptoms

(3)   the substance is often taken in larger amounts or over a longer period than was intended

(4)   there is a persistent desire or unsuccessful efforts to cut down or control substance use

(5)   a great deal of time is spent in activities necessary to obtain the substance (e.g., visiting multiple doctors or driving long distances), use the substance (e.g., chain-smoking), or recover from its effects

(6)   important social, occupational, or recreational activities are given up or reduced because of substance use

(7)   the substance use is continued despite knowledge of having a persistent or recurrent physical or psychological problem that is likely to have been caused or exacerbated by the substance (e.g., current cocaine use despite recognition of cocaine-induced depression, or continued drinking despite recognition that an ulcer was made worse by alcohol consumption)

Specify if:

    With Physiological Dependence: evidence of tolerance or withdrawal (i.e., either Item 1 or 2 is present)

    Without Physiological Dependence: no evidence of tolerance or withdrawal (i.e., neither Item 1 nor 2 is present)

Table 7–2. DSM-IV-TR diagnostic criteria for substance dependence *(continued)*

Course specifiers (see text of DSM-IV-TR for definitions):

Early Full Remission

Early Partial Remission

Sustained Full Remission

Sustained Partial Remission

On Agonist Therapy

In a Controlled Environment

Source. Reprinted from American Psychiatric Association: *Diagnostic and Statistical Manual of Mental Disorders,* 4th Edition, Revised. Washington, DC, American Psychiatric Association, 2000. Copyright 2000, American Psychiatric Association. Used with permission.

gene products, as well as specific patterns of use. If a moderate drinker is homozygous for the slow-oxidizing ADH3 genotype, she or he may have higher high-density lipoprotein (HDL) cholesterol levels and a lower risk of having a myocardial infarction compared with a nonhomozygotic individual (Hine et al. 2001). Protective factors such as increased HDL cholesterol, inhibition of platelets, enhanced insulin sensitivity, and reduction in fasting insulin could also play a role through a person's lifetime. However, excessive alcohol intake increases one's chances for cardiovascular risk factors such as high blood pressure, elevated low-density lipoprotein cholesterol levels, and increased clotting factors. Of course, these risk factors apply to individuals older than 40 years, given that coronary artery disease is rare before that age. Despite potential health benefits of low to moderate alcohol intake in adulthood, alcohol is often considered the second most common factor related to preventable death in the United States (Zahler and Piselli 1992). Psychiatrists and other health care professionals are in a difficult position weighing the potential protective effects of alcohol use in moderation alongside the risks of alcohol abuse and dependence.

Drug Abuse and Dependence: Always a Problem

The widespread effects of alcohol can also be seen with illicit substances. About 40% of persons in the United States have used an illicit substance at least once, and a drug use disorder is found in more than 15% of individuals who are more than 18 years old (Johnston et al. 2006). Substance-induced disorders can mimic and contribute to the full range of psychiatric disorders, including mood, anxiety, cognitive, psychotic, sexual, and sleep disorders. SUDs (abuse and dependence) must be considered in clinical practice for nearly every patient with regard to differential diagnosis and comorbidity. Depending on the substance's medical or psychological effects, nearly every organ system can be affected.

Substances must be available to people in order for them to use them. As sellers aim to increase the availability of drugs because of their profitability, public health agencies, other governmental organizations, religious/faith-based communities, and the medical community are attempting to diminish availability and consumption. Use of illicit drugs and nicotine in the young has declined in recent years, largely because of these efforts.

The series of Monitoring the Future surveys has revealed the alarmingly high nonmedical use of prescription drugs (e.g., stimulant medications, opiate analgesics, and benzodiazepines) (Johnston et al. 2006). The frequent portrayal and acceptance of such drug use in the media influences use in society. Such agents are more available due to Internet access and increasing numbers of prescriptions from physicians. The desire is not always to get "high" but to increase performance. For example, stimulant medications are sometimes used by students to perform better when studying and taking exams, by girls to lose weight to achieve an unrealistic or idealized body image, and by adults to manage in a highly competitive job environment. However, positive trends have shown decreased use of illicit drugs among high school students.

The costs of illicit SUDs are far reaching. Adverse health effects, morbidity and premature mortality, direct costs of use, lost productivity, crime, incarceration, drug enforcement and legal services costs, and rehabilitation and treatment costs are lofty. All segments of the U.S. populace have experienced improved health over the last 30 years except for adolescents. This is partly because teens are disproportionately affected by drug abuse (B. L. Cook and Abreu 1998). Unintentional injury, homicide, and suicide cause more than 77% of deaths in adolescents, and drug abuse has been implicated in more than half of these deaths. Moreover, there is a noteworthy link between intravenous drug use and seropositivity for the human immunodeficiency virus (HIV) and other blood-borne infections (B. L. Cook and Abreu 1998).

Prevention Is Crucial

The prevention of alcohol and drug abuse is crucial to bring about significant mental and physical health improvements and financial savings, in addition to improving the quality of life for those living with or around an individual with an SUD. Psychiatrists and other mental health professionals must think preventively on a daily basis to avert morbidity and mortality arising from substance abuse. A person could begin to use a substance, whether it is alcohol, illicit, or prescribed, at any time, and we need to track its use.

Psychiatrists and other mental health professionals must also be familiar with SUDs and ask all of their patients about substance use. In order to provide the appropriate help, health care providers need to be aware of a person's risk and protective factors and address these in each interview (see "Risk and Protective Factors" in both the "Prevention of Alcohol Abuse and Dependence" section and the "Prevention of Drug Abuse and Dependence" section). Given that the diagnosis of an SUD does not address etiology, clinicians should follow the established diagnostic criteria. For instance, whether a person is more prone to alcohol dependence because of a genetic predisposition or an adverse social environment or troubled peer group, the diagnosis is still applicable and the patient is still in need of treatment. Moreover, an SUD diagnosis is not based on the quantity or frequency of use, but on the consequences of use. Mental health professionals should keep in mind that a person could begin to use a substance at any time during a therapeutic relationship. Therefore, they must always assess patients for new or different substance abuse, especially if the patient's psychosocial status is declining and there is no other obvious reason for the decline. After the assessment, health care providers need to advise patients on decreasing or stopping their use of the substance. Even if a person needs to be advised 10 times that she or he should stop smoking, for example, and a given professional is the seventh to do so, then the patient is one step closer to quitting.

Prevention can be implemented at several different levels in society. Some prevention programs, including community-based and legal efforts, affect the population as a whole. Some more directly affect the person on an individual level. Psychiatrists and other mental health professionals can be involved in all levels of preventive interventions, as well as treatment.

Prevention of Alcohol Abuse and Dependence

Given the previously discussed potential health benefit of low to moderate alcohol intake in adulthood ("Alcohol Use as a Problem and a Benefit: The Paradox"), if a person is consuming a small amount of alcohol each day, unless there is a specific health reason to quit, a physician need not alter the behavior. However, if a person is abstinent or drinks infrequently, the clinician should not instigate beginning or increasing alcohol intake. Individuals vary in their vulnerability to alcohol dependence, depression, and alcohol-related pathologies and physicians cannot reliably predict a patient's path before he or she begins or escalates drinking.

Adverse psychosocial or health consequences can begin quickly after a person starts a problematic pattern of alcohol use, and detection is not always easy. If a heavy drinker has heart disease, she or he needs to immediately reduce consumption. Alcohol abuse, not even necessarily dependence, can worsen psychiatric disorders including the risk of suicide. Physicians always must ask about patterns of alcohol use no matter what the current amount of intake. Clinicians must be aware of the risk and protective factors associated with problematic alcohol drinking in order to help prevent alcohol abuse and dependence.

Risk and Protective Factors

Genetics and Alcohol Dependence

Some 40%–60% of the risk of alcohol dependence comes from genetic factors. If one has a relative with alcohol dependence, one is at 3–5-times greater risk of developing alcohol dependence compared with the general population. This risk increases based on the number and biological relatedness of relatives with alcohol dependence (Schuckit 2002). Even genetically prone children who are adopted into a nondrinking family can easily develop alcohol drinking problems. Genetics contributes to an enhanced brain reward pathway, decreased initial impairment, altered alcohol metabolism, and tolerance. Tolerance can cause a varied level of response such that a low level of response at an early age is a factor that increases the risk of alcohol dependence later in life (Krystal and Tabakoff 2002). Sons of alcoholic fathers rate themselves lower than sons of nonalcoholics in feelings of drunkenness, dizziness, drug effects, and sleepiness after using alcohol (Schuckit 2000). This low reaction to alcohol reveals more tolerance, and therefore a higher tendency toward dependence.

In general, American Indians have an increased risk of alcohol dependence because of their inherited lower response to alcohol. On the other hand, individuals of Asian descent often have a more intense response to alcohol because of variants in the ADH metabolic enzyme that can cause a higher level of acetaldehyde. This intensified response to alcohol leads to a lower risk of alcohol dependence. Personality-based inherited factors include a high level of impulsivity, sensation seeking, and disinhibition, all of which influence the risk of alcohol abuse and dependence (Schuckit 2002).

Social/Environmental and Psychological Risk Factors

If even one parent has alcohol dependence, a child may have more struggles socializing, and may join peer groups in which drinking and other risky behaviors are accepted or even supported. Some children who are monitored minimally by parents with alcohol dependence often begin drinking before the age of 15 years (Goodwin et al. 1974). The American Academy of Pediatrics recommends that patients and their families be advised that even casual use of alcohol by children and adolescents, regardless of amount or frequency, is illegal and has potential adverse health consequences (Agency for Healthcare Research and Quality 2008c).

Temperamental differences in children can affect inner distress and reactions to alcohol consumption. When anxious or depressed children take their first drink, their inner distress may dissipate for a short while, which could lead to more problematic drinking through negative reinforcement. If a child is moody, negative, or provocative, parents and teachers may be more critical. This could lead to strained reactions, which could cause a child to turn to alcohol. Sensitivity to the effects of alcohol in regard to sedative or stimulating properties vary from person to person. For example, studies suggest that heavy drinkers may have less sedation and cortisol response compared with light drinkers. In terms of risk, children with attention-deficit/hyperactivity disorder (ADHD), conduct disorder, or aggression problems are at increased risk for an alcohol use disorder. Males are generally at greater risk than females. Females with depression or anxiety, or who exhibit social avoidance, are at higher risk than their counterparts without those traits. Parents are overwhelmingly the most important factor influencing an adolescent's decision to drink.

A child living in adverse home conditions is more likely to develop an alcohol use disorder later in life than those in stable, supportive homes. Conditions in the home that are risk factors for teens to abuse alcohol include a crowded, noisy, and disorderly home without rules or religion. Other risk factors for teens' use include perceiving themselves as highly stressed, being easily angered, feeling resentful of absent parents, or having conflictual homes. Moreover, women from physically abusive homes are 1½–2 times more likely to abuse alcohol than nonabused adults, so childhood abuse is also a significant risk factor (Schuck and Widom 2001).

Physicians who treat children need to assess parental alcohol use and then ensure that parents receive adequate treatment when indicated. Children of parents with an untreated alcohol use disorder score lower on measures of family cohesion, intellectual and cultural orientation, active recreational orientation, and independence. There is also a greater risk of family conflict and even domestic violence when a parent has an alcohol use disorder. Children's development can be hampered because they cannot communicate well with other family members. A child may also be affected in a negative way by the abnormal behavior of the nonalcoholic spouse of an alcoholic parent, who may inadvertently support the drinking member of the family. There is a much greater chance of separation and divorce in couples in which one has alcohol dependence, and of course this negatively affects the children in those families as well. Children of alcoholic parents benefit from support groups such as Children of Alcoholics.

Protective Factors Against Alcohol Use Disorders

Nearly 12,000 students in grades 7–12 were given lengthy interviews timed 1 year apart in the National Longitudinal Study on Adolescent Health (Resnick et al. 1997). The researchers discovered two factors that kept children from taking health risks over the previous year in four major areas: substance abuse (tobacco, alcohol, and cannabis), sexuality, violence, and emotional health. These two protective factors were parent-family connectedness and school connectedness. Parent-family connectedness meant that they felt that they were close to a parent, felt that a parent cared about them, felt satisfied with their parent relationships, and felt loved by their family. School connectedness referred to feeling that they were a part of their school and that they were treated fairly by their teachers (Resnick et al. 1997).

Preventive Interventions

Universal Preventive Interventions

Universal preventive interventions in the community can affect patterns of use, availability of alcohol (including legal restrictions and cost), and peer-group behavior. Some studies have addressed changing the behavior of individuals rather than the environment. But limiting availability, increasing enforcement of laws, legislating stricter laws, influencing community standards, and increasing the cost of alcohol through taxation is sometimes easier and may be more effective. The cultural climate of some communities and their acceptance of alcohol use vary from place to place. Increased consumption in an area is associated with increased rates of alcohol problems in that area (Popham et al. 1976). Price increases via taxation have been shown to reduce cirrhosis mortality and automobile fatalities (P. J. Cook 1981). Moderate and heavy alcohol drinking can be reduced with controls on availability (B. L. Cook and Abreu 1998). Availability factors associated with consumption include the level of restrictions on times of sales permitted, particular types of stores that sell alcohol, number of outlet stores, unique characteristics and location of the stores, and the distribution system (Ryan and Segars 1987). Age restrictions represent an effective legal barrier to alcohol use, because it has been shown that the lower the legal age to drink, the higher the rate of consumption and associated problems (Moser 1980).

Holder (2000) showed how a strong community effort implementing the following diminished the misuse of alcohol:

- Community organization and support
- Responsible beverage services at alcohol outlets, bars, and restaurants
- Increased drunken driving enforcement efficiency
- Reduction of alcohol availability to minors
- Use of local zoning powers and other municipal controls

This extensive community project reduced alcohol-involved motor vehicle crashes, reduced sales to minors, increased responsible serving practices in bars and restaurants, and increased community support and awareness of alcohol-related problems (Holder 2000). The Lifestyle Management Class is another example of a universal prevention program, in this case among voluntary and mandated college students, utilizing peer- and professional-led group interventions. It has been shown to decrease driving after drinking and change heavy drinking patterns in some individuals (Fromme and Corbin 2004). Cardiovascular wellness programs on the worksite are another example; these programs help prevent alcohol abuse because they attract a large part of the working population and the accompanying alcohol education is well accepted in this format (Heirich and Sieck 2000).

Selective Preventive Interventions

Selective preventive interventions are tailored for individuals with a greater than average risk of developing alcohol use problems. The strongest predictor may be genetic influences. Alcohol dependence is familial, so if a strong family history is discovered, education should be provided for the unaffected persons in the family.

Screening detects those with hazardous drinking patterns or early symptoms of alcohol abuse or dependence that are still undetected. These individuals are the targets of selective or indicated preventive interventions. Screening also uncovers those with abuse or dependence who are not yet diagnosed (for secondary or tertiary prevention efforts). Screening is also necessary because time constraints limit a clinician from going down the list of DSM-IV-TR criteria for each SUD. The most commonly used screening tools are the MAST (Michigan Alcoholism Screening Test) (Selzer 1971), abbreviated MAST (Pokorny et al. 1972), CAGE (control, others annoyed, guilt, eye opener) questions (Mayfield et al. 1974), and T-ACE (tolerance, others annoyed, control, eye opener) questions (Sokol et al. 1989). However, these tools do not screen adolescents and the elderly adequately. The Adolescent Drinking Index is used for teens (Harrell and Wirtz 1989), whereas the elderly need questions about quantity and frequency in addition to the CAGE questions (Adams et al. 1996). Some of these recommended screening tests are provided in the appendix to this chapter.

Indicated Preventive Interventions

Indicated interventions are measures for individuals who have been found on screening to demonstrate a very high risk of developing alcohol abuse or dependence. The screening measures noted above can be used repeatedly in assessments. Laboratory screening tests include blood alcohol levels, liver enzyme elevations, erythrocyte mean corpuscular volume (MCV), lipid profiles, and carbohydrate-deficient transferrin (CDT). The MCV, like elevations in liver enzyme levels, is relatively specific to heavy alcohol intake and provides supporting evidence of heavy alcohol use (Skinner et al. 1984). CDT, although still under investigation, may serve as a laboratory marker to help distinguish alcoholic patients who consume large quantities of alcohol from light drinkers or nondrinkers (Allen et al. 1994). For pregnant women, the Michigan Quality Improvement Consortium (2008) recommends that health care professionals screen by history for substance use at every health maintenance exam or initial pregnancy visit (repeat as indicated), using a validated screening tool, such as the Alcohol Use Disorders Identification Test (AUDIT [see Appendix]; Babor et al. 1992), TWEAK questions (tolerance, worried, eye opener, amnesia, "kut down" [*sic*]) (Russell et al. 2006), MAST, and CAGE. Once clinical screening measures suggest problematic drinking or early alcohol abuse or dependence, treatment efforts should be initiated immediately.

How Do Mental Health Professionals Assess and Then Advise Patients About Problematic Alcohol Use?

A patient may ask us directly about our beliefs regarding healthy versus risky alcohol use. If a patient drinks a small to moderate amount of alcohol, physicians do not need to suggest a change, as there are some known health benefits. Exceptions are if that small amount has led to negative consequences or other risk factors for abuse exist. If a patient is abstinent or drinks occasionally, we should not recommend to begin or increase alcohol use. There are several other variables where the potential risks outweigh any benefits. Of course, some alcohol use is not the only way to reduce the risk of cardiovascular disease. Patients may be aware of a relative who has a history of problem drinking and has other reasons not to imbibe that we may not be aware of. Providers cannot predict which alcohol drinkers could be associated with an increased amount of depression, dependence, or other pathologies if they increase their use. Health or behavioral consequences can come much later than at the beginning of disproportionate or inappropriate use.

Alcohol abuse, as defined in the DSM-IV-TR, is a maladaptive pattern of use with one or more particular criteria occurring over a 1-year period of time (Table 7–1). The criteria are summarized as problems with fulfilling obligations, dangerous use (driving), legal problems, or interpersonal or social problems. Individuals with alcohol abuse can respond successfully to brief interventions in which they are given information about problems associated with excessive drinking and advised to cut down or abstain if such a recommendation is appropriate. If there is not an intervention at this stage, 10% will likely go on to become dependent on alcohol and 50%–60% will continue to experience problems from abuse over the next 5 years (Schuckit 2000). The acronym FRAMES can be used to describe the six key elements of brief intervention as defined by Miller and Sanchez (1994):

- Feedback of personal risks and findings
- Responsibility of the patient
- Advice to change
- Menu of strategies
- Empathetic counseling style
- Self-efficacy or optimism of the patient

In addition to the principles of FRAMES, goal setting and follow-up are important elements of brief intervention.

Alcohol dependence is a chronic disorder that can progress over time and damage emotional, physical, social, occupational, and relational aspects of a patient's life. If it is untreated, the person can have substantial morbidity, and even mortality, from progressive heart, liver, brain, or other organ failure. There is also an elevated risk of suicide, motor vehicle crashes, violence, and other traumatic events. Early identification and treatment is crucial. The DSM-IV-TR criteria for dependence are shown in Table 7–2. Denial is a common distortion among those with alcohol dependence, but it is not part of the diagnostic criteria. Most mental health professionals are familiar with the specific withdrawal and tolerance symptoms, but it should be noted that symptoms of withdrawal—including irritability, emotional lability, insomnia, anxiety, and elevated vital signs—can occur even after a person has abstained from alcohol for days to weeks. These symptoms of the *dry drunk* easily could be mistaken as another illness. Another clinical pearl is that even though it may be easy to identify tolerance as requiring increasing amounts of alcohol to feel the same effect, it may not be as easy to identify the late stages of alcohol dependence. This is when reverse-tolerance occurs, which means the person becomes intoxicated more quickly and with less alcohol. One should not rely on liver function tests as definitive markers of dependence.

Again, brief intervention can be successful if applied early enough, but the skill and competencies necessary by the clinician are often lacking to detect an emerging or frank alcohol use disorder and then appropriately treat it. If the person has become dependent already, he or she needs more comprehensive treatment. If there is any doubt about the diagnosis or treatment, a referral needs to be made to a local expert or treatment facility. The U.S. Preventive Services Task Force recommends screening and behavioral counseling interventions to reduce alcohol misuse by adults, including pregnant women, in primary care settings (Agency for Healthcare Research and Quality 2008b) (see Appendix).

Prevention of Drug Abuse and Dependence

Drug abuse and dependence affect much of the population with varying degrees of severity. Though highly prevalent, these disorders have received less attention and resources for prevention and treatment compared with other psychiatric disorders. Rates of drug use are on the rise again over the last several years, but are not quite as high as the historic rates of cannabis (*Cannabis spp.*, hereafter referred to by its common knickname, *marijuana*) use in the 1970s and cocaine use in the 1980s. Prevention is necessary so that rates of drug use in society do not reach those high rates again. Universal preventive interventions started with school-based programs to target smoking in the 1970s. Research has expanded to programs in a variety of settings, aimed at cigarette, alcohol, and illicit drug use. Bukoski (1991) supports the use of a combination of prevention strategies based on the level of the person's psychosocial development and the extent of her or his drug use. Prevention strategies are designed to focus on the individual, family, peer group, and community. Risk factors, protective factors, developmental factors, social influences, and community-specific factors are integrated in comprehensive prevention programs. Dorfman and Smith (2002) recommended six effective preventive behavioral health interventions out of 54 studies evaluated for use in managed care; these interventions could have a major public health impact.

Adults do not receive as much preventive attention as children and adolescents do, as it has been discovered that adults who abuse drugs typically began use in adolescence. Thus, most prevention efforts are geared toward children and adolescents. Peers have been successfully used to influence, teach, and counsel others and to facilitate delivery of universal prevention programs directed toward youths. Studies have assessed various types of programs such as those designed to improve knowledge only; those designed to enhance general self-esteem or competency; those designed to teach refusal, social, or life skills; those pertaining to both knowledge and self-esteem/competency enhancement; or alternative programs that address social activities. A meta-analysis of 143 drug prevention programs aimed at adolescents (Tobler 1986) showed that even though changes in knowledge or attitudes did not contribute greatly to drug use prevention, the use of peers as facilitators produced positive outcomes for the average student. Special populations, such as minority ethnic groups, adolescents who perform poorly in school, and those already using drugs, require high-intensity strategies (Tobler 1986). Interactive compared to noninteractive programs have been shown to increase knowledge about drug use. The Drug Abuse Resistance Education (DARE) project is the most commonly implemented school-based drug use prevention program. Expert instruction is necessary, along with group discussion and role playing, thus utilizing some interactive measures. The DARE intervention is superior to noninteractive programs in enhancing drug knowledge, changing attitudes about drug use, and improving social skills. However, this intervention does not decrease the use of tobacco, alcohol, and marijuana as effectively as interactive programs involving peer-delivered information (West and O'Neal 2004).

Prevention of drug use is facilitated using basic social learning and persuasive communication, including training in social assertiveness, cognitive-behavioral skills, decision skills, and life skills. Many such programs have helped prevent escalation of drug use in those already using drugs to some extent (Schuster and Kilbey 1998). A comprehensive program developed by Pentz and colleagues (1989) involving mass media, resistance training in schools, parental involvement and education, community organization, and health policies has had high impact and at a reasonable cost. This program guides communities in cost-effective, efficient prevention measures in school-age children, who constitute one of the largest populations at risk for drug abuse. Programs often need modification to target various subpopulations. Frequency of use has been found to be an important variable in predicting whether or not a drug abuse or dependence problem will develop in those who already have used illicit substances (Kandel et al. 1986). Kandel and colleagues (1986) found that a large number of people, especially males, who use illicit drugs 10 or more times are likely to continue use. Therefore, studies must address those already using drugs. Other programs, including those in the workplace such as the PeerCare program, train workers to recognize, intervene, and refer coworkers whom they suspect have a problem (Spicer and Miller 2005).

Of the types of prevention programs mentioned, DARE is the most heavily financed drug prevention program in U.S. schools, but after more than 15 years of evaluations the impact is minimal to none according to some. Although substantial money has gone to drug-related law enforcement and supply reduction programs, they have been studied only minimally. Drug prevention programs within routine clinical practice have also received little empirical study. Perhaps delaying the onset of drug use will reduce the risk of drug dependence, given that it is known that the earlier the onset of drug use, the more likely one is to develop problematic drug use later (Anthony 2007). It is unclear whether early onset drug use is just a marker of increased vulnerability to later drug dependence or whether it is causal in terms of increasing the risk of later drug dependence (Anthony 2007).

Prevention of Substance Abuse in Children and Adolescents

Most adults with SUDs can remember the first time they used substances when they were young. They also commonly report that the problem started during adolescence and wish that it had been prevented at that time. The emergence of substance abuse in the pediatric population is dependent on many different factors in the behavioral, emotional, and environmental arenas. Effective prevention and intervention programs consider the current evidence base and the cultural context, applying social resistance skills training and education in an interactive school-based program. Risk and protective factors must also be considered. The younger a child is when she or he initiates alcohol and other drug use, the higher the risk of serious health consequences and substance abuse in adulthood. Treatment professionals need to have the skills to detect drug-related problems in young patients, as well as in their parents and other family members. Health care providers also need to have knowledge of local trends in drug use, the availability of drugs in the community, and local treatment resources.

Overview of the Problem

SUDs in adolescents are linked to motor vehicle accidents, suicide, violence, sexual risk-taking behavior, poor academic performance, difficulties with social relationships, and even an increased risk of involvement in crimes. As youths get older, their use of tobacco, alcohol, and other drugs increases. Research indicates that at any given time, nearly half of all twelfth graders have consumed alcohol within the last 30 days, and that illicit drugs have been used by 10% of eighth graders and one-quarter of twelfth graders within the prior 30 days. Sedatives and barbiturates are increasing in use among high school students, as is inhalant use by eighth graders, while marijuana use actually decreased between 2001 and 2005. Nearly half of college students use tobacco and alcohol, and 32% have used marijuana in the previous year. Furthermore, one-fifth of college students are high-risk drinkers. It is also estimated that about 11 million adolescents ages 12 and older have tried 3,4-methylenedioxymethamphetamine (MDMA; *ecstasy*) (Johnston et al. 2006).

The series of Monitoring the Future surveys began including eighth through tenth graders in 1991, because of the extension of substance abuse to these young groups. Trends in drug use in the young have shown an increase in the monthly use of marijuana, cocaine, stimulants, sedatives, hallucinogens, and heroin among children in grades 6 through 8 (Johnston et al. 2006). Although the use of illicit drugs has leveled off in the adolescent population, the increase in early use places younger children on a dangerous trajectory for future use. A child who smokes tobacco or drinks alcohol is 65 times more likely to use marijuana than a child who never smokes or drinks. Children who use marijuana are 104 times more likely to use cocaine compared with their counterparts who never used marijuana (National Institute on Drug Abuse 1995).

The new "party drugs" for teenagers are prescription and over-the-counter drugs. One in five teens has abused prescription drugs and a similar proportion has abused prescription pain medicines, such as hydrocodone (Vicodin) and oxycodone (OxyContin). One in 10 has abused prescription stimulants, commonly methylphenidate (Ritalin) or amphetamine and dextroamphetamine mixed salts (Adderall, or "A" on the streets). Additionally, one in 10 teens has abused cough medicine (Partnership for a Drug Free America 2006). Usually such medicines are in the family medicine cabinet. They also can be obtained easily from Internet sites devoted to how to obtain and abuse medicines. Cough or cold medicines containing dextromethorphan found in adolescents' belongings when they haven't had a recent illness may be a sign of abuse. Other usual signs that need to be monitored include falling grades; loss of interest in hobbies and usual activities; changes in friends, physical appearance, hygiene, or general behavior; and disrupted eating or sleeping habits.

Another easily accessible substance is inhalants. They are commonly found in household supplies including items such as glue, shoe polish, spray paints, and correction fluid. Abuse of inhalants is an important public health issue, and prevention is crucial given their toxic and possibly fatal effects (Leonard 2006).

Risk and Protective Factors

The National Institute on Drug Abuse (1999) summarized important risk and protective factors related to substance abuse in youth. Risk factors depend on the developmental phase, and those involving the family are probably the most important, including:

- Chaotic home environments, particularly in which parents abuse substances or suffer from mental illnesses
- Ineffective parenting, especially with children with difficult temperaments and conduct disorders
- Lack of mutual attachments and nurturing

Other risk factors that are important to the developing child but involve the community, school, and peers are:

- Inappropriately shy or aggressive behavior in the classroom
- Failure in school performance
- Poor social coping skills
- Affiliations with deviant peers

- Perceptions of approval of drug-using behaviors in school, peers, and the community
- The availability of drugs, trafficking patterns, and beliefs that drug use is generally tolerated

Vulnerable periods for the young include times of transition. Growing from one developmental stage to the next, changing from one grade to the next, experiencing difficult life events, moving to a new home or school, and experiencing parental discord or divorce elevate risk. Leaving the security of the family and beginning school is the first major transition. Developing a wider base of peers as when changing schools, or going from elementary to middle or middle to high school, can be intense transitions. In high school, preparing for the future can be stressful. Going off to college, getting married, or entering the workforce causes young adults to face increased risks as well.

Most youths who use drugs begin to do so at about age 12 or 13. Young teens often move from the use of alcohol, cigarettes, and inhalants to the use of generally illegal substances, marijuana usually being the first. Social attitudes, norms, and availability contribute to this common progression. Although drinking and smoking experimentally at a young age are not necessarily the cause of drug use later in life, sequencing data show that for a youth who has smoked tobacco or drunk alcohol, the risk of moving on to marijuana use is *65 times higher* than for a youth who has never done so (National Institute on Drug Abuse 1995). For someone who has smoked marijuana, the risk of progressing to cocaine is *104 times higher* compared with someone who has never smoked marijuana. Factors that contribute to these alarming data could involve biological, social, behavioral, or peer-association factors.

Cigarette use is still considered the gateway to alcohol and drug use disorders in the young. A key indicator for SUD risk is the use of cigarettes before the age of 18 years. ADHD is also a risk factor for smoking. The earlier the onset of smoking and the greater the frequency, the higher the chance of advancement from tobacco to other substances (Riala et al. 2004). Therefore the importance of curbing early use of tobacco is paramount.

Risk factors related to drug use during the teenage years also include poor self-image, a low level of religiosity, poor school performance, parental rejection, family dysfunction, abuse, undercontrolling or overcontrolling by parents, and divorce (Belcher and Shinitzky 1998). Externalizing disorders (conduct disorder, oppositional defiant disorder, and ADHD) are associated with substance abuse (McMahon 1994) if not treated early and appropriately. Temperamental difficulties can affect attachment with caregivers and lead to coercive parenting that is associated with later substance abuse and delinquency (McMahon 1994). Hyperactivity in a child also is a risk factor for SUDs (Kramer and Loney 1982). ADHD is an independent risk factor for the development of SUDs, with a threefold higher risk of SUDs (and, among those who do develop an SUD, earlier onset) than in children without ADHD (Katusic et al. 2003). Alcohol abuse begins earlier and lasts into adulthood 20 years longer in those with ADHD than in those without ADHD. Children treated for ADHD are less likely to initiate drug and alcohol use in adolescence (Greenfield et al. 1988) compared with those who remain untreated. Aggressive behaviors (Brook et al. 1996) and high levels of novelty-seeking and low levels of harm-avoidance behaviors in boys (Masse and Tremblay 1997) also put them at risk for developing an SUD.

Peer pressure is a factor not only in drug use but also in drug abstinence. Peer pressure studies find that adolescents believe that their peers' general attitude is against drug use (Robin and Johnson 1996). With the exception of alcohol, the lower the perceived acceptance rate, the higher the perceived risk of drugs, and the less frequent the drug use (Johnston 2005). Poor coping mechanisms in adverse situations and a lack of self-control during early childhood are associated with a greater risk of both marijuana use and the use of harder drugs in adolescence. The association of substance abuse with childhood antisocial behavior is well established (Stanford 2001). Child abuse is also a significant risk factor for a later SUD (Bennett and Kemper 1994). Significantly more alcohol, tobacco, and marijuana use was found in eighth graders who took care of themselves after school, especially in those with a longer duration of self-care (Richardson et al. 1989).

The role of peer groups in shaping the behavior of adolescents is central. As an adolescent begins engaging in substance use, he or she becomes drawn into a culture that often engages in other risk-taking behaviors. The adolescent can then become involved in illegal acts and end up entangled in the criminal justice system. Risky sexual behaviors may lead to an increased risk of exposure to HIV, hepatitis, and other sexually transmitted diseases. In 2005, the Centers for Disease Control and Prevention estimated that about one-half of the new cases of HIV occur in youths less than 25 years old. Early exposure to stress and/or trauma is a known risk factor for substance abuse and other mental health disorders, so any preventive interventions must utilize resources for youths who experience high stress and trauma.

Protective factors are characteristics within the individual, the family, and the environment that help one to resist using alcohol or other substances. Protective factors include growing up in a nurturing home with open communication between children and parents and positive parental support (Climent et al. 1990). Having committed teachers, positive self-esteem, a positive self-concept, self-control, assertiveness, social competence, and a high level of academic achievement all promote resilience (Belcher and Shinitzky 1998). Regular church attendance is also protective (Hawkins et al. 1992). Adolescent resiliency is also associated with high intelligence, low levels of novelty-seeking behaviors, and avoidance of friendships with delinquent peers (Fergusson and Lynskey 1996).

Important protective factors, which are not always the opposites of risk factors, include the following (National Institute on Drug Abuse 1999):

- Strong bonds with one's family
- Experience of parental monitoring with clear rules of conduct within the family unit and a high level of involvement of parents in their children's lives
- Success in school performance
- Strong bonds with prosocial institutions such as school and religious organizations
- Adoption of conventional norms about drug use

Understanding the risk factors and the protective factors that influence substance abuse is crucial for the early identification and prevention of SUDs in youth. Keeping these in mind during each evaluation of a child or adolescent, and her or his family members, will direct more suitable and comprehensive care and treatment in the long term.

Local leaders could promote the tailoring of prevention efforts by assessing the risk in their particular area. Drug use epidemiologists have suggested using household and school surveys and collecting data from health departments, hospitals, drug abuse treatment facilities, law enforcement agencies, and school systems. Ethnographic studies assess behaviors of use in natural settings to document the perspectives of the people under observation. Focus groups can be convened to represent subpopulations of persons who use substances, to investigate use in the general community population. Multiple strategies are needed because each has advantages and disadvantages. Taken together, a community can make informed decisions about the most appropriate type of prevention programs and policies for their area.

Preventive Interventions

The primary targets for preventive interventions must take into consideration risk and protective factors within each domain of functioning:

1. *Family relationships.* Effective programs need to help parents learn skills for better family communication and discipline, including firm and consistent enforcement of family rules. Parents need to be active in their children's lives by discussing drug use with them, monitoring their activities closely, getting to know their children's friends and their families, and understanding any problems that arise and their children's personal concerns.

2. *Peer relationships.* Important skills to teach the young include social competency skills, improved communication skills, enhancement of positive peer relationships and social behaviors, and resistance skills to refuse drug-pushing efforts by others.

3. *The social and school environment.* A child's sense of identity and achievement is necessary to enhance academic performance and strengthen his or her bond to school, which can reduce the likelihood of dropping out of school. Schools should foster curricula that support positive peer relationships and teach the norm that most people do not use drugs (see subsection "Examples of Preventive Interventions" below). The avoidance of initiating drug use is achieved by children understanding the negative aspects of drug use and perceiving social disapproval of drug use from their friends and families. The importance of educating the young about the negative impact of drug use in their lives is paramount. Success in school behavior and academics helps to strengthen prosocial bonds.

4. *The community environment.* Programs for prevention in the community often involve civic, religious, law enforcement, and governmental organizations. These groups must promote antidrug norms and prosocial behav-

ior through changes in policy and regulations, mass media efforts, and far-reaching awareness programs. Laws and enforcement, advertising restrictions, and drug-free school zones all can be designed to provide a cleaner, safer, drug-free environment.

The most promising prevention measures focus on psychosocial etiological issues. Issues of particular importance include parental, peer, media, and other pressures, and the teaching of coping mechanisms to deal with those pressures. Special considerations for adolescents (Powers 1998) are:

- Assessing and treating predisposing psychiatric disorders
- Providing proper education regarding knowledge and attitudes about substances of abuse
- Encouraging the development of proper social and problem-solving skills
- Treating problems in family functioning
- Increasing opportunities for activities with prosocial peers and in the community
- Limiting early access to the use of gateway drugs such as nicotine and alcohol

Examples of preventive interventions.   Project STAR (Students Taught Awareness and Resistance) is a universal drug abuse prevention program that reaches the entire community with a comprehensive school program, mass media efforts, a parental program, community organization, and a component aimed at changing local health policy. Research has shown positive long-term results based on student assessments when starting the program in junior high and then in high school. Significantly less use of marijuana (30% less), tobacco (~25% less), and alcohol (~20% less) was found in those who participated compared with those who did not. The most influential factor was the perception of friends' intolerance of drug use (Pentz 1995).

The Strengthening Families Program is a selective, multicomponent, family-focused preventive intervention for the 6- to 10-year-old children of parents who abuse substances. The parents are taught to strengthen their parenting skills and reduce their children's risk factors. In addition to parental training, children's skills training and family skills training are components of the intervention. The program has also been modified and found effective in several different cultures, in various settings and in different racial and ethnic groups. Overall results indicate reductions in family conflict, improvements in family communication and organization, and reductions in youth conduct disorder, aggressiveness, and substance abuse (Kumpfer et al. 1996).

The Reconnecting Youth program is a school-based, indicated prevention program that targets adolescents in grades 9–12 who show signs of poor school achievement and potential for dropping out of school. They may also have other behavioral problems such as substance abuse, depression, and suicidal ideation. Skills to build resiliency with regard to risk factors and moderating early signs of drug use are taught. Adolescents enter the program if they have fewer credits than recommended for their age, have high absenteeism, or have grades that drop significantly over time. If they already have dropped out or show a substantial risk of dropping out, they may also enter the program. Social support and life skills training incorporating personal growth classes, social activities, and school bonding, as well as school system crisis response, are components of the intervention. Improvements have been seen in program participants in terms of better school performance, less involvement with drugs, and less deviant peer bonding. Increases in self-esteem, personal control, school bonding, and social support have been demonstrated. Researchers also reported less aggression, anger, depression, hopelessness, stress, and suicidal behavior among program participants (Eggert et al. 1994).

The Seattle Social Development Project is a school-based, universal preventive intervention for students in grades 1–6 that seeks to diminish shared childhood risks for delinquency and drug abuse by enhancing protective factors. Elementary school teachers are taught to use active classroom management, interactive teaching strategies, and cooperative learning techniques. Parents are also involved in the curriculum. Prosocial involvement in school and home is promoted by enhancing opportunities, skills, and rewards for the youths in the program. The researchers found an increased bond to school and family and a commitment to the norm of not using drugs. Some of the results found were: reductions in antisocial behavior, improved academic skills, greater commitment to school, reduced levels of alienation and better bonding to prosocial others, less misbehavior in school, and fewer incidents of drug use in school (Hawkins et al. 1992).

Most prevention studies have been conducted with predominantly white, middle-class youths. Botvin and colleagues (2001) also showed significant protective effects using a school-based prevention program with binge-drinking, minority, inner-city youths. This 3-year prevention curriculum for middle school students covered three major areas: drug resistance skills and information, self-management skills, and general social skills. The program utilized the cognitive-behavioral approach called *Life Skills Training.* Some evaluations have shown it to be effective with implementation under different scheduling formats and with different levels of project staff involvement (Botvin 2001). Studies have also shown its effectiveness whether the program providers were adults or peer leaders. More research needs to involve teens from all socioeconomic classes, cultural backgrounds, and ethnicities (Botvin 2001).

The Adolescent Training and Learning to Avoid Steroids (ATLAS) and Athletes Targeting Healthy Exercise and Nutrition Alternatives (ATHENA) programs have revealed that sports teams are useful vehicles for delivering gender-specific, peer-led curricula that promote a healthy lifestyle. Results demonstrate a reduction in steroid and other drug use among high school athletes after participation in these programs (Elliot et al. 2004). The ATLAS program is a universal program for male high school athletes that promotes healthy sports nutrition and strength-training alternatives to steroids and reduces known risk factors for substance abuse. Scripted materials are used by coach and peer facilitators of small learning groups. Classroom sessions, physical training periods, role playing, student-created campaigns, instructional aids, exercise guides, easy-to-follow workbooks, and educational games are some of the techniques used. Learning about steroids and other drugs, resistance training, ethics, drug use norms, vulnerability to drug use, media images, intolerance of use by the team, goal setting regarding weight, nutrition, and exercise are components of the educational portion. Safe training practices at school decrease the use of commercial gyms, where drugs are more available. Parent participation is also part of the program. Students have reported a greater understanding of the negative effects of drugs and steroids, personal vulnerability to the use of drugs, and intolerance of use by coaches and parents. They had improved drug refusal skills, less belief in steroid-promoting mass media images, more confidence in their abilities to build muscle strength and mass without the use of drugs, greater self-esteem, and less desire to use drugs. Even 1 year after the intervention, the youths involved in the study were still resisting the temptation to use anabolic steroids and maintained better nutrition and exercise habits compared with those who were not in the study. Booster sessions were provided each subsequent year of high school (Goldberg et al. 1996).

Pediatric visits should include assessments of substance use from birth to 21 years. In utero exposure to tobacco affects about 11% of newborns, and 10%–13% of newborns have been exposed to alcohol. About 40,000 babies are born each year with fetal alcohol syndrome and many more with fetal alcohol effects. Screenings must include parents' and other family members' use of substances because parental behavior and heritability of SUDs affect risk in the children. Besides the direct risk to the child of parents with SUDs, at least one-third of confirmed child abuse cases involve a parent with an SUD (Johnston et al. 2006). Attitudes about drugs and alcohol are formed in middle childhood, so clinicians should begin counseling by this age. Clinically important problems associated with drug or alcohol use can occur without a DSM-IV-TR diagnosis, especially around the time of separation and individuation in middle to late adolescence as other high-risk behaviors may emerge.

Research in the area of effective treatment of substance abuse and dependence has led to most of the efforts in research of prevention. Unfortunately, most of these products of research are not necessarily effective for prevention, so we need to focus on what is useful and effective and also accepted and practically useful in the community. The blend of research and practice shows that there is a close inverse correlation between the longitudinal trends of substance abuse and the perceived risk of harm; therefore, as the perception of the harmfulness drops, the use of addicting substances rises. Moreover, there are noticeable socioeconomic and cultural factors that can partially compromise or enhance a person's resistance to use and misuse. Keeping in mind the importance of reliable research to substantiate prevention efforts, vulnerabilities for addiction are complicated in nature, comorbidities influence the vulnerabilities, and the long-lasting neurobehavioral impact of the drugs of abuse on the brain all should help shape any prevention attempts.

Relapse Prevention

Relapse, a return to the use of alcohol or drugs after a period of abstinence, is a serious problem for patients who temporarily recover from SUDs. Even with effective initial treatment of addiction, only 20%–50% of patients remain abstinent during their first year of recovery (Hunt et al. 1971). High-quality specialty aftercare decreases the rate of relapse. Continued screening must persist for each patient, to determine whether treatment is warranted again. A supportive and nonjudgmental therapeutic relationship is necessary. Awareness of the recovering patient's ongoing struggle, constant monitoring of the patient's progress, providing all-inclusive continuity of care, reinforcing positive behavioral change and maintenance, working with families, and rapid intervention for the first signs of relapse are crucial. Other ways that a physician can help prevent relapse (Friedmann et al. 1998) are:

- Have regular follow-up appointments
- Encourage family support
- Facilitate involvement in 12-step recovery groups
- Assist with recognition and coping strategies concerning relapse precipitants and craving
- Assist with a plan to manage early relapse
- Facilitate positive lifestyle changes
- Manage depression, anxiety, and other comorbid conditions
- Consider adjunctive pharmacotherapy
- Collaborate with addiction specialists

Marijuana abuse/dependence relapse prevention may need to be specialized to be successful, because the traditional 12-step approaches appear not to be as effective as they are for other types of abuse or dependence. Stephens and colleagues (1994) hypothesized that a learning-based conceptualization of excessive use and treatment may be more useful. This stems from the idea that relapse is a failure of behavioral and cognitive coping skills rather than a physiologically based loss of control over that particular substance. Lifestyle balance is also promoted. As compared with the traditional social support model, this relapse prevention approach displayed few significant differences in outcome. Both groups lead to large reductions in the amount of marijuana use and related problems (Stephens et al. 1994).

The reduction of drug craving and the prevention of relapse into compulsive drug taking can be aided with some medications, when used in combination with psychotherapy and other psychosocial treatments. Such medicines include methadone, buprenorphine, clonidine, and naltrexone for opioid dependence; and naltrexone, acamprosate, and disulfiram for alcohol dependence. Rimonabant, a cannabinoid receptor antagonist, had been advancing through the U.S. Food and Drug Administration (FDA) approval process but its application was withdrawn due to adverse side effects (Johansson et al. 2009); however, ondansetron still holds potential for use treating alcohol addiction. Five medications with FDA approval for other purposes may help in treating cocaine dependence, including disulfiram, topiramate, modafinil, propranolol, and baclofen (O'Brien 2005). Further research on these and other promising agents is needed.

Integrated Substance Abuse and Mental Health Treatment

Comorbidities between SUDs and mental illnesses are highly prevalent. Substance abuse in patients with chronic mental illnesses negatively affects treatment. Unfortunately, clinicians have few successful models for treating individuals with dual diagnoses. Such patients are also at greater risk for suicide, homicide, destructiveness, and irresponsibility compared with psychiatric patients without a comorbid SUD.

The integration of therapeutic approaches used in the field of SUD treatment with those traditionally used in psychiatric care, such as self-help models (12-step programs) and the token economy program, has been found to be useful (Franco et al. 1995). In a study that compared integrating mental health care, substance abuse treatment, and housing interventions versus standard treatment for homeless individuals with dual diagnoses, the interventions led to fewer days spent in an institution, more days in stable housing, and more successful recovery from SUDs, including greater improvement in alcohol use disorders (Drake et al. 1997). Specialized hospital dual-diagnosis treatment programs (day programs) can improve treatment adherence, hospital utilization, and drug abstinence. These programs are based on the little research that is available on existing successful programs, and on observations that traditional cognitive-behavioral and 12-step approaches are less successful in the dual-diagnosis population. Specialized programs must be instituted for these patients (Ho et al. 1999). Mobile and continuous community treatment programs for urban homeless adults with serious mental illnesses and SUDs improve long-term outcomes if integrated into an ongoing service package that includes assertive outreach, intensive case management, individual and group counseling, mutual self-help, and social control (Meisler et al. 1997).

Evaluation of Prevention Efforts Is a Difficult Task

The task of assessing current prevention efforts is daunting given the growing problems of drug use, changing patterns of use over time, shrinking resources for research, prevention and treatment, and limited expertise in many settings. The National Institutes of Health devised a comprehensive checklist to determine whether specific programs include research-based prevention principles in the domains of community, school, and family (National Institute on Drug Abuse 1999). Community coalitions should instigate community-wide meetings, public education campaigns, and the attraction of sponsors for comprehensive prevention strategies. Any plan should involve the assessment of a community's specific needs, the identification of a community's risk and protective factors, the resources identified to sustain future planning, and the designation of key stakeholders. Sometimes adapting a preexisting program is most economical, and benefits may be derived from enhancing law enforcement, policies, school programs, and interventions already in place.

Shaping interventions that have been shown to be effective through research (e.g., Life Skills Training, the Strengthening Families Program, and Project STAR) to fit into individual communities to address differences while maintaining the programs' original effectiveness is a challenge, but an important goal. When evaluating current programs, problems can arise in study designs, so findings may not show a clear relationship between the program and outcomes. Other factors may complicate evaluations in each community, such as unique community events or the maturation of target groups. Always important in the evaluations are:

- Using tested data collection instruments
- Obtaining reliable baseline information
- Using control or comparison groups

- Monitoring the quality of program implementation, making sure that postimplementation follow-up includes a large percentage of the target population that was part of the program, and using appropriate analytical techniques

Conclusion

The emotional and physical costs associated with SUDs are immense for everyone involved. However, the economic burden of these disorders has forced managed care organizations to look closely at prevention programs. It has been estimated that almost 90% of privately insured persons in the United States are enrolled in managed care plans; therefore, a large number of people could benefit from prevention efforts. It is difficult to quantify the extensive costs and pain borne by individuals with SUDs and their families, as well as loss of productivity at work and home. Prevention potentially could reduce the toll of mental disorders and SUDs to a large extent. In its assessment of preventive mental health and substance abuse programs and services in managed care, the Substance Abuse and Mental Health Services Administration concluded that "prevention programs have been shown to increase the latency of first alcohol, tobacco, or drug use; to reduce alcohol, tobacco, and drug use; and to decrease risk factors related to late alcohol, tobacco, and drug use" (Dorfman and Smith 2002).

Prevention of SUDs can help alleviate or decrease much pain and suffering in psychiatric patients. Whether the SUD is part of the etiology for a mental illness, or vice versa, comorbidity is highly prevalent. Psychiatrists and other mental health professionals see patients who are affected directly or indirectly by substance use every day. When evaluating individual patients, the effects of the SUD on family members must be considered. Continuous evaluation of patients for any new occurrence of an SUD is necessary. Alcohol and drug abuse prevention perhaps has taken a back seat to the treatment of these disorders in routine psychiatric care settings. More research is needed to find the most effective, time- and cost-efficient, and practical prevention techniques for mental health professionals to use.

SUDs develop over time and in the context of each individual and her or his environment, so in addition to individual-level efforts, prevention techniques could range from environmental controls to limiting supply to education. Combined approaches are best because the problem is complex and there is no single solution. Interpretation of risk and protective factors is necessary to help with any prevention effort, but caution must be taken not to assume causal links without examining the full range of available information. Skinner (1987) has summarized why early detection and effective intervention strategies deserve focused emphasis:

- Most heavy drinkers do not seek treatment for their problem; rather, others usually bring them to treatment because of the consequences of misuse.
- Socially stable persons at early stages of problem drinking have a better prognosis with treatment than at later stages.
- Health care professionals in practice are in excellent positions to identify problem drinkers and those using illicit drugs.
- Brief interventions by health care professionals can be effective in reducing heavy alcohol or drug use.

Unfortunately, there is widespread pessimism among health care professionals about the ability to intervene effectively. There also exists confusion about who has responsibility and about the best manner of nonjudgmental confrontation. Many providers lack knowledge about the first step toward early detection and treatment. Being prevention-minded will help psychiatrists and other mental health professionals incorporate efforts to institute ongoing prevention techniques in practice.

Key Points

- SUDs (substance use disorders) are highly prevalent conditions that are associated with diverse complications, consequences, and disabilities. Prevention of SUDs benefits individuals, families, and the community.
- Alcohol abuse is more common than any other SUD. The consequences of alcohol abuse and dependence can be all-encompassing and insidious. However, research suggests that low to moderate alcohol intake may decrease cardiovascular disease

risk, which may lead to a reduction in all-cause mortality. Psychiatrists and other health professionals must weigh the potential protective effects of alcohol use in moderation alongside the risks of alcohol abuse and dependence.

- Risk factors associated with problematic alcohol drinking include genetics and a family history of alcohol use disorders, as well as social/environmental factors and psychological factors. Protective factors should also be considered.

- The use of illicit substances is nearly always problematic and can affect all areas of a person's functioning.

- Universal, selective, and indicated preventive interventions have been designed and studied for alcohol use disorders and SUDs.

- Among people with SUDs, substance use typically began during adolescence. For this reason, prevention efforts are commonly focused on the adolescent population. Preventive interventions should take into account risk and protective factors within several domains of functioning, including family relationships, peer relationships, the social and school environment, and the community.

- In the mental health setting, clinicians should focus on relapse prevention in patients with a history of an SUD that is in remission. For patients with comorbidities involving serious mental illnesses and SUDs, integrated substance abuse and mental health treatment should be provided.

References

Adams WL, Barry KL, Fleming MF: Screening for problem drinking in older primary care patients. JAMA 276:1964–1967, 1996

Agency for Healthcare Research and Quality: Fetal alcohol syndrome. Guidelines for referral and diagnosis. 2008a. Available at: http://www.guideline.gov/summary/summary.aspx?doc_id=5960. Accessed March 14, 2008.

Agency for Healthcare Research and Quality: Screening and behavioral counseling interventions in primary care to reduce alcohol misuse. 2008b. Available at: http://www.ahrq.gov/clinic/uspstf/uspsdrin.htm. Accessed March 14, 2008.

Agency for Healthcare Research and Quality: Tobacco, alcohol, and other drugs: the role of the pediatrician in prevention, identification, and management of substance abuse. 2008c. Available at: http://www.guidelines.gov/summary/summary.aspx?doc_ id=6631. Accessed March 14, 2008.

Allen JP, Litten RZ, Anton RF, et al: Carbohydrate-deficient transferring as a measure of immoderate drinking: remaining issues. Alcohol Clin Exp Res 8:799–808, 1994

American Psychiatric Association: Diagnostic and Statistical Manual of Mental Disorders, 4th Edition, Text Revision. Washington, DC, American Psychiatric Association, 2000

Anthony JC: Five facts about preventing drug dependence, in Recognition and Prevention of Major Mental and Substance Use Disorders. Edited by Tsuang M, Stone W, Lyons M. Washington, DC, American Psychiatric Publishing, 2007, pp 329–346

Babor TF, Biddle-Higgins JC, Saunders JB, et al: AUDIT: The Alcohol Use Disorders Identification Test. Guidelines for Use in Primary Care (WHO Publ No WHO/MSD/MSB/01.6a). Geneva, Switzerland, World Health Organization, 1992

Belcher HME, Shinitzky HE: Substance abuse in children: prediction, protection, and prevention. Arch Pediatr Adolesc Med 152:952–960, 1998

Bennett EM, Kemper KJ: Is abuse during childhood a risk factor for developing substance abuse problems as an adult? J Dev Behav Pediatr 15:426–429, 1994

Botvin GJ, Griffin KW, Diaz T, et al: Preventing binge drinking during early adolescence: one- and two-year follow-up of a school-based preventive intervention. Psychol Addict Behav 15:360–365, 2001

Brook JS, Whiteman M, Finch SJ, et al: Young adult drug use and delinquency: childhood antecedents and adolescent mediators. J Am Acad Child Adolesc Psychiatry 35:1584–1592, 1996

Bukoski WJ: A definition of drug abuse prevention research, in Persuasive Communication and Drug Abuse Prevention. Edited by Donohew L, Sipher HE, Bukoski WJ. Hillsdale, NJ, Erlbaum, 1991, pp 3–19

Climent CE, de Aragon LV, Plutchik R: Prediction of risk for drug use in high school students. Int J Addict 25:545–556, 1990

Cook BL, Abreu JA: Alcohol-related health problems, in Maxcy-Rosenau-Last Public Health and Preventive Medicine, 14th Edition. Edited by Wallace RB. Stamford, CT, Appleton & Lange, 1998, pp 847–860

Cook PJ: The effect of liquor taxes on drinking, cirrhosis and auto accidents, in Alcohol and Public Policy: Beyond the Shadow of Prohibition. Edited by Moore MH, Gerstein DR. Washington, DC, National Academy Press, 1981

Dorfman SL, Smith SA: Preventive mental health and substance abuse programs and services in managed care. J Behav Health Serv Res 29:233–258, 2002

Drake RE, Yovetich NA, Bebout RR, et al: Integrated treatment for dually diagnosed homeless adults. J Nerv Ment Dis 185:298–305, 1997

Eggert LL, Thompson EA, Herting JR, et al: Preventing adolescent drug abuse and high school dropout through an intensive school-based social network development program. Am J Health Promot 8:202–215, 1994

Elliot DL, Goldberg L, Moe EL, et al: Preventing substance use and disordered eating: initial outcomes of the ATHENA (Athletes Targeting Healthy Exercise and Nutrition Alternatives) program. Arch Pediatr Adolesc Med 158:1043–1049, 2004

Fergusson DM, Lynskey MT: Adolescent resiliency to family adversity. J Child Psychol Psychiatry 7:281–292, 1996

Franco H, Galanter M, Castaneda R, et al: Combining behavioral and self-help approaches in the inpatient management of dually diagnosed patients. J Subst Abuse Treat 12:227–232, 1995

Friedmann PD, Saitz R, Samet JH: Management of adults recovering from alcohol or other drug problems: relapse prevention in primary care. JAMA 297:1227–1231, 1998

Fromme K, Corbin W: Prevention of heavy drinking and associated negative consequences among mandated and voluntary college students. J Consult Clin Psychol 2:1038–1049, 2004

Goldberg L, Elliot D, Clarke GN, et al: Effects of a multi-dimensional anabolic steroid prevention intervention: the A.T.L.A.S. (Adolescents Training and Learning to Avoid Steroids) program. JAMA 276:1555–1562, 1996

Goodwin DW, Schulsinger F, Moller N, et al: Drinking problems in adopted and nonadopted sons of alcoholics. Arch Gen Psychiatry 31:164–169, 1974

Grant KA: Emerging neurochemical concepts in the action of ethanol at ligand-gated ion channels. Behav Pharmacol 5:383–404, 1994

Greenfield B, Hechtman L, Weiss G: Two subgroups of hyperactives as adults: correlation of outcome. Can J Psychiatry 33:505–508, 1988

Harrell AV, Wirtz PW: Screening for adolescent problem drinking: validation of a multidimensional instrument for case identification. Psychol Assess 1:61–63, 1989

Harwood HJ: Updating estimates of the economic costs of alcohol abuse in the United States: estimates, update methods and data (NIH Publ No 98-4327). Rockville, MD, National Institutes of Health, 1998

Harwood HJ: Updating estimates of the economic costs of alcohol abuse in the United States: estimates, update methods and data. Report prepared by the Lewin Group for the National Institute on Alcohol Abuse and Alcoholism, 2000

Harwood HJ: The economic cost of drug abuse in the United States: 1992–2002 (Publ No 207303). Washington, DC, Executive Office of the President, Office of National Drug Control Policy, 2004

Hawkins JD, Catalano RF, Miller JY: Risk and protective factors for alcohol and other drug problems in adolescence and early adulthood: implications for substance abuse prevention. Psychol Bull 112:64–105, 1992

Heirich M, Sieck CJ: Worksite cardiovascular wellness programs as a route to substance abuse prevention. J Occup Environ Med 42:47–65, 2000

Hine LM, Stampfer MJ, Ma J, et al: Genetic variation in alcohol dehydrogenase and the beneficial effect of moderate alcohol consumption on myocardial infarction. N Engl J Med 244:549–555, 2001

Ho AP, Tsuang JW, Liberman RP, et al: Achieving effective treatment of patients with chronic psychotic illness and comorbid substance dependence. Am J Psychiatry 156:1765–1770, 1999

Holder HD: Community prevention of alcohol problems. Addict Behav 25:843–859, 2000

Hunt WA, Barnett W, Branch LG: Relapse rates in addiction programs. J Clin Psychol 27:455–456, 1971

Johansson K, Neovius K, Desantis SM, et al: Discontinuation due to adverse events in randomized trials of orlistat, sibutramine and rimonabant: a meta-analysis. Obes Rev May 12, 2009 (Epub ahead of print)

Johnston LD: Monitoring the Future Study (press release): National Results on Adolescent Drug Use: Overview of Key Findings 2004. National Institute on Drug Abuse, 2005. Ann Arbor, MI, NewsInfo, 2005

Johnston LD, O'Malley PM, Bachman JG, et al: Monitoring the Future: national results on adolescent drug use: overview of key findings 2005 (NIH Publ No 06-5882). Bethesda, MD: National Institute on Drug Abuse, 2006. Available at: http://monitoringthefuture.org/pubs/monographs/overview2005.pdf. Accessed December 15, 2008.

Kandel DB, Simcha-Fagan O, Davies M: Risk factors for delinquency and illicit drug use from adolescence to adulthood. J Drug Issues 16:67–90, 1986

Katusic S, Barbaresi W, Colligan R: Substance abuse among ADHD cases: a population-based birth cohort study. Presentation at the annual meeting of the Pediatric Academic Societies, May 2003, Seattle, WA

Knight JR, Wechsler H, Kuo M, et al: Alcohol abuse and dependence among U.S. college students. J Stud Alcohol 63:263–270, 2002

Kramer J, Loney J: Childhood hyperactivity and substance abuse: a review of the literature, in Advances in Learning and Behavioral Disabilities, Vol 1. Edited by Gadow KD, Bialer I. Greenwich, CT, JAI Press, 1982

Krystal JH, Tabakoff B: Ethanol abuse, dependence, and withdrawal: neurobiology and clinical implications, in Neuropsychopharmacology: The Fifth Generation of Progress. Edited by Davis KL, Charney D, Coyle JT, et al. Philadelphia, PA, Lippincott Williams & Wilkins, 2002

Kumpfer KL, Molraard V, Spoth R: The "Strengthening Families Program" for the prevention of delinquency and drug use, in Preventing Childhood Disorders, Substance Abuse, and Delinquency. Edited by Peters R, McMahon R. Thousand Oaks, CA, Sage, 1996

Leonard HL (ed): Treating inhalant abuse: prevention is key, in Brown University Child and Adolescent Psychopharmacology Update. Hoboken, NJ, Wiley, 2006

Masse LC, Tremblay RE: Behavior of boys in kindergarten and the onset of substance use during adolescence. Arch Gen Psychiatry 54:62–68, 1997

Mayfield D, McLeod G, Hall P: The CAGE questionnaire: validation of a new alcoholism screening instrument. Am J Psychiatry 131:1121–1123, 1974

McMahon RL: Diagnosis, assessment and treatment of externalizing problems in children: the role of longitudinal data. J Consult Clin Psychol 62:901–917, 1994

Meisler N, Blankertz L, Santos AB, et al: Impact of assertive community treatment on homeless persons with co-occurring severe psychiatric and substance use disorders. Community Ment Health J 33:113–122, 1997

Michigan Quality Improvement Consortium: Michigan Quality Improvement Consortium Web site. Available at: http://www.mqic.org/guid.htm. Accessed December 8, 2008.

Miller WR, Sanchez VC: Motivating young adults for treatment and lifestyle change, in Alcohol Use and Misuse by Young Adults. Edited by Howard G, Nathan P. Notre Dame, IN, University of Notre Dame Press, 1994

Moser J: Prevention of Alcohol-related Problems: An International Review of Preventive Measures, Policies, and Programmes. Toronto, ON, Canada, Alcoholism and Drug Addiction Research Foundation (published on behalf of the World Health Organization), 1980

National Institute on Alcohol Abuse and Alcoholism: The Physicians' Guide to Helping Patients With Alcohol Problems (NIH Publ No 95-3769). Bethesda, MD, U.S. Department of Health and Human Services, 1995

National Institute on Drug Abuse: Drug use among racial/ethnic minorities (NIH Publ No 95-3888). Rockville, MD, National Institute of Drug Abuse, 1995

National Institute on Drug Abuse: Preventing drug use among children and adolescents: a research-based guide (NIH Publication No. 04-4212B). Rockville, MD, National Institute of Drug Abuse, 1999

O'Brien CP: Anticraving medications for relapse prevention: a possible new class of psychoactive medications. Am J Psychiatry 162:1423–1431, 2005

Partnership for a Drug-Free America and Consumer Healthcare Products Association: Preventing Teen Cough Medicine Abuse: A Parent's Guide. 2006. Available at: http://www.drugfree.org/Files/Preventing_Teen_Cough_Medicine_Abuse/. Accessed December 16, 2008.

Pentz MA: The school-community interface in comprehensive school health education, in 1996 Institute of Medicine Annual Report, Committee on Comprehensive School Health Programs. Edited by Stansfield S. Washington, DC, National Academy Press, 1995

Pentz MA, Dwyer JH, MacKinnon DP, et al: A multicommunity trial for primary prevention of adolescent drug use: effects on drug use prevalence. JAMA 261:3259–3266, 1989

Pokorny AD, Miller BA, Kaplan HB: The brief MAST: a shortened version of the Michigan Alcoholism Screening Test. Am J Psychiatry 129:342–345, 1972

Popham RE, Schmidt W, de Lint J: The effects of legal restraint on drinking, in The Biology of Alcoholism, Vol 4: Social Aspects of Alcoholism. Edited by Kissin B, Begleiter H. New York, Plenum, 1976, pp 579–625

Powers RA: Substance abuse, in Clinical Child Psychiatry. Edited by Klykylo WM, Kay J, Rube D. Philadelphia, PA, WB Saunders, 1998, pp 234, 235, 261

Resnick MD, Bearman PS, Blum RW, et al: Protecting adolescents from harm: findings from the National Longitudinal Study on Adolescent Health. JAMA 278:823–832, 1997

Riala K, Hakko H, Isohanni M, et al: Teenage smoking and substance use as predictors of severe alcohol problems in late adolescence and in young adulthood. J Adolesc Health 35:245–254, 2004

Richardson JL, Dwyer K, McGuigan K: Substance use among eighth-grade students who take care of themselves after school. Pediatrics 84:556–566, 1989

Robin SS, Johnson EO: Attitude and peer cross pressure: adolescent drug and alcohol use. J Drug Educ 26:69–99, 1996

Russell M, Martier SS, Sokol RJ, et al: Screening for pregnancy risk-drinking. Alcohol Clin Exp Res 18:1156–1161, 2006

Ryan BE, Segars L: Mini-marts and maxi-problems: the relationship between purchase and consumption levels. Alcohol Health Res World 12:26–29, 1987

Schuck AM, Widom CS: Childhood victimization and alcohol symptoms in females: causal inferences and hypothesized mediators. Child Abuse Negl 25:1069–1092, 2001

Schuckit MA: Drug and Alcohol Abuse: A Clinical Guide to Diagnosis and Treatment, 5th Edition. New York, Kluwer Academic/Plenum, 2000

Schuckit MA: Vulnerability factors for alcoholism, in Neuropsychology: The Fifth Generation of Progress. Edited by Davis KL, Charney D, Coyle JT, et al. Philadelphia, PA, Lippincott Williams & Wilkins, 2002

Schuster CR, Kilbey MM: Prevention of drug abuse, in Maxcy-Rosenau-Last Public Health and Preventive Medicine, 14th Edition. Edited by Wallace RB. Stamford, CT, Appleton & Lange, 1998, pp 861–879

Selzer ML: Michigan Alcoholism Screening Test: the quest for a new diagnostic instrument. Am J Psychiatry 127:89–94, 1971

Skinner HA: Early detection of alcohol and drug problems—why? Australian Drug and Alcohol Review 6:293–301, 1987

Skinner HA, Holt S, Schuller R, et al: Identification of alcohol abuse using laboratory tests and a history of trauma. Ann Intern Med 101:847–851, 1984

Sokol RJ, Martier SS, Ager JW: The T-ACES questions: practical prenatal detection of risk drinking. Am J Obstet Gynecol 160:863–870, 1989

Spicer RS, Miller TR: Impact of a workplace peer-focused substance abuse prevention and early intervention program. Alcohol Clin Exp Res 29:609–611, 2005

Stanford M: The relationship between antisocial behavior and substance abuse in childhood and adolescence: implications for etiology, prevention and treatment. Curr Opin Psychiatry 14:317–323, 2001

Stephens RS, Roffman RA, Simpson EE: Treating adult marijuana dependence: a test of the relapse prevention model. J Consult Clin Psychol 62:92–99, 1994

Substance Abuse and Mental Health Services Administration: Results from the 2006 National Survey on Drug Use and Health: national findings (DHHS Publ No SMA 07-4293). Rockville, MD, U.S. Department of Health and Human Services, 2007

Tizabi Y, Copeland RL Jr, Louis VA, et al: Effects of combined systemic alcohol and central nicotine administration into ventral tegmental area on dopamine release in the nucleus accumbens. Alcohol Clin Exp Res 26:394–399, 2002

Tobler NS: Meta-analysis of 143 adolescent drug prevention programs: quantitative outcome results of program participants compared to a control or comparison group. J Drug Issues 16:537–567, 1986

West SL, O'Neal KK: Project D.A.R.E. outcome effectiveness revisited. Am J Public Health 94:1027–1029, 2004

World Health Organization: Diet, nutrition, and the prevention of chronic diseases: report of a joint WHO/FAO expert consultation (WHO Technical Report Series, No 916). 2002. Available at: http://whqlibdoc.who.int/trs/WHO_TRS_916.pdf. Accessed February 14, 2008.

Zahler R, Piselli C: Smoking, alcohol and drugs, in Yale University School of Medicine Heart Book. Edited by Zaret BL, Moser M, Cohen LS. New York, Hearst Books, 1992

Appendix: Screening Tests for Alcohol-Related Problems

When is screening for alcohol-related problems appropriate?

- As part of a routine health examination
- Before prescribing a medication that interacts with alcohol
- In response to presenting problems that may be related to alcohol use

Ask all patients:

- Do you drink alcohol, including beer, wine, liquor, or spirits?

Ask current drinkers about alcohol consumption:

- On average, how many days per week do you drink alcohol?
- On a typical day when you drink, how many drinks do you have?
- What is the maximum number of drinks you had on any given occasion during the last month?

CAGE (Cut Down, Annoyed, Guilty, and Eye Opener) Questions

CAGE is one of the most commonly used screening tools in medicine. It is easy to remember and fast and easy to use, even with limited time.

- Have you ever felt that you should **cut down** on your drinking?
- Have people **annoyed** you by criticizing your drinking?
- Have you ever felt bad or **guilty** about your drinking?
- Have you ever had a drink first thing in the morning to steady your nerves or get rid of a hangover (**eye opener**)?

CAGE Scoring

If there is a positive response to any of these questions: Ask whether this occurred during the past year.

A patient may be at risk for alcohol-related problems IF:

- Alcohol consumption is:

Men: >14 drinks per week or >4 drinks per occasion

Women: >7 drinks per week or >3 drinks per occasion

OR

- One or more positive responses to the CAGE have occurred in the past year.
- One *yes* to the CAGE suggests an alcohol use problem. More than one *yes* strongly suggests that a problem exists (U.S. Department of Health and Human Services 1995).

Alcohol Use Disorders Identification Test

Use the Alcohol Use Disorders Identification Test (AUDIT; copyright © 2001 World Health Organization) if the CAGE assessment is positive or if clinical suspicions of an alcohol-related problem are high. The AUDIT was developed by the World Health Organization to identify people whose alcohol consumption has become problematic to their health (Babor et al. 1992). This test has 10 screening questions, as shown below: 3 on the frequency and amount of drinking, 3 on dependence, and 4 on problems associated with alcohol use. The patient circles the most appropriate response for each question.

1. How often do you have a drink containing alcohol?

    0. Never
    1. Monthly or less
    2. 2–4 times a month
    3. 2–3 times a week
    4. ≥4 times a week

2. How many drinks containing alcohol do you have on a typical day when you are drinking?

    0. 1 or 2
    1. 3 or 4
    2. 5 or 6
    3. 7 or 8
    4. ≥10

3. How often do you have ≥6 or more drinks on one occasion?

   0. Never
   1. Less than monthly
   2. Monthly
   3. Weekly
   4. Daily or almost daily

4. How often during the past year have you found that you were not able to stop drinking once you had started?

   0. Never
   1. Less than monthly
   2. Monthly
   3. Weekly
   4. Daily or almost daily

5. How often during the past year have you failed to do what was normally expected from you because of drinking?

   0. Never
   1. Less than monthly
   2. Monthly
   3. Weekly
   4. Daily or almost daily

6. How often during the past year have you needed a first drink in the morning to get yourself going after a heavy drinking session?

   0. Never
   1. Less than monthly
   2. Monthly
   3. Weekly
   4. Daily or almost daily

7. How often during the past year have you had a feeling of guilt or remorse after drinking?

   0. Never
   1. Less than monthly
   2. Monthly

3. Weekly
4. Daily or almost daily

8. How often during the past year have you been unable to remember what happened the night before because you had been drinking?

0. Never
1. Less than monthly
2. Monthly
3. Weekly
4. Daily or almost daily

9. Have you or someone else been injured as a result of your drinking?

0. No
2. Yes, but not in the past year
4. Yes, during the past year

10. Has a relative or friend, or a doctor or other health worker, been concerned about your drinking or suggested you cut down?

0. No
2. Yes, but not in the past year
4. Yes, during the past year

AUDIT Scoring

The minimum score is 0 and the maximum possible score is 40. A score of 8 or more indicates a strong likelihood of hazardous or harmful alcohol consumption (Babor et al. 1992).

Michigan Alcohol Screening Test

The Michigan Alcohol Screening Test (MAST) is a good screening tool for alcohol use disorders, but one also needs to ask about amount and frequency of alcohol use as well (Hirata et al. 2001).

1. Do you think you are a normal drinker? (By normal we mean you drink less than or as much as most other people.)
   No = 1   Yes = 0
2. Does your wife, husband, or parent, or other near relative ever worry or complain about your drinking?
   No = 0   Yes = 1

3. Do you feel guilty about your drinking?
   No = 0   Yes = 1
4. Do friends or relatives think you are a normal drinker?
   No = 1   Yes = 0
5. Are you able to stop drinking when you want to?
   No = 1   Yes = 0
6. Have you ever attended a meeting of Alcoholics Anonymous?
   No = 0   Yes = 1
7. Has drinking ever created problems between you and your wife, husband, a parent, or other near relative?
   No = 0   Yes = 1
8. Have you ever gotten into trouble at work because of your drinking?
   No = 0   Yes = 1
9. Have you ever neglected your obligations, your family, or your work for 2 or more days in a row because you were drinking?
   No = 0   Yes = 1
10. Have you ever gone to anyone for help about your drinking?
    No = 0   Yes = 1
11. Have you ever been in a hospital because of drinking?
    No = 0   Yes = 1
12. Have you ever been arrested for drunken driving, driving while intoxicated, or driving under the influence of alcoholic beverages?
    No = 0   Yes = 1
13. Have you ever been arrested, even for a few hours, because of drunken behavior?
    No = 0   Yes = 1

MAST Scoring

1. Seltzer definition:

   a. 0–1 points = nonalcoholic
   b. 2 points = possibly alcoholic
   c. ≥3 points or *Yes* answer to items 6, 10, or 11 = alcoholic

2. Ross definition:

   5 points = alcohol abuse

Tests for Alcohol Use

Recent Use (Hours)

The liver and metabolism of alcohol in the liver are the basis for many tests that can identify recent use of alcohol. The markers that can be used to detect recent use are urine/breath/blood, dermal patch, methanol, ethylglucuronide, and the urinary ratio of 5-hydroxytryptophol (5-HTOL) to 5-hydroxyindole-3-acetic acid (5-HIAA) (Arndt et al. 2000).

Less Recent Use (Weeks)

The carbohydrate-deficient transferrin (CDT) test was approved by the U.S. Food and Drug Administration for the detection of alcohol dependence and alcohol-related disorders. Elevated levels of CDT are detected even several weeks after drinking has ceased, so the test can access prolonged ingestion of alcohol (more than 50–60 g/day). The CDT test is reliable, and results can be obtained within 4 hours with automation (Sorvajarvi et al. 1996). It is often used in combination with other screening tests, such as gamma-glutamyl-transferase (GGT), to increase the sensitivity over one of the tests used alone.

Chronic Use (Years)

Classic markers to evaluate for alcohol left in the body with long-term use are liver funtion tests, glucose challenge test, aspartate transaminase (AST), alanine transaminase (ALT), red blood cell count (RBC), and mean cell volume (MCV).

References

Arndt T, Gilg T, Soyka M: Diagnosis of alcoholism: CDT rest does help. MMW Fortschr Med 146:10–11, 2000

Babor TF, Biddle-Higgins JC, Saunders JB, et al: AUDIT: The Alcohol Use Disorders Identification Test. Guidelines for Use in Primary Care (WHO Publ No WHO/MSD/MSB/01.6a). Geneva, Switzerland, World Health Organization, 1992

Hirata ES, Almeida OP, Funari RR, et al: Validity of the Michigan Alcoholism Screening Test (MAST) for the detection of alcohol-related problems among male geriatric outpatients. Am J Geriatr Psychiatry 9:30–34, 2001

Mayfield D, McLeod G, Hall P: The CAGE questionnaire: validation of a new alcoholism screening instrument. Am J Psychiatry 131:1121–1123, 1974

National Institute on Alcohol Abuse and Alcoholism: The Physicians' Guide to Helping Patients With Alcohol Problems (NIH Publ No 95–3769). Bethesda, MD, U.S. Department of Health and Human Services, 1995

Sorvajarvi K, Blake JE, Israel Y, et al: Sensitivity and specificity of carbohydrate-deficient transferrin as a marker of alcohol abuse are significantly influenced by alterations in serum transferrin. Alcohol Clin Exp Res 20:449–454, 1996

8

Suicide Prevention

Michael F. Grunebaum, M.D.
Laili Soleimani, M.Sc., M.D.

T he statistician George Box is credited with the quote, "Essentially, all models are wrong, but some are useful." In a similar vein, there is no single correct model of suicide prevention. However, many approaches to the prevention of suicide overall suggest reasons for clinicians to be optimistic about reducing the risk of this worst of psychiatric outcomes in their patients. In this chapter we attempt to review concisely the evidence regarding many different models of suicide prevention. We first briefly review the epidemiology, risk, and protective factors for suicide. Next, we review evidence on primary prevention efforts, which seek to reduce suicide rates by decreasing the development of suicidal risk

This work was supported by National Institute of Mental Health Grant K23 MH076049.

in people and populations. Such efforts include public education, gatekeeper education, education of healthcare professionals, screening and treatment, and multi-level prevention programs. We next review the evidence regarding secondary prevention approaches, those designed to reduce repeat suicidal behavior in vulnerable groups. We discuss the evidence related to suicide prevention with pharmacotherapy, electroconvulsive therapy, and psychotherapies, as well as other social interventions such as telephone hotlines, community outreach, restrictions on the means of suicide, and issues related to media reporting. Tertiary prevention, which aims to reduce the long term effects of suicidal behavior, is reviewed with respect to use of safer medications, the importance of follow-up, and the identification of persons at risk. We then review evidence specifically related to suicide prevention in adolescents. The chapter concludes with a section on clinical suicide prevention advice for practitioners.

Overall, we hope to convey that suicide is a behavioral phenomenon that is an outcome of a complex interplay of biopsychosocial stress and vulnerability and, therefore, that prevention should be similarly multi-faceted. There are many potentially modifiable risk and protective factors for suicide, and targeting as many as possible will have the best chance of reducing the overall risk.

Epidemiology of Suicidal Behavior: A Brief Overview

Suicide Around the World

Worldwide, suicide is among the top three leading causes of death among people 15–44 years old. There were approximately one million suicides worldwide in 2000, roughly one suicide every 40 seconds. An estimated 10–20 suicide attempts occur for each completed suicide. In the last 45 years, global suicide rates have increased 60%. It was estimated that suicide accounted for approximately 1.8% of the global burden of disease in 1998. Young people constitute an increasing percentage of suicides, with approximately 100,000 adolescents dying by suicide annually (World Health Organization 2008).

Suicide in the United States

Approximately 30,000 people die by suicide every year in the United States. In 2005, suicide was the eleventh leading cause of death for people of all ages and for both sexes, with 32,629 deaths. Suicide accounts for 2.6 times more deaths annually than human immunodeficiency virus (HIV)–associated illnesses do and 1.8 times more than homicide does (National Center for Injury Prevention and Control 2008).

The epidemiology of suicide varies greatly across sociodemographic groups. For example, it was the eighth leading cause of death in males in the United States in 2005, but the seventeenth leading cause for females. The male to female ratio of suicides is approximately 4:1. The most common suicide method among males is handguns (~55%) and among females is poisoning (~40%). Among people less than 34 years old, suicide is the third leading cause of death. Elderly, white men have the highest rates of suicide in the United States; in 2005, the suicide rate among white men, 65 years or older, was approximately 32 per 100,000 population (National Center for Injury Prevention and Control 2008). In terms of racial and ethnic groups, the highest rates are among non-Hispanic whites (~13 per 100,000) and American Indian/Alaska natives (~14 per 100,000). The lowest rates are among non-Hispanic blacks (~5.4 per 100,000), Asian and Pacific Islanders (~5.2 per 100,000), and Hispanics (~5.6 per 100,000) (National Center for Injury Prevention and Control 2008).

Risk Factors for Suicide

Although many risk factors for suicide have been identified empirically in research samples (Table 8–1) (for review, see Michel 2000; Plutchik 2000), it is very difficult to predict suicide at the individual level. For example, a meta-analysis of four studies with follow-up on more than 2,500 patients for 5–12 years tested whether the Beck Hopelessness Scale (BHS) score, an established indicator of risk, could predict completed or attempted suicide (McMillan et al. 2007). Results for predicting completed suicide showed that, at the standard cutoff score of 9 on the BHS, the pooled sensitivity was 80% and specificity was 42%, which would yield a 20% false-negative rate, but an almost 60% false-positive rate. Results for nonfatal suicide attempt prediction were very similar. Thus, although higher risk groups can be identified, the nonspecificity of even established risk factors such as hopelessness means that there are as yet no clinic-ready methods to predict which individuals will attempt or commit suicide.

Table 8–1. Evidence-based risk factors for suicide

Prior suicide attempt

Psychiatric illness, especially a mood disorder, schizophrenia, substance abuse or dependence, or borderline personality disorder

Recent loss or separation

Family history of a mood disorder, suicide, or alcoholism

Access to lethal means of suicide

Social isolation

Demographic characteristics, including being white, male, or elderly

Hopelessness

Preparatory acts such as obtaining means or writing a note

Recent psychiatric or medical hospitalization

A useful framework for understanding suicide risk is the *stress-diathesis model* (Mann and Arango 1992). This model proposes that suicide is the result of complex interactions between intrinsic traits predisposing an individual toward suicidal behavior (Mann et al. 2009), and stressors such as environmental triggers, personal crises, or acute episodes of a psychiatric illness. Based on this model, genetic and neurochemical factors, as well as aggressive or impulsive personality traits, may decrease an individual's threshold to self-harm in response to stress. See Table 8–2 for examples of stress (trigger) and diathesis (lowered threshold) risk factors.

Psychiatric Illnesses and Comorbidity

Psychological autopsy studies, in which friends, family members, and caretakers of the person who died by suicide are interviewed, show that approximately 90% of individuals who commmit suicide have a diagnosed or diagnosable psychiatric illness at the time of death and 70%–80% have comorbidity involving more than one psychiatric disorder (Mann and Currier 2007). Major depression associated with unipolar or bipolar mood disorders constitutes up to 60% of these cases and most of the individuals are either untreated or taking subtherapeutic doses of antidepressants at the time of death (Isacsson et al. 1999; Isometsä et al. 1994; Marzuk et al. 1995; Rich and Isacsson 1997). This suggests a need for better recognition and treatment of depressed and suicidal patients. Cluster B personality disorders, alcohol or drug

Table 8–2. Stress-diathesis factors that may affect risk of suicidal behavior

Stress (trigger)	Diathesis (lowered threshold)
Acute psychiatric illness such as a major depressive episode, or a medical illness	Genetic factors, which may be evidenced by a family history of depression or suicidality
Substance abuse or intoxication	Impulsive or aggressive personality traits
Acute loss, such as of relationship or job	Trauma history, such as child abuse or being a war veteran
	Early-onset major depressive disorder
	Neurocognitive dysfunction
	Dysfunctional cortisol response to psychosocial stress
	Serotonergic system alterations

abuse, anxiety, and psychosis are among other mental disorders associated with suicide. Co-occurrence of depression with these disorders increases the risk of suicide (for review, see Mann and Currier 2007).

Family History of Suicide

Various studies provide evidence for the familial transmission of suicide (for review, see Brent and Melhem 2008). Both suicide attempts and completed suicides are more common in people with a family history of suicide. Nongenetic factors (e.g., exposure to family violence, hostility and discord, low parental involvement, imitation of suicidal behavior) can influence familial aggregation, and genetic transmission of suicide risk may also be involved. Twin studies and adoption studies both support the role of genetic factors in suicide. Meta-analysis of studies involving monozygotic and dizygotic twin pairs has found significantly greater concordance for suicide in monozygotic than in dizygotic twins. Adoptees who committed suicide had a sixfold higher rate of suicide in their biological families than matched adoptees who had not committed suicide. Studies attempting to find specific genetic variants associated with suicidal behavior have focused on neurotransmitter systems, especially the serotonin system, and to a lesser extent the noradrenergic, dopamine, and hypothalamic-pituitary-adrenal systems (for review, see Currier and Mann 2008).

Biological Traits

A large amount of literature investigates the relationship between suicide, impulsivity and aggression, and cerebrospinal fluid levels of the serotonin metabolite 5-hydroxyindoleacetic acid (5-HIAA) that are lower than those in control groups. Studies suggest a brain serotonergic function deficit in suicide attempters (e.g., reduced levels of 5-HIAA in cerebrospinal fluid), and that such deficiency is correlated with severity and lethality of attempts. Autopsy studies on suicide victims also reveal abnormalities in serotonin receptor binding in the brain stem and prefrontal cortex (for review, see Oquendo et al. 1997).

Early Life Adversity

A history of child abuse and early parental loss increases the likelihood of suicidal behavior. Victims of child abuse are more likely to develop aggressive or impulsive traits or psychiatric disorders, which may increase the risk of self-harm (Mann and Currier 2007). These risk factors are concordant with biological studies showing associations between a reported history of child abuse and developmental impairment in neurobiological systems, including the serotonergic system and the hypothalamic-pituitary-adrenal axis stress response system (for review, see Brodsky et al. 2001).

Individual Characteristics

Although situation-dependent processes may trigger suicidality, some of the predisposing as well as protective factors lie in the structure of one's personality (Brezo et al. 2006). Personality traits that may increase the risk of suicidal behavior include helplessness, pessimism, aggression, impulsivity, anxiety, and neuroticism. Protective traits are thought to include resilience, hardiness, agreeableness, and stable self-esteem. Personality disorders, which represent dysfunctional extremes of normative personality traits, are associated with an increased risk of suicidal ideation and attempts. This is particularly true of cluster B personality disorders, especially borderline personality disorder (Suominen et al. 2000). Aggression has been shown to be associated with highly lethal suicide attempts across psychiatric disorders (Mann et al. 1999; Placidi et al. 2001). Impulsive people, on the other hand, tend to make more frequent but less lethal suicide attempts (Baca-García et al. 2001). Traits might be the mediators of genetic variation and/or of early environmental and family influences. For example, an impulsive-aggressive trait has been suggested to be an intermediate phenotype associated with both serotonergic genes and vulnerability to suicidality (for review, see Brezo et al. 2006).

Environmental Factors

Among environmental factors, having a social support network (measured by marital status, interaction with family members, and number of close friends), is a protective factor against suicide. On the other hand, psychosocial crises, such as interpersonal losses or conflicts, financial crisis, and job problems, may act as triggers of suicidal behavior, possibly through increased stress from disruption of the individual's social support network (for review, see Goldney 2005a; Oquendo et al. 1997).

Protective Factors for Suicide

Reduction of risk factors, such as effective treatment of psychiatric illness, substance abuse, aggression, and impulsivity, is likely to be protective. A number of studies have also identified characteristics that may themselves confer protection against suicidal behavior. These include family and marriage (especially for white males) (for review, see Bongar et al. 2000), more self-reported reasons for living (Malone et al. 2001), religious affiliation mediated by moral objections to suicide (Dervic et al. 2004), and family cohesion (for review, see Gould 2003).

Primary Prevention of Suicidal Behavior

Primary prevention aims to reduce suicide rates by improving the physical, mental, or emotional health or well-being of a population. Interventions targeted at primary prevention of suicide include public education, mental health screening programs for depression and other disorders, enhancement of life skills, parenting programs, and training of health professionals and other gatekeepers in the early diagnosis and management of depression (Oquendo et al. 1997).

Public Education

When the general public is informed about the facts of mental illnesses and suicide, members of the population are better able to support a friend or family member at high risk or encourage him or her to seek professional help (for review, see Mann et al. 2005). Several campaigns have been carried out and studied in different countries aiming to destigmatize mental illnesses, increase general public awareness about depression and other mental illnesses, and promote recognition of suicide risk factors. The studies show that the programs have modest effects on public attitudes toward mental illnesses and depression but overall do not demonstrate strong effects on suicidal behavior (for review, see Mann et al. 2005).

Gatekeeper Education

Gatekeepers are individuals in the community (including clergy, first responders, pharmacists, geriatric caregivers, hospital staff and school teachers) who may be in contact with potentially suicidal individuals and are in a position to identify them and refer them for treatment. A key component of gatekeeper education is learning about warning signs for suicide, then asking persons who show these signs whether they are thinking of suicide (C. H. Brown et al. 2007). Systematic studies on the effectiveness of gatekeeper education are mostly limited to components of multilevel interventions such as those in the United States Air Force (Knox et al. 2003); studies of these programs reported reductions in suicide rates with the interventions (for review, see Mann et al. 2005). The United States Air Force in 2006 began a population-based prevention program following an increase in the suicide rate, especially among staff members between ages 24 and 35. This multimodal program emphasized community-wide training to enhance awareness of mental health, destigmatize help-seeking behaviors, enhance social networks, and facilitate help seeking. The program affects more than five million U.S. Air Force personnel and has been associated with a 33% relative risk reduction for suicide, as well as decreased accidental deaths, homicides, and family violence at the moderate-severe level (Knox et al. 2003).

Education of Health Professionals and Early Detection and Treatment of Depression

Studies show that three of four persons who commit suicide had contact with a primary care physician within a year of their death (Luoma et al. 2002). Up to 66% of these contacts were within a month of the suicide (Andersen et al. 2000). These data indicate the importance of primary care providers as a target for suicide prevention efforts (Mann et al. 2005). The fact that depressed patients tend to express suicidal behavior early in the course of the illness further emphasizes the significance of early detection of high-risk patients, and the key role of primary care physicians in inquiring about suicidal thoughts and diagnosing and properly treating underlying disorders such as depression, substance abuse, and other psychiatric illnesses (Isometsä et al. 1994; McGirr et al. 2008).

Education of primary care clinicians not only may improve the care of patients but also may reduce the public-health burden of depressive symptoms. An influential study was done on the Swedish island of Gotland (with 18 physicians and a population of 60,000), where a special postgraduate training program for general practitioners about mood disorders led to an increase in antidepressant prescriptions and a decrease in sickness-related absence from work, hospital referrals, and suicide rates. However, the effects lasted only for 3 years after the program ended, suggesting that such educational efforts should be repeated at regular intervals (Rutz et al. 1992). Other studies have confirmed the impact of training primary care physicians on the prevention of suicidal behavior. These interventions represent some of the most striking ones available to lower suicide rates (Mann et al. 2005).

Multilevel Intervention Programs

Considering these results and the complexity of factors affecting rates of detection and treatment of depression, a multilevel program would appear to be the most promising for primary prevention of suicide (for review, see Goldney 2005b; Hegerl et al. 2006; Knox et al. 2004). A 2-year intervention was performed in Nuremberg (480,000 inhabitants) at four levels: training and support of family doctors, a public relations campaign about depression, cooperation with community facilitators (teachers, priests, local media, etc.), and support for self-help activities involving high-risk groups. Results after 2 years showed a statistically significant, greater than 27% reduction in the frequency of suicide attempts in Nuremberg compared with a control region. Differences in rates of completed suicides did not reach statistical significance (Hegerl et al. 2006).

Secondary Prevention

Secondary prevention efforts aim to decrease the likelihood of repeat suicidal behavior in high-risk patients by intervening either during or after a suicidal crisis. Interventions may include crisis counseling for, close supervision of, and treatment of individuals who have expressed suicidal thoughts (including pharmacotherapy and psychotherapy for underlying psychiatric disorders), and reducing availability of the means to commit suicide.

Pharmacotherapy

Antidepressants

Logically, treatment of underlying psychiatric disease should have a positive impact on the prevention of suicide. Ecological studies of antidepressant prescribing and suicide rates in different countries (for review, see Mann et al. 2005) suggest that antidepressants may protect against suicide. Studies in Sweden, Australia, Hungary, Japan, and the United States have reported a correlation between greater numbers of antidepressant prescriptions and lower suicide rates, though this was not found in Italy or Iceland. Although ecological studies cannot make a causal connection between antidepressant prescribing and suicide rates, the pattern seen in most countries is consistent with a protective effect of antidepressants.

Unlike large, population-based studies, randomized, controlled trials have failed to demonstrate a significant effect of antidepressant use on suicide rates (Fergusson et al. 2005; Gunnell et al. 2005; Khan et al. 2003). Some have even detected a slight increase in the risk of self-harm, but not suicide, associated with selective serotonin reuptake inhibitors (SSRIs) (Gunnell et al. 2005). A randomized clinical trial to test rigorously whether antidepressants, or SSRIs specifically, may prevent suicide would be challenging to undertake. Given the relative infrequency of suicide—about 11 per 100,000 persons in the United States—such a trial would require a sample of many thousands and/or long-term follow-up to determine whether treatment significantly reduces suicidal behavior (for review, see C. H. Brown et al. 2007; Grunebaum and Mann 2007).

The U.S. Food and Drug Administration conducted a meta-analysis of antidepressant clinical trial data for adults (Stone et al. 2006). This analysis included data pooled from 372 trials of 11 currently used antidepressants (bupropion, citalopram, duloxetine, escitalopram, fluoxetine, fluvoxamine, mirtazapine, nefazodone, paroxetine, sertraline, and venlafaxine), involving almost 100,000 individuals. With 15,505 subject-years of observation used, there were 8 suicides and 134 subjects who only attempted suicide. As few as one suicidal ideation or behavior event occurred in 59% of the trials, with no events in 41%. The statistically nonsignificant ($P = 0.08$) overall odds ratio for suicidality (ideation or behavior) with test drugs versus placebo found in this meta-analysis was 0.85 (95% CI: 0.71–1.02); this is consistent with a protective (antisuicidal) effect on adults overall. The estimated odds ratio for suicidal behavior (preparatory acts, attempts, and suicide) associated with antidepressant drug treatment versus placebo was 1.12 (95% CI: 0.79–1.58), a statistically nonsignificant increased risk. No difference was seen with SSRIs versus non-SSRIs (Stone et al. 2006). When the analysis was stratified by age group, the benefit of antidepressants was greater for patients older than 25 years. There was a suggestion of an elevated risk of suicidal ideation or behavior among adults younger than 25 years, a neutral or possibly protective effect for adults between ages 25 and 64, and a protective effect in those age 65 and older. For 18- to 24-year-olds with psychiatric disorders, the rate of suicide was 0.03% (~1 per 3,810) and the rate of suicide attempts was 0.55% (~21 per 3,810) (Stone et al. 2006). By comparison, in a meta-analysis of patients with mood disorders, the lifetime prevalence of suicide was 2.2%–8.6%, depending partly on illness severity (Bostwick and Pankratz 2000).

Studies of depression treatment in members of a group health plan demonstrate that suicide attempt rates in adolescents, younger adults (<25 years), and older adults are highest in the month preceding treatment and decline steadily after initiation of treatment with either antidepressant medication or psychotherapy (Simon et al. 2006). The pattern was the same whether antidepressant treatment was with a primary care physician or a psychiatrist.

Most people who commit suicide and are found to have had major depression at the time of death were untreated or were taking subtherapeutic doses of antidepressants (Isacsson et al. 1999; Isometsä et al. 1994; Marzuk et al. 1995; Rich and Isacsson 1997). Therefore, the evidence suggests overall that untreated or undertreated depression is a greater contributor to suicide rates than infrequent adverse reactions to antidepressant medications.

Lithium

Lithium has been used for more than half a century to treat mood disorders, particularly bipolar disorder. Its preventive effect on bipolar relapse has been shown (for review, see Burgess et al. 2001); however, its reported antisuicidal effect has been more challenging to prove. The low rates of suicide make it difficult to conduct adequately powered trials (because of small population sizes) testing the preventive effects of lithium and other interventions (Cipriani et al. 2005).

Some studies support a preventive effect of lithium on suicidal behavior. Baldessarini and colleagues (2006) conducted a meta-analysis of 31 lithium studies, including 33,340 subjects and 85,229 person-years of lithium treatment (average = 2.08 years). They found that lithium treatment of patients with bipolar and other major affective disorders consistently decreased the risk of completed and attempted suicide by approximately 80% compared with the risk in patients not treated with lithium. This benefit was sustained in randomized as well as open clinical trials. The preventive effect was more pronounced in patients with unipolar and bipolar II disorders than in patients with bipolar I disorder, and reduced suicide rates to those seen in the general population. Proposed mechanisms of lithium's effect included lowering of the risk of depressive relapse; a serotonin-mediated reduction in impulsivity or aggressive behavior; and a nonspecific benefit arising from the long-term monitoring provided during lithium therapy (Baldessarini et al. 2003). It is noteworthy that lithium discontinuation, particularly if abrupt, has been reported to lead to mood instability and suicidal behavior (Baldessarini et al. 1999).

Some argue that reports of an antisuicidal effect of lithium are mostly based on nonrandomized, retrospective data, and thus biased toward individuals who respond positively to lithium (Burgess et al. 2001). Of note, higher quality, randomized, controlled trials usually involve shorter exposures, making the testing of lithium's putative antisuicidal effects difficult (Baldessarini et al. 2006).

Antipsychotics

Among patients diagnosed with schizophrenia or schizoaffective disorder, suicide is a major contributor to mortality, with a 50% lifetime risk of a suicide attempt, and suicide accounts for about 10% of deaths in these patients (Meltzer 2002). Because antipsychotic treatment remains the mainstay of pharmacological treatment for schizophrenia, it is critical to know whether and how these drugs influence suicidal behavior. First-generation antipsychotics such as fluphenazine, thiothixene, and haloperidol have not been demonstrated to reduce the overall risk of suicidal behavior among patients with schizophrenia. It has even been suggested that some troubling side effects of older-generation antipsychotics, such as akathisia and secondary depression (*neuroleptic dysphoria*), might contribute to suicide attempts (for review, see Caldwell and Gottesman 1990).

Among antipsychotic drugs, clozapine is the best studied with respect to suicidal behavior. As a second-generation antipsychotic, it has several advantages over the first-generation drugs, including fewer extrapyramidal neurological side effects (Baldessarini and Tarazi 2001) and efficacy in the treatment of refractory schizophrenia ("Practice Guideline for the Assessment and Treatment of Patients With Suicidal Behaviors" 2003, p. 135). Retrospective analysis of clozapine registry data has mostly shown a decrease in suicidality. In some studies, such as the retrospective analysis of the U.S. Department of Veterans Affairs dataset, the decrease was not statistically significant ("Practice Guideline for the Assessment and Treatment of Patients With Suicidal Behaviors" 2003, p. 135). Although these studies provide some evidence for the ability of clozapine therapy to reduce suicidal behavior, they have limitations; for example, they are not adjusted for possible differences in suicide risk, relative differences in clozapine dosages, use of concomitant medications, or clinical contacts (which are usually more frequent in patients treated with clozapine than in patients treated with other antipsychotics due to the requirement of regular monitoring of blood tests for neutropenia) (Meltzer et al. 2003).

In an international, multicenter, 2-year, randomized, controlled trial, which controlled for clinical contact across treatments, Meltzer and colleagues (2003) demonstrated an advantage to using clozapine versus olanzapine for reducing suicidal behavior. Fewer clozapine recipients attempted suicide, required hospitalization or rescue interventions to prevent suicide, or required concomitant treatment with antidepressants (Meltzer et al. 2003). Because the risk of suicide is one of the chief indicators for hospitalization of patients with schizophrenia or schizoaffective disorder, these results suggest that wider use of clozapine in suicidal schizophrenia patients could reduce treatment costs as well as prevent suicide. This consideration suggests a more favorable risk-benefit profile than is usually associated with clozapine, especially in patients at risk for suicide (Meltzer et al. 2003). A meta-analysis of six relatively heterogeneous studies also yielded a pooled risk ratio (3.3; 95% CI: 1.7–6.3) favoring clozapine versus other treatments in terms of suicide attempt/completion rates in patients with schizophrenia or schizoaffective disorder (Hennen and Baldessarini 2005).

Electroconvulsive Therapy

Electroconvulsive therapy (ECT) has been used in the treatment of mental illnesses for more than 60 years (Challiner and Griffiths 2000). Many textbooks and guidelines suggest ECT as the first choice for marked suicidality. Much of the rationale for this clinical practice is indirect and based primarily on the established efficacy of ECT in treating severe depression, which itself often underlies suicidal ideation and behavior. As reviewed in the American Psychiatric Association's "Practice Guideline for the Assessment and Treatment of Patients With Suicidal Behaviors" (2003, pp. 138–139), ECT may provide a more rapid response than psychopharmacological, psychosocial, or other treatments, especially in severe, acute depression with or without psychotic features.

In several ECT studies that included depressed patients (for review, see "Practice Guideline for the Assessment and Treatment of Patients With Suicidal Behaviors" 2003, pp. 138–139), patients have shown a rapid and robust decline in suicidality, as measured by the suicide item of the Hamilton Rating Scale for Depression. One major limitation of these studies was the reliance on a single scale item. Furthermore, the effects related only to the short-term efficacy of ECT. Failure to find enduring effects on suicide rate after short-term ECT by some studies may be explained by their methodological limitations (i.e., retrospective, nonrandomized, uncontrolled, and with small sample sizes).

Some who object to the claim that ECT can prevent suicide suggest that there is anecdotal evidence that the confusion and memory loss associated with ECT may increase suicide risk in some patients. Critics document the fate of Ernest Hemingway, who shot himself only days after being released from a hospital following more than 20 ECT treatments (Challiner and Griffiths 2000).

To evaluate the long-term effect of ECT on suicidality, some naturalistic studies compared the rate of suicide before and after the introduction of ECT. O'Leary and colleagues (2001) systematically reviewed 75 studies with a minimum follow-up duration of 6 months and calculated the suicide rates from 1966 to 1995. Their analysis indicated a 41% decrease in suicide rate, from 1.33% to 0.77% per year, from before the introduction of ECT and antidepressants to after their introduction. However, the interpretation of this information is obscured by uncertain reliability in identifying persons who died by suicide in different eras, by the effect of multiple therapeutic developments across the decades, and by potential confounding variables not adjusted for in the analyses.

On the other hand, an earlier study comparing patients from a registry in Monroe County, New York, did not show a significant difference in suicide mortality between those who received ECT and those who received other treatments. One possible explanation could be the selection of more severely ill patients for ECT treatment (Babigian and Guttmacher 1984).

The available data thus suggest that ECT may quickly provide a short-term benefit in reducing suicidal thinking, but do not provide evidence of sustained reduction of suicide risk following short-term ECT (for review, see "Practice Guideline for the Assessment and Treatment of Patients With Suicidal Behaviors" 2003, pp. 138–139). As with antidepressant therapy, there is little information from systematically applied and evaluated long-term treatment with ECT that is comparable to that for lithium and clozapine. It may not be reasonable to expect a long-term effect on suicide risk from short-term treatments.

Psychotherapy

Psychotherapy plays an important role in the management of suicidal behavior in clinical practice. Reviewing the current literature on the effect of psychotherapy indicates promising results in the treatment of those who have attempted suicide and people with borderline personality disorder. Cognitive therapy, problem-solving therapy, intensive treatment plus outreach, and interpersonal psychotherapy have been shown to improve treatment adherence and also to decrease the rate of repetition of deliberate self-harm (G.K. Brown et al. 2005; Guthrie et al. 2001; Hawton et al. 1999). G.K. Brown and colleagues (2005) compared cognitive therapy versus enhanced usual care with tracking and referrals after a suicide attempt in a randomized trial and found that the reattempt rate was 50% lower after cognitive therapy than after enhanced usual care during an 18-month follow-up period. In patients with borderline personality disorder, rates of suicidal behavior were lower after dialectical behavioral therapy, psychoanalytically oriented partial hospitalization, and transference-focused psychotherapy (Bateman and Fonagy 2001; Clarkin et al. 2007; Linehan et al. 2006). In addition, suicidal ideation was decreased with interpersonal psychotherapy, cognitive-behavioral therapy, or dialectical behavioral therapy compared with usual care (for review, see Gaynes et al. 2004). The apparent superiority of combination treatment with psychotherapy and pharmacotherapy in individuals with depression also suggests a need for further study of such combined treatment in individuals with suicidal behavior (for review, see "Practice Guideline for the Assessment and Treatment of Patients With Suicidal Behaviors" 2003, pp. 139–142; Mann et al. 2005).

Societal Interventions

Crisis Hotlines

Crisis centers and hotlines use trained volunteers or paid staff, often linked to mental health services, who provide telephone or other types of counseling services for those in emotional distress or experiencing suicidal crises (King et al. 2003). Such counseling services are based on the fact that suicidal behavior is often associated with a stressful life event such as an interpersonal loss. Often, coexisting ambivalent feelings of wishing to die and to be rescued may lead suicidal persons to seek help (Gould et al. 2007). Crisis centers and hotlines have been active in many parts of the world including the United States and many European countries since the 1950s and 1960s (Goldney 2005b). They are now sources of help for high-risk individuals in many developed countries. Despite their theoretical and practical significance there are inconsistent empirical data regarding their effectiveness in preventing suicides.

One method of measuring the effectiveness of telephone crisis services has been ecological comparisons of suicide rates in areas with and without or before and after a crisis program. In an early study, Bagley (1968) found a significant effect of the Samaritans crisis group on suicide prevention in England. Later studies using more elaborate statistical techniques failed to replicate this (Barraclough and Jennings 1977). Many researchers suggested that the decrease in suicide rates observed was due to other societal changes during the same time period, including the detoxification of domestic gas (Krutman 1976) and the change from sedatives with a relatively low therapeutic index (e.g., barbiturates) to those with a higher safety margin (e.g., benzodiazepines) (Miller et al. 1984).

Recent reviews are more promising. A meta-analysis of 14 studies by Lester (1997) concluded that crisis centers and hotlines have a small preventive effect. Gould and colleagues (2007) found decreases in callers' suicidal ideation after consultation (Gould et al. 2007; King et al. 2003; Lester 1997). Significant decreases in suicidality were found during the course of the telephone session, with continuing decreases in hopelessness and psychological pain in the following weeks (Gould et al. 2007). Without a control group, however, these effects cannot be definitively attributed to the crisis intervention. This is an important obstacle in this series of studies. Ethical concerns do not allow compromising services to high-risk individuals (Gould et al. 2007). King and colleagues (2003) also found decreases in suicidality between the beginning and end of telephone counseling sessions for adolescents. These studies highlight the importance of outreach, follow-up, and referrals to mental health specialty care in suicidal callers, especially those with a history of suicide attempts.

Enhanced Ongoing Contact With High-Risk, Elderly Individuals

A case-control study of data from 1988–1998 from a telephone-based outreach and support service for the elderly in the Veneto region of Italy found a suicide preventive effect (De Leo et al. 2002). Suicide rates were lower among 18,641 users of this service, which attempted to foster "connectedness," relative to a comparable general population control group. Tele-Help consisted of a portable device that enabled patients to send an alarm signal if they needed help, and Tele-Check was a regular biweekly check of patients by telephone. Longitudinal data collected between 1988 and 1998 indicated that the telephone help line and social support for these individuals had a positive impact on their psychosocial functioning and was associated with a 71% reduction in the suicide rate (observed vs. expected) when data on individuals of both sexes were analyzed. However, the effect was statistically significant only for females (with an 83% reduction) (De Leo et al. 2002). Active outreach, continuity of care, and an increased level of emotional support seem to be key elements in providing protection against suicide, at least in females. The results corroborate previous findings that connection and response to services are influenced by the gender of the patient (De Leo et al. 2002). De Leo et al. (2002) highlighted the need for innovative efforts to prevent suicide in males.

Restriction of Means

Restricting access to common methods of suicide has been shown to decrease suicide by those specific means (Mann et al. 2005). Removing access to the means of committing suicide has a considerable impact on suicide rates due to the association with impulsivity (Baca-García et al. 2001). However, it is not as clear whether means restriction decreases overall suicide rates or whether suicidal individuals tend to switch to other methods of self-harm. Examples of means restriction that appeared to reduce suicide rates include: banning firearms in Canada and in Washington, D.C.; restricting access to barbiturates in Australia; detoxifying domestic gas in Switzerland and the United Kingdom; and reducing carbon monoxide concentrations in vehicle exhaust by requiring the use of catalytic converters in England (for reviews, see Hawton 2005; Mann et al. 2005).

Legislation in 1998 reducing the package size of paracetamol and salicylate analgesics in England had a marked and sustained effect on reducing suicide rates by these methods (Hawton et al. 2004). While there was some evidence of switching to ibuprofen as a means of suicide, this is a less lethal method and appeared to be associated with few deaths (Hawton et al. 2004). This evidence supports the practice, commonly used by clinicians, of prescribing smaller amounts of potentially dangerous medicines to patients who appear to be at risk of suicide.

Media Campaigns

It has been suggested that the media play a dual role in the prevention of suicide. Although a major means of public education, the media may also increase the risk of subsequent suicides by glamorizing dramatic suicide reports (Mann et al. 2005). Restricting the reporting of suicides may reduce suicide rates. Sonneck and colleagues (1994) reported that a sustained 75% decrease in the number of subway suicides in Vienna occurred for 5 years following initiatives to abstain from reporting on such suicides (Goldney 2005b; Sonneck et al. 1994). What the data have shown, however, is only that suicides at a particular site (such as a bridge or a train platform) have been reduced. It is not clear whether such changes can affect overall suicide rates (Paris 2006).

Tertiary Prevention

Tertiary prevention aims to diminish the long-term consequences of suicidal behavior through efforts to reduce the severity of injuries or disabilities. Tertiary interventions also increase support for bereaved friends and family members who are at risk for distress and psychiatric morbidity, including the development of suicidal thoughts and behaviors (Maris 2002).

Use of Safer Medications

One aspect of tertiary prevention is decreasing the lethality of suicide attempts by using safer medications. The availability of antidepressants and hypnotics/anxiolytics that are relatively safe in high doses has made the treatment of the depressed, suicidal patient on an outpatient basis more feasible. SSRIs, for example, have the advantage of a greater margin of safety in overdose compared to tricyclic antidepressants, which are associated with cardiotoxicity (for review, see Oquendo et al. 1997).

Follow-Up

As previously noted, the strongest risk factor for suicide is a history of a previous attempt, particularly in the period shortly following psychiatric hospitalization (for review, see McMillan et al. 2007). Given the chronic and recurring nature of psychiatric disorders such as depression, it is logical to consider continuous follow-up and maintenance care, including psychiatric hospitalization when necessary, for high-risk patients (for review, see Mann et al. 2005). However, a heightened risk of suicide may be present both before and immediately after psychiatric hospitalization. A special challenge to mental health care is presented by high-risk patients who decline continued outpatient treatment or, having accepted such treatment, quickly discontinue the planned program (Motto and Bostrom 2001).

In a randomized, controlled trial, Motto and Bostrom (2001) studied 843 patients who had been hospitalized for depression or suicidality but refused follow-up after discharge. Patients were randomly assigned to no contact ($n=454$) or a simple follow-up intervention of sending patients a letter four times a year ($n=389$). Survival analysis showed a lower suicide rate during the first 2 years for the intervention group that was marginally significant ($P=0.043$; one-tailed). An example of the letters (Motto and Bostrom 2001, p. 829), which were individually typed, worded differently, and included a self-addressed return envelope, is, "Dear . . . , It has been some time since you were here at the hospital, and we hope things are going well for you. If you wish to drop us a note we would be glad to hear from you." Other studies have found no effect of interventions—including telephone follow-up, intensive psychosocial follow-up, and video education plus family therapy—on repeated attempts or reemergent suicidal ideation in persons who had attempted suicide (for review, see Goldney 2005b).

Some authors posit that interventions may paradoxically increase the risk of repeat suicide attempts in certain patient subgroups, such as those with borderline personality disorder, by providing positive reinforcement after suicidal behavior (for review, see Pitman 2007). However, researchers and clinicians generally agree that, in most cases, intensive interventions are indicated after any form of suicidality.

Identification of Family Members at Risk

Another tertiary prevention modality includes the assessment of family members who may be affected by a relative's suicide attempt and might attempt suicide themselves. The clinician may want to either directly evaluate family members after an attempted or completed suicide or refer them for evaluation. Evaluation should focus on the family member's view of suicidal behavior and assess for the presence of suicidal ideation (for review, see Oquendo et al. 1997).

Adolescent Suicidality

In 2006, suicide accounted for 10.3% of all deaths in 10- to 19-year-olds, making it the third leading cause of death in this age group in the United States, after accidents and homicide (National Center for Injury Prevention and Control 2008). Attempts are 10–20 times as prevalent as actual suicides, indicating the magnitude of the problem (World Health Organization 2008). Suicide is rare before puberty. Suicide rates increase markedly in the late teenage years and continue to rise until the early twenties, reaching a level that is maintained throughout adulthood until the sixth decade, when the rate increases markedly among men (for review, see Anderson 2002; Steele and Doey 2007a). As in other age groups, suicidal ideation and attempts in adolescents tend to be more common among females, whereas completed suicides, which are often associated with aggressive behavior and substance abuse, are more common in males (for review, see Gould et al. 2003).

Risk factors associated with suicide in youths can be classified into those related to characteristics of the attempter; family factors, socioeconomic and contextual conditions they are exposed to; and stressful life experiences (for review, see Gould et al. 2003). Longitudinal retrospective and prospective studies show that most suicides in youths are associated with previous suicide attempts or ideation, psychiatric hospitalization, and preexisting mental illnesses, especially depression, substance abuse, psychosis, borderline personality, and, to a lesser extent, conduct disorder (for review, see C. H. Brown et al. 2007). Youths may also be influenced by the suicide of a peer or family member or by media reporting of suicides (C. H. Brown et al. 2007). Certain subgroups are classified as being at high risk for engaging in suicidal behavior, including gay, lesbian and bisexual youths; homeless and runaway youths; and incarcerated adolescents (for review, see Spirito and Esposito-Smythers 2006).

In youth suicide prevention, special attention has been given to schools as a main point of access to the adolescent population. Evidence supporting school-based suicide awareness programs, which prepare teenagers to identify peers who may be at risk and to know how to respond, has been largely inconclusive (Gould et al. 2003). However, a study of the school-based suicide prevention program called the *Signs of Suicide,* in which high school students received education and screening and were referred for help when appropriate, was found to significantly lower rates of self-reported suicide attempts and to increase adaptive attitudes about depression and suicide in students (Aseltine et al. 2007). Although most studies confirm the role of such school-based programs in increasing knowledge about suicide and improving attitudes about mental illnesses, the results overall have been insufficient to support their having a preventive role. Some even report negative effects, such as hopelessness and maladaptive coping responses in males and adolescents with a history of suicidal behavior (for review, see Gould et al. 2003; Spirito and Esposito-Smythers 2006; Steele and Doey 2007b).

Gatekeeper programs for adolescents aim to train school personnel to identify suicidal youth. Research examining the effectiveness of gatekeeper training is limited. However, findings show improvement in personnel's knowledge, attitudes, intervention skills, crisis preparation, and referral practices (Gould et al. 2003). The *Question, Persuade, and Refer* (QPR) method of gatekeeper training teaches school staff about the signs of depression and risk factors for suicide, and recommends steps to take to refer someone who needs help. Preliminary evidence suggests that QPR training increases self-reported knowledge, appraisals of efficacy, and service access (Wyman et al. 2008). However, it is not clear whether the effects are sufficient to reduce rates of suicide (for review, see C. H. Brown et al. 2007; Gould et al. 2003; Steele and Doey 2007b).

Suicide Prevention Advice for Practitioners

Overall, the evidence on suicide prevention suggests that practitioners should take a risk-reduction approach when treating individuals who may be at risk for suicidal behavior. There are well-established, evidence-based risk factors for suicidal behavior. The informed clinician can intervene in multiple ways to target several risk factors simultaneously with the goal of reducing overall suicide risk. There is encouraging evidence that some interventions, such as means restriction and certain pharmacotherapies and psychotherapies, may help prevent suicidal behavior. However, further clinical trials are needed to test promising suicide preventive interventions. Innovative study designs will likely be required given that the relative infrequency of suicide makes it a challenge to conduct studies large enough (e.g., with sufficient statistical power) to detect preventive effects. With individual patients, practitioners must assess risk, formulate treatment plans considering relative risks and benefits, and document their decision-making process. With the goal of suicide prevention through risk reduction in mind, the advice below is not intended to be comprehensive, but to review some potentially helpful practices for clinicians.

a. Suicide assessment is an essential part of a comprehensive psychiatric evaluation. The first step is to establish a rapport and constructive working relationship with the patient. Many studies demonstrate that better relationships protect against suicide and this includes that between clinician and patient. We recommend a supportive, straightforward, honest, and practical approach. Practitioners should not be afraid to ask patients directly about current suicidal ideation, intent, plans, reasons for living, and sources of support. Beyond psychiatric signs and symptoms, practitioners should focus on history of prior suicide attempts or self-harm including frequency, lethality, and recency as well as alcohol and/or drug abuse. Other important factors include past treatment, history of family dysfunction, family history of mental illness or suicide, recent stressors, and psychological strengths and vulnerabilities.

b. Clinicians should inquire specifically about suicidal ideation and/or plans and availability of the means to carry out the plan.

c. Clinicians should estimate suicide risk in the individual patient based on the presence of both risk factors and protective factors. Although research has tended to emphasize risk factors, there is increasing attention toward protective factors and it is essential to inventory both in clinical practice.

d. As with treatment of any medical illness, clinicians must balance potential risks and benefits of somatic or psychosocial therapies, including hospitalization, for each individual patient. Patients should be educated about potential risks and benefits of therapy in order to make informed decisions about treatment. Clinical monitoring should be frequent (e.g., weekly or biweekly), especially during early treatment, dosage adjustments, or periods of stress. The first weeks after initiating use of an antidepressant medication may be associated with an elevated risk of agitation and irritability, which may increase suicidal risk. If logistics, such as distance or insurance coverage, preclude frequent in-person visits, then brief telephone checks can be very helpful.

e. With potentially suicidal patients, practitioners should pay special attention to collaboration and communication with other members of a treatment team, particularly in *split treatments* (involving both a pharmacologist and a therapist). Education of patients and, where possible, family members and friends, is also important (for review, see "Practice Guideline for the Assessment and Treatment of Patients With Suicidal Behaviors" 2003, pp. 57–58). In some clinical situations it may help to have joint sessions with a suicidal patient and her or his significant other or a family member.

f. Clinicians should bear in mind that different sociodemographic groups have different patterns of suicidal behavior and prevention efforts should differ accordingly. Adolescent and young adult suicidality may be associated with interpersonal/psychosocial triggers, impulsivity, and substance abuse more often than in older individuals. Adult suicidality among women may occur during pregnancy and with postpartum mood disorders, whereas among men it may be especially associated with job or relationship loss. Late-life suicidality is often associated with medical and functional disability, social isolation, and well-planned, more lethal methods. Persons living in poor or crime-ridden communities may have easier access to firearms. Clinicians should be alert to the unique patterns of risks among different population subgroups and should tailor prevention efforts accordingly.

g. Means restriction at the individual patient level—such as reducing access to firearms, drugs that are dangerous in overdose, or car keys by removing them from the home of a suicidal person—is also an important area where a practitioner can and often should intervene.

h. Practitioners should always document their evaluations, discussions with other caregivers or close contacts of the patient, decision-making process, and treatment plans, as well as patient response and progress, in the patient's chart.

i. Every individual patient has a unique mixture of risk and protective factors. These dictate specific targets for intervention by the clinician. For example, social isolation should prompt consideration of outreach to family and/or friends of the patient or exploration of possibilities for socialization such as support groups. Severe depression or melancholia, the latter itself a risk factor for suicidal behavior (Grunebaum et al. 2004), warrants aggressive antidepressant pharmacotherapy, possibly with adjunctive psychotherapy. Relational dysfunction and/or signs of personality pathology with suicidality may warrant a specific psychotherapy such as dialectical behavioral therapy. Psychotic symptoms, bipolarity, anxiety, and/or substance abuse require specific somatic or psychosocial therapies. Failure to establish an adequate working relationship with an outpatient clinician, lack of social supports, impaired judgment, or acute suicidal plans or intent often require inpatient hospitalization. These are only some examples intended to illustrate the multimodal approach that clinicians should follow. By analogy, any tributary whose flow can be lessened will reduce the risk of the river flooding downstream.

Key Points

- Suicide is an important public health problem globally and in the United States, where it outnumbers HIV-related illnesses and homicide as an annual cause of death. Suicide rates vary markedly by sociodemographic group and are highest among elderly, white males.

- Evidence supports numerous risk factors for suicide, such as a prior attempt, psychiatric illness, social isolation, substance abuse, aggression, and impulsivity. However, while suicide is commonly associated with one or more such risk factors, the presence of any one factor is often not useful for predicting suicide by an individual patient. This is because of the low specificity, or high false positive rates, of such risk factors. In other words, most patients with any specific risk factor or even combinations thereof do not commit suicide.

- Primary prevention aims to prevent suicidal behavior before it occurs. The most effective methods appear to be multilevel interventions, which have been carried out in settings like the United States Air Force. These usually include training and support for primary care practitioners and other gatekeepers in the detection and treatment of depression and suicidality, as well as efforts to destigmatize and facilitate help seeking in the community. The reported success of these efforts may relate to published research demonstrating that most persons who commit suicide have contact with a primary care clinician not long before death.

- Secondary prevention aims to prevent the repetition of suicidal behavior. Interventions include
  - counseling during suicidal crises, such as through telephone hotlines
  - treatment of underlying psychiatric disorders with somatic or psychotherapeutic modalities
  - outreach to isolated elderly persons
  - restrictions on access to means of suicide, such as firearms, drugs, and domestic gas regulations
  - cooperation with media: 1) to restrict reporting of suicides (because dramatic reports can promote suicides); and 2) to enhance public education.

  Evidence supporting the effectiveness of these interventions varies.
- Tertiary prevention involves efforts to reduce the longer-term sequelae of suicidal behavior. Examples include minimizing injury and disability by prescribing suicidal individuals drugs known to be relatively safe in overdose, such as SSRIs, and supporting the suicidal person's family members, who themselves may be at risk.
- Suicide is one of the top causes of death among adolescents. Numerous risk factors have been identified. Certain youth subgroups may be at particularly high risk. School-based prevention efforts appear to improve knowledge about and attitudes toward mental illnesses, but it is unclear whether suicidal behavior rates are reduced.
- Suicide prevention by clinicians with individual patients requires comprehensive evaluation of risk and protective factors, weighing the relative risks and benefits of alternative treatments, collaboration with other caregivers (including the patient's family and friends), close follow-up, and careful documentation.

References

Andersen VA, Andersen M, Rosholm JV, et al: Contacts to the healthcare system prior to suicide: a comprehensive analysis using registers for general and psychiatric hospital admissions, contacts to general practitioners and practicing specialists and drug prescriptions. Acta Psychiatr Scand 102:126–134, 2000

Anderson RN: Deaths: leading causes for 2000. Natl Vital Stat Rep 50:1–85, 2002

Aseltine RH Jr, James A, Schilling EA, et al: Evaluating the SOS suicide prevention program: a replication and extension. BMC Public Health 7 (July 18):161, 2007

Babigian HM, Guttmacher LB: Epidemiologic considerations in electroconvulsive therapy. Arch Gen Psychiatry 41:246–253, 1984

Baca-García E, Diaz-Sastre C, Basurte E, et al: A prospective study of the paradoxical relationship between impulsivity and lethality of suicide attempts. J Clin Psychiatry 62:560–564, 2001

Bagley C: The evaluation of a suicide prevention scheme by an ecological method. Soc Sci Med 2:1–14, 1968

Baldessarini RJ, Tarazi FI: Drugs and the Treatment of Psychiatric Disorders: Psychosis and Mania, 10th Edition. New York, McGraw-Hill, 2001

Baldessarini RJ, Tondo L, Hennen J: Effects of lithium treatment and its discontinuation on suicidal behavior in bipolar manic-depressive disorders. J Clin Psychiatry 60 (suppl 2):77–84, discussion 111–116, 1999

Baldessarini RJ, Tondo L, Hennen J: Lithium treatment and suicide risk in major affective disorders: update and new findings. J Clin Psychiatry 64 (suppl 5):44–52, 2003

Baldessarini RJ, Tondo L, Davis P, et al: Decreased risk of suicides and attempts during long-term lithium treatment: a meta-analytic review. Bipolar Disord 8:625–639, 2006

Barraclough BM, Jennings C: Suicide prevention by the Samaritans: a controlled study of effectiveness. Lancet 2:237–239, 1977

Bateman A, Fonagy P: Treatment of borderline personality disorder with psychoanalytically oriented partial hospitalization: an 18-month follow-up. Am J Psychiatry 158:36–42, 2001

Bongar B, Goldberg L, Cleary K, et al: Marriage, family, family therapy, and suicide, in Comprehensive Textbook of Suicidology. Edited by Maris RW, Berman AL, Silverman MM. New York, Guilford, 2000, pp 222-239

Bostwick JM, Pankratz VS: Affective disorders and suicide risk: a reexamination. Am J Psychiatry 157:1925–1932, 2000

Brent DA, Melhem N: Familial transmission of suicidal behavior. Psychiatr Clin North Am 31(2):157–177, 2008

Brezo J, Paris J, Turecki G: Personality traits as correlates of suicidal ideation, suicide attempts, and suicide completions: a systematic review. Acta Psychiatr Scand 113:180–206, 2006

Brodsky BS, Oquendo M, Ellis SP, et al: The relationship of childhood abuse to impulsivity and suicidal behavior in adults with major depression. Am J Psychiatry 158:1871–1877, 2001

Brown CH, Wyman PA, Brinales JM, et al: The role of randomized trials in testing interventions for the prevention of youth suicide. Int Rev Psychiatry, 19:617–631, 2007

Brown GK, Ten Have T, Henriques GR, et al: Cognitive therapy for the prevention of suicide attempts: a randomized controlled trial. JAMA 294:563–570, 2005

Burgess S, Geddes J, Hawton K, et al: Lithium for maintenance treatment of mood disorders. Cochrane Database Syst Rev Issue 3, Art No: CD003013. DOI: 10.1002/14651858, 2001

Caldwell CB, Gottesman II: Schizophrenics kill themselves too: a review of risk factors for suicide. Schizophr Bull 16:571–589, 1990

Challiner V, Griffiths L: Electroconvulsive therapy: a review of the literature. J Psychiatr Ment Health Nurs 7:191–198, 2000

Cipriani A, Pretty H, Hawton K, et al: Lithium in the prevention of suicidal behavior and all-cause mortality in patients with mood disorders: a systematic review of randomized trials. Am J Psychiatry 162:1805–1819, 2005

Clarkin JF, Levy KN, Lenzenweger MF, et al: Evaluating three treatments for borderline personality disorder: a multiwave study. Am J Psychiatry 164:922–928, 2007

Currier D, Mann JJ: Stress, genes and the biology of suicidal behavior. Psychiatr Clin North Am 31:247–269, 2008

De Leo D, Dello Buono M, Dwyer J: Suicide among the elderly: the long-term impact of a telephone support and assessment intervention in northern Italy. Br J Psychiatry 181:226–229, 2002

Dervic K, Oquendo MA, Grunebaum MF, et al: Religious affiliation and suicide attempt. Am J Psychiatry 161:2303-2308, 2004

Fergusson D, Doucette S, Glass KC, et al: Association between suicide attempts and selective serotonin reuptake inhibitors: systematic review of randomised controlled trials. BMJ 330:396–400, 2005

Gaynes BN, West SL, Ford CA, et al; U.S. Preventive Services Task Force: Screening for suicide risk in adults: a summary of the evidence for the U.S. Preventive Services Task Force. Ann Intern Med 140:822–835, 2004

Goldney RD: Risk factors for suicidal behaviour: translating knowledge into practice, in Prevention and Treatment of Suicidal Behaviour: From Science to Practice. Edited by Hawton K. Oxford, UK, Oxford University Press, 2005a, pp 161–162

Goldney RD: Suicide prevention: a pragmatic review of recent studies. Crisis 26:128–140, 2005b

Gould MS, Greenberg T, Velting DM, et al: Youth suicide risk and preventive interventions: a review of the past 10 years. J Am Acad Child Adolesc Psychiatry 42:386–405, 2003

Gould MS, Kalafat J, Harrismunfakh JL, et al: An evaluation of crisis hotline outcomes: part 2: suicidal callers. Suicide Life Threat Behav 37:338–352, 2007

Grunebaum MF, Mann JJ: How strong is evidence for new suicide warning? Curr Psychiatr 6:27–43, 2007

Grunebaum MF, Galfalvy HC, Oquendo MA, et al: Melancholia and the probability and lethality of suicide attempts. Br J Psychiatry 184:534–535, 2004

Gunnell D, Saperia J, Ashby D: Selective serotonin reuptake inhibitors (SSRIs) and suicide in adults: meta-analysis of drug company data from placebo controlled, randomised controlled trials submitted to the MHRA's safety review. BMJ 330:385–390, 2005

Guthrie E, Kapur N, Mackway-Jones K, et al: Randomised controlled trial of brief psychological intervention after deliberate self poisoning. BMJ 323:135–138, 2001

Hawton K, Townsend E, Arensman E, et al: Psychosocial and pharmacological treatments for deliberate self harm. Cochrane Database Syst Rev Issue 4, Art No: CD001764. DOI: 10.1002/14651858, 1999

Hawton K, Simkin S, Deeks J, UK legislation on analgesic packs: before and after study of long term effect on poisonings. BMJ 329(7474):1076, 2004

Hawton K: Restriction of access to methods of suicide as a means of suicide prevention, in Prevention and Treatment of Suicidal Behavior: From Science to Practice. Edited by Hawton K. Oxford, UK, Oxford University Press, 2005, pp 279–291

Hegerl U, Althaus D, Schmidtke A, et al: The alliance against depression: 2-year evaluation of a community-based intervention to reduce suicidality. Psychol Med 36:1225–1233, 2006

Hennen J, Baldessarini RJ: Suicidal risk during treatment with clozapine: a meta-analysis. Schizophr Res 73:139–145, 2005

Isacsson G, Holmgren P, Druid H, et al: Psychotropics and suicide prevention: implications from toxicological screening of 5281 suicides in Sweden 1992–1994. Br J Psychiatry 174:259–265, 1999

Isometsä ET, Henriksson MM, Aro HM, et al: Suicide in major depression. Am J Psychiatry 151:530–536, 1994

Khan A, Khan S, Kolts R, et al: Suicide rates in clinical trials of SSRIs, other antidepressants, and placebo: analysis of FDA reports. Am J Psychiatry 160:790–792, 2003

King R, Nurcombe B, Bickman L, et al: Telephone counselling for adolescent suicide prevention: changes in suicidality and mental state from beginning to end of a counselling session. Suicide Life Threat Behav 33:400–411, 2003

Knox KL, Litts DA, Talcott GW, et al: Risk of suicide and related adverse outcomes after exposure to a suicide prevention programme in the US Air Force: cohort study. BMJ 327:1376–1380, 2003

Knox KL, Conwell Y, Caine ED: If suicide is a public health problem, what are we doing to prevent it? Am J Public Health 94:37–45, 2004

Krutman N: The coal gas story. Br J Prev Soc Med 30:86–93, 1976

Lester D: The effectiveness of suicide prevention centers: a review. Suicide Life Threat Behav 27:304–310, 1997

Linehan MM, Comtois KA, Murray AM, et al: Two-year randomized controlled trial and follow-up of dialectical behavior therapy vs therapy by experts for suicidal behaviors and borderline personality disorder. Arch Gen Psychiatry 63:757–766, 2006

Luoma JB, Martin CE, Pearson JL: Contact with mental health and primary care providers before suicide: a review of the evidence. Am J Psychiatry 159:909–916, 2002

Malone KM, Oquendo MA, Haas GL, et al: Protective factors against suicidal acts in major depression: reasons for living. Am J Psychiatry 157:1084-1088, 2000

Mann JJ, Arango V: Integration of neurobiology and psychopathology in a unified model of suicidal behavior. J Clin Psychopharmacol 12 (suppl 2):2S–7S, 1992

Mann JJ, Currier D: Prevention of suicide. Psychiatr Ann 37:331–339, 2007

Mann JJ, Waternaux C, Haas GL, et al: Toward a clinical model of suicidal behavior in psychiatric patients. Am J Psychiatry 156:181–189, 1999

Mann JJ, Apter A, Bertolote J, et al: Suicide prevention strategies: a systematic review. JAMA 294:2064–2074, 2005

Mann JJ, Arango VA, Avenevoli S, et al: Candidate endophenotypes for genetic studies of suicidal behavior. Biol Psychiatry 65:556–563, 2009

Maris RW: Suicide. Lancet 360:319–326, 2002

Marzuk PM, Tardiff K, Leon AC, et al: Use of prescription psychotropic drugs among suicide victims in New York City. Am J Psychiatry 152:1520–1522, 1995

McGirr A, Renaud J, Séguin M, et al: Course of major depressive disorder and suicide outcome: a psychological autopsy study. J Clin Psychiatry 69:966–970, 2008

McMillan D, Gilbody S, Beresford E, et al: Can we predict suicide and non-fatal self-harm with the Beck Hopelessness Scale?: a meta-analysis. Psychol Med 37:769–778, 2007

Meltzer HY: Suicidality in schizophrenia: a review of the evidence for risk factors and treatment options. Curr Psychiatry Rep 4:279–283, 2002

Meltzer HY, Alphs L, Green AI, et al: Clozapine treatment for suicidality in schizophrenia: International Suicide Prevention Trial (InterSePT). Arch Gen Psychiatry 60:82–91, 2003

Michel K: Suicide prevention and primary care, in The International Handbook of Suicide and Attempted Suicide. Edited by Hawton K, van Heeringen K. West Sussex, England, Wiley, 2000, pp 662–665

Miller HL, Coombs DW, Leeper JD, et al: An analysis of the effects of suicide prevention facilities on suicide rates in the United States. Am J Public Health 74:340–343, 1984

Motto JA, Bostrom AG: A randomized controlled trial of postcrisis suicide prevention. Psychiatr Serv 52:828–833, 2001

National Center for Injury Prevention and Control: Web-based Injury Statistics Query and Reporting System [WISQARS™ Web site]. Available at: http://www.cdc.gov/ncipc/wisqars/. Accessed November 14, 2008.

O'Leary D, Paykel E, Todd C, et al: Suicide in primary affective disorders revisited: a systematic review by treatment era. J Clin Psychiatry 62:804–811, 2001

Oquendo MA, Malone KM, Mann JJ: Suicide: risk factors and prevention in refractory major depression. Depress Anxiety 5:202–211, 1997

Paris J: Predicting and preventing suicide: do we know enough to do either? Harv Rev Psychiatry 14:233–240, 2006

Pitman A: Policy on the prevention of suicidal behaviour; one treatment for all may be an unrealistic expectation. J R Soc Med 100:461–464, 2007

Placidi GP, Oquendo MA, Malone KM, et al: Aggressivity, suicide attempts, and depression: relationship to cerebrospinal fluid monoamine metabolite levels. Biol Psychiatry 50:783–791, 2001

Plutchik R: Aggression, violence, and suicide, in Comprehensive Textbook of Suicidology. Edited by Maris RW, Berman AL, Silverman MM. New York, Guilford, 2000, pp 413-415

Practice guideline for the assessment and treatment of patients with suicidal behaviors. Am J Psychiatry 160 (11, suppl):1–60, 2003

Rich CL, Isacsson G: Suicide and antidepressants in south Alabama: evidence for improved treatment of depression. J Affect Disord 45:135–142, 1997

Rutz W, von Knorring L, Wålinder J: Long-term effects of an educational program for general practitioners given by the Swedish Committee for the Prevention and Treatment of Depression. Acta Psychiatr Scand 85:83–88, 1992

Simon GE, Savarino J, Operskalski B, et al: Suicide risk during antidepressant treatment. Am J Psychiatry 163:41–47, 2006

Sonneck G, Etzersdorfer E, Nagel-Kuess S: Imitative suicide on the Viennese subway. Soc Sci Med 38:453–457, 1994

Spirito A, Esposito-Smythers C: Attempted and completed suicide in adolescence. Annu Rev Clin Psychol 2:237–266, 2006

Steele MM, Doey T: Suicidal behaviour in children and adolescents: part 1: etiology and risk factors. Can J Psychiatry 52 (suppl 1):21S–33S, 2007a

Steele MM, Doey T: Suicidal behaviour in children and adolescents: part 2: treatment and prevention. Can J Psychiatry 52 (suppl 1):35S–45S, 2007b

Stone M, Jones L, Levenson M, et al: Clinical review: relationship between antidepressant drugs and suicidality in adults: statistical evaluation of suicidality in adults treated with antidepressants. U.S. Food and Drug Administration, Center for Drug Evaluation and Research. November 16, 2006. Available at: http://www.fda.gov/ohrms/dockets/ac/06/briefing/2006-4272b1-01-FDA.pdf. Accessed July 13, 2009.

Suominen KH, Isometsä ET, Henriksson MM, et al: Suicide attempts and personality disorder. Acta Psychiatr Scand 102:118–125, 2000

World Health Organization: Suicide prevention (SUPRE). 2008. Available at: http://www.who.int/mental_health/prevention/suicide/suicideprevent/en/. Accessed September 10, 2008.

Wyman PA, Brown CH, Inman J, et al: Randomized trial of a gatekeeper program for suicide prevention: 1-year impact on secondary school staff. J Consult Clin Psychol 76:104–115, 2008

9

Prevention of Family Violence

Kenneth Rogers, M.D., M.S.H.S.

Barbara Baumgardner, Ph.D., R.N.

Kathleen Connors, L.C.S.W.-C.

Patricia Martens, Ph.D.

Laurel Kiser, Ph.D., M.B.A.

Families are the basic social unit of our society to provide for and meet the fundamental needs of all of their individual members. Most families are able to successfully accomplish this, but an alarming number are unable to create or maintain a safe environment due to family violence.

Family violence encompasses physical, sexual, and psychological aggression between or among any members of a family. Physical aggression, such as pushing, slapping, scratching, kicking, or using weapons to hurt a family member, is the easiest to detect, although it often remains hidden from those outside the family. Witnessing violence or being victimized by sexual assault, neglect, threats of harm, coercion, and degradation also constitute forms of family violence.

Most commonly, family violence occurs within spousal or parent-child relationships. Within the parent-child relationship, violence is typically parent to child (child abuse), although children can become violent toward their parents as in cases of adolescent aggression or elder abuse. Interpersonal violence can also occur between siblings of any age. Unfortunately, the violence within families often occurs across multiple subsystems. For example, studies demonstrate the propensity for mothers who are in abusive relationships to be more abusive toward their children than mothers in nonviolent relationships are, with child maltreatment co-occurring with intimate partner violence in 30%–70% of families affected by intimate partner violence (Mahoney et al. 2003). Generally, family violence is not a single act of aggression but rather is revealed as repeated patterns of family interactions (Gelles and Maynard 1987). Intergenerational transmission of violence is evident in the fact that about one-third of children who were abused become perpetrators in adulthood (Kaufman and Zigler 1987). As Jaffe and Wolfe (1986, p. 142) observed, "Each generation learns to be violent by being a participant in a violent family."

Prevalence

The following statistics reveal the extent of family violence in the United States (Emery and Laumann-Billings 1998; U.S. Department of Justice 2005):

- Twenty-seven percent of all violent crimes occur among family members.
- Almost 20% of adult women have been physically abused (excluding sexual assault) by a male partner.
- Twenty-two percent of women and 7.5% of men report that they have been raped and/or physically assaulted by an intimate partner (i.e., spouse, partner, or date) at some time in their life.
- Between 3.3 and 10 million children witness domestic violence yearly.

- More than 1,500 women were murdered in 1995 by their husband or boy-friend. And more than 60% of women murdered in 2004 were killed by a spouse or intimate partner.
- Ninety-three to ninety-seven percent of children experience physical discipline ranging from spankings to beatings.
- 2.5 million reports of child abuse are made yearly, with 20%–35% of these children suffering a serious injury and 1,200–1,500 children dying annually as a result.
- Almost 900,000 cases of neglect and abuse are substantiated yearly in this country, with 300,000 youths placed in care outside the home.

The consequences of family violence are well documented. Although direct victims are at greatest risk of harm, the effects are systemic. They include physical injuries and death of victims, increased risk of short- and long-term mental and physical health problems, and practical consequences such as the break-up of the family unit.

Women are more often the victims of domestic violence than men and are more likely to suffer injuries and health consequences such as sexually transmitted diseases, gastrointestinal and gynecological diseases, and mental health consequences such as depression, substance use disorders, eating and sleeping problems, chronic panic, and posttraumatic stress disorder (Campbell 2002). Children often have been considered the unseen victims of domestic violence; the negative sequelae of psychological trauma associated with domestic violence impact all aspects of their development (Groves 2002). Children exposed to domestic violence exhibit higher rates of emotional and behavioral problems, including low self-esteem; unresolved feelings of anger, guilt, and fear; and depression, anxiety, and aggression toward both peers and those considered weaker (Goodman 2006; McCloskey et al. 1995). Growing up in a violent home is one of the greatest risk factors for the development of antisocial behavior. The child exposed to violence is more likely to attempt suicide, abuse drugs and alcohol, run away from home, engage in teenage prostitution, and commit sexual assault crimes (Wolfe et al. 1995). These children are also more likely to have physical problems including allergies, asthma, gastrointestinal problems, headaches, and influenza (Graham-Bermann and Seng 2005).

Etiologies of Family Violence

Herron and colleagues noted that a family has "the potential for becoming a violent place due to both the individual personality characteristics of its members and their systemic interaction, as well as the impact of social-structural violence on the family. Family members need the personal resources to cope with the potential for violence that surrounds them and exists within them. When these resources are lacking, then violence is likely to occur" (Herron et al. 1994, p. 222).

A variety of theories and models have been proposed to explain how and why violence disrupts families. Table 9–1 provides an overview of the various theories. Each of the theories espoused has been empirically tested and all have data supporting them. All of the theories also have significant limitations, and in reality the causes of family violence are multiple (Herron et al. 1994). Family violence occurs in the context of sociopsychological stressors embedded within the microsystem of the family, the mesosystem of the family in the community, and the macrosystem of the norms of society (Belsky 1993).

Individual (Microsystem) Risks

Individual characteristics of family members make independent contributions to the occurrence of family violence. The biology of the stress response, including the fight response and the genetic pathways through which aggressive tendencies are inherited, must be considered in the dynamics underlying family violence. Further, high incidences of parental distress, psychopathology, and substance abuse are linked to heightened risks for violence within the family (Emery and Laumann-Billings 1998; Herron et al. 1994). Dominance and its counterpoint, vulnerability or dependency, are related to domestic violence and child abuse (Bornstein 2006). The child must also be seen as an active participant in the relationship dynamics, though not at fault when maltreatment occurs. This may be seen in the relationship between maltreatment and early child stressors such as premature birth, developmental delays, or congenital malformations. The underlying assumption seems to be that the child may elicit different responses from the parent (i.e., maltreatment) than the child would if development assumed a normal trajectory. However, the consensus regarding bidirectionality of effects is that the young child has little effect on the quality of parenting over time or on the overall quality of rela-

Table 9–1. Etiological theories of family violence

Individual-driven	Family-driven	Society/culture-driven
Psychopathology	Intergenerational transmission	Culture of violence
Substance use or abuse	Family stress theory	Patriarchy
Previous victimization	Family regulation	Feminist theory
Vulnerability of the victim	Family processes	Resource theory
Biology of aggression	Learning theory or modeling	

tionships with caregivers, particularly at the extreme end of the parenting distribution where abuse lies (Pianta et al. 1997).

For example, as mentioned earlier, child abuse co-occurs with intimate partner violence in a significant number of interpersonally violent homes. Witnessing violence is stressful and confusing for children, particularly if those involved with violence, either as the perpetrator or the victim (or both), are the people the child normally depends on for protection and resources. The confusion will likely result in either withdrawal (deactivation and internalization) or increased attempts at seeking attention (hyperactivation and externalization) by the child. The child's atypical behavior is likely to require additional effort on the part of the parent to understand and to choose how to respond. This places additional stress on the already stressed environment and could result in child maltreatment. Although the child's characteristics (e.g., temperament, regulatory skills, clarity of cues, cognitions) interact dynamically with the caregiver's responses, the child's contribution to the overall effect is relatively minor.

Family (Mesosystem) Risks

Families are systems organized around structures including roles, rules, and patterned interactions. Structural factors that influence family violence include the abuse of relationship power that often coincides with the hierarchical nature of families and the traditional role of the male as the head of the family. Low family income and geographical isolation increase the risk of multiple forms of family violence.

As systems, families seek to regulate the emotions and behaviors of family members to maintain balance. These attempts to regulate stressful situations can be understood through the ABCX model. This model posits that a family's available coping resources and interpretation of the stressful event will lead to an eventual outcome. Based on the ABCX family crisis model (Hill 1958), if family violence is seen as the outcome of a family experiencing a mismatch between demands and resources, it is predictable that when the normal levels of everyday difficulties encountered by families are compounded by stressors that affect their economic and human resources, then violence becomes more likely.

An additional group of theories focuses on learned behavior in family violence. Studies that have attempted to demonstrate common traits (e.g., anger or aggression) among maltreating parents have largely failed (Pianta et al. 1997). Instead, current theory suggests that when family interactions involve aggression, such behavior becomes normalized and becomes an acceptable form of interpersonal relatedness (Fosco et al. 2007). Family violence may thus have a pervasive influence on the representation of close interpersonal relationships; consistent failure of adults to provide protection and control their anger is internalized.

Society (Macrosystem) Risks

At the societal level, family violence is influenced by structural factors, values and beliefs, and norms. Structural factors consist of the male-female inequality in our culture, poverty, racial/ethnic segregation, and community disintegration. Values and beliefs that support family violence take account of the acceptability of aggression as a means of solving problems and the sovereignty of the family unit (Fosco et al. 2007). Family violence is also influenced by the widespread use of physical punishment in the United States.

Interaction of Risk and Protective Factors

Several researchers suggest that the risk factors for family violence are cumulative rather than merely additive (Biederman et al. 1995). Tables 9–2 and 9–3 summarize the risks for child abuse and domestic violence, the two most common forms of family violence.

Risks also interact with protective factors, those qualities that promote resilience. In general, research has found that emotionally satisfying and nurturing relationships—dependable and meaningful social networks available during stressful life events—are protective factors. In children who have expe-

Table 9–2. Risk factors for child abuse

Caregiver factors	Early developmental experiences (including having been a victim of child abuse)
	Internal working model
	Low level of education
	Poor social skills
	Insufficient knowledge about child development
	History of mental illness
	Substance abuse
	Having a criminal record
	Perception of increased stress
	Adolescent parenting
	Single parenting
	Poor prenatal care
	Harsh parenting style (e.g., curses at child when upset)
	Known history of abusing a child
Child factors	Temperament
	Decreased clarity of cues
	Poor regulatory ability
	Physical health problems
	Disability or developmental delay
	Prematurity or low birth weight
	Child ≤3 years old
Family and social factors	Domestic violence in the home
	Poverty
	Social isolation
	High levels of local unemployment
	Inadequate community resources
	Multiple young children
	Unwanted pregnancy or denial of pregnancy
	Being unprepared for stress of newborn
Sociopolitical factors	Disparity in access to health care
	Disparity in educational opportunities
	High crime neighborhoods/communities
	Tolerance of some types of interpersonal violence
	Unequal treatment due to gender
	High proportion of neighborhood poverty

Table 9–3.   Risk factors for domestic violence

Individual factors	African American or American Indian race/ethnicity; age 16–24 years; being female; being pregnant, divorced or separated; living in rental housing
Family and social factors	Experiencing or witnessing abuse as a child; unemployment; alcohol use by perpetrator; criminal behavior
Sociopolitical factors	Attitudes of patriarchy or entitlement

rienced abuse, those who were able to resolve family conflict and develop a supportive, nonabusive, and stable relationship with their parents or, later, an intimate partner, are able to go on to develop a secure attachment with their own children. Protective factors may also be developed through intervention. An understanding of the etiologies and risk and protective factors for family violence provides the foundation for determining effective prevention strategies.

Child Maltreatment

Enormous sums of time and money have been spent developing and implementing programs to prevent child abuse. However, only a small fraction of these efforts has included outcome assessments. Child maltreatment prevention programs have focused either on physical abuse and neglect or on sexual abuse. Although emotional and psychological maltreatment is commonly accepted as a type of abuse, little can be found in the literature on prevention efforts to address it.

Child Physical Abuse and Neglect

Primary Prevention

Among primary prevention programs for child physical abuse and neglect, there are two broad types. Some target a mass audience (universal preventive interventions) and commonly include some form of media that can reach all members of society. Various types of legal action also fall in this category. Others are characterized by a more personal approach (selective and indicated preventive interventions) and commonly include home visits by a professional or paraprofessional. Table 9–4 provides a summary of these efforts as well as treatment for children who have experienced sexual abuse.

Table 9–4.   Child maltreatment prevention efforts: summary of outcomes

Efforts to prevent	Outcomes
Child physical abuse and neglect	
Mass media campaigns (electronic and printed media)	Public awareness of child abuse and its consequences increased approximately ninefold from the mid 1970s to the early 1980s.
Home visitation programs, including parental education and modeling and rehearsing techniques	A large body of outcome data exist; however, only one RCT has shown reductions in actual child abuse (13 years after services), as opposed to child abuse proxies or more distal risk variables. Presence of domestic violence seems to attenuate potential benefits of home visitation programs on child abuse risk.
AF-CBT, a form of family therapy with cognitive-behavioral and psychoeducational underpinnings	One RCT showed reductions in parents' abuse potential, use of physical discipline, anger overexpression, psychological distress and drug use; reductions in child behavioral problems and family conflict; and increased family cohesion.
PCIT, widely tested with young children with behavioral problems; adapted for use with older children and children who have experienced physical abuse	One RCT showed reduction in abuse by improving parent-child interactions.
Child sexual abuse	
School-based primary prevention (classroom-based psychoeducation and rehearsal)	A substantial research base exists but no data address whether sexual abuse rates are affected. Children have increased knowledge and risk-reducing skills are improved. Possible iatrogenic effects have been reported.
TF-CBT, treatment with a cognitive-behavioral basis and psychoeducation	Numerous RCTs have shown reductions in childrens' symptoms of posttraumatic stress disorder, depression, and anxiety; externalizing behaviors; sexual behaviors; and feelings of shame and mistrust. Also reductions in parental depression and distress about the child's abuse, and improved parenting practices and support of child.

Note.   AF-CBT = abuse-focused cognitive-behavioral therapy; PCIT = parent-child interaction therapy; RCT = randomized, controlled trial; TF-CBT = trauma-focused cognitive-behavioral therapy.

Universal preventive interventions.   Mass media campaigns about child abuse and neglect were implemented beginning in the late 1970s, via advertisements and special segments through radio, television, and printed publications. Shortly before this, state-mandated reporting laws were put into effect, requiring certain professionals to report suspicions of child abuse. These efforts have been effective in raising awareness of the existence of child maltreatment and its harm to victims, from an awareness level of approximately 10% in the mid 1970s to approximately 90% in the early 1980s based on survey reports data (for a review, see Daro and McCurdy 2007). They have also been associated with an increase in the identification of maltreatment, as evidenced by a 225% increase in reports from 1976 to 1987 (Zellman and Fair 2002). Although mass media campaigns and reporting laws appear to have been effective educational and abuse identification strategies, they have not been proven to reduce the incidence or prevalence of child maltreatment.

Although not yet passed in the United States, laws prohibiting the use of corporal punishment (all forms, regardless of severity level) have been enacted in more than 20 countries around the world. Sweden was the first to pass such laws, in 1979, following a series of legislative reforms taking place over several decades that were designed to reduce the use of corporal punishment in schools and to discourage its use by parents. The ban on corporal punishment was enacted in tandem with a mass educational campaign (Durrant and Olsen 1997, as cited in Durrant and Janson 2005). Data suggest that parental use of corporal punishment subsequently declined in Sweden. Whereas nearly all mothers used physical discipline and 13% used object implements in Sweden in the 1950s, only one-third of 13- to 15-year-old youths reported ever being corporally disciplined in 1996, and 86% of 11- to 13-year-old youths reported no history of corporal punishment. Only 3% reported having been punished with an object in 2000 (Janson 2001; Statistiska Centralbyrån [SCB] 1996, as cited in Durrant and Janson 2005). Although corporal punishment rates appear to have declined in response to legislative action and mass education, rates of children's deaths at the hands of parents do not appear to have been affected (Beckett 2005).

Selective and indicated preventive interventions.   Several home visitation programs have been implemented on a large scale (e.g., Healthy Families America and the Nurse-Family Partnership [formerly called the *Nurse Home*

Visitation Program]) and evaluated, as discussed below. These interventions can vary widely regarding the visitors' credentials (professional or paraprofessional), program duration, participant selection criteria, and focus of the intervention (increasing social support vs. knowledge of child development). Nevertheless, they have a common conceptual base in the notion that parents are at risk for perpetrating child physical abuse because they are deficient in certain areas, and if those deficiencies can be remedied the parents will be at substantially lower risk. Home visitation programs usually begin perinatally or prenatally and continue through the child's first 2–3 years of life.

A large body of research on home visitation programs exists. Although evaluation has yielded inconsistent findings (for a review, see Daro and McCurdy 2007), some apparent benefits of home visitation include the following:

- Improved parental behavior and attitudes
- Increased parental use of community resources
- Increased maternal education, employment rates, and economic viability

These outcome variables are believed to be protective factors for child maltreatment. Home visitation programs have revealed small but significant effects of home visitation on child abuse and neglect reports (Geeraert et al. 2004; Sweet and Appelbaum 2004). However, few studies in the literature base employed randomized, controlled designs and used hard data on abuse and neglect reports following intervention. A qualitative review (see Chaffin 2005) of 12 randomized, controlled studies using protective services data as the child maltreatment outcome revealed only one with significant positive results: roughly one-third of home-visited families versus more than half of control families had state-verified reports of abuse or neglect 13 years after home visitation services (Olds et al. 1997). Moreover, a potential limitation is the presence of extensive domestic violence, which can interfere with participants' ability to benefit from home visitation programs (Eckenrode et al. 2000).

Secondary Prevention

Secondary prevention programs have incorporated home visitation and have sought to improve parenting skills, anger management, and social skills, as well as reduce depression (DePanfilis et al. 2008; Peterson et al. 2003); thus, they resemble primary prevention home visitation programs. However, they recruit families that evidence risk factors that are closer proxies to child maltreatment, such as use of physical discipline or unsubstantiated reports of neglect, rather than recruiting them based on demographic risk factors. Preliminary data from these programs suggest no significant effects on rates of child abuse and neglect based on child protective services reports, but did find improvements in protective factors (parenting attitudes, use of inductive discipline methods, developmentally based problem solving, and social support) and reductions in other risk factors (parental depression, anger, and stress; use of harsh discipline) (DePanfilis et al. 2008; Peterson et al. 2003).

Tertiary Prevention

Home visitation models have also been used with abusive families to prevent recurrence of physical abuse and/or neglect. However, a relatively recent randomized, controlled trial examining child protective services records after treatment revealed no benefits of adding a nurse home visitation component to standard treatment (consisting of recidivism risk assessment, parental education, and providing community-based referrals for various services) with these families (MacMillan et al. 2005). Various psychotherapy models with a cognitive-behavioral orientation are more commonly used and recognized as effective with child maltreatment victims and their families. The National Child Traumatic Stress Network (http://www.nctsnet.org) has identified several tertiary prevention methods as promising practices or empirically supported treatments for child maltreatment; synopses of their research can be found on their Web site. Two are discussed briefly below:

- Abuse-focused cognitive-behavioral therapy (AF-CBT) is a leading empirically based treatment for families who have been involved with child physical abuse. AF-CBT is designed to be relatively short-term and emphasizes skills teaching, behavior modification, and CBT principles. Benefits associated with AF-CBT include parental factors, such as reduced use of physical discipline, abuse potential, problematic anger expression, psychological distress, and drug use; child factors such as reduced externalization of problems; and family variables, such as reduced conflict and improved cohesion (results seen in AF-CBT recipients compared with a treatment-as-usual control group; Kolko 2002).

- Parent-child interaction therapy (PCIT) is another evidence-based therapy for child physical abuse. PCIT is conducted via a transmitter-receiver system through which a therapist coaches parents in relationship-building skills and effective behavior management. Compared with a standard community group treatment, PCIT has been associated with significantly lower rates of repeat physical abuse (19% vs. 49%, respectively; Chaffin et al. 2004).

Child Sexual Abuse

Whereas prevention efforts for physical abuse and neglect target potential or actual perpetrators, prevention programs for child sexual abuse usually target potential victims (and in the course of doing so, may reach actual victims). Most programs aiming to prevent sexual abuse have been either primary and universal in nature or tertiary and targeted for the prevention of future abuse and/or treatment of the abuse sequelae.

Primary Prevention

Primary prevention of sexual abuse typically has taken place in the school setting, and includes a knowledge and skills component emphasizing body ownership, interpersonal/physical boundaries, distinguishing appropriate versus inappropriate physical contact, declining inappropriate advances by others, and reporting to trusted adults any abuse or inappropriate advances. Changes in children's knowledge and skills have been measured using questionnaires or vignettes. Evaluations of these programs have found that children who participate in these programs, compared with those who do not participate, demonstrate increased knowledge and improvement in skills that would lower their risk of sexual abuse victimization (Zwi et al. 2007). Most studies that have examined retention in knowledge and skills have done so within 3 months posttreatment, and generally have found that treatment gains are retained; two studies have found that treatment gains remained stable at 6 and 12 months posttreatment (Zwi et al. 2007).

Disclosures of sexual abuse following school-based primary prevention trials have not been greater in treated versus control groups (Zwi et al. 2007). Whether these programs yield decreases in child sexual abuse incidence or prevalence is not known.

Most studies of child maltreatment prevention efforts do not assess iatrogenic effects. However, of the studies reviewed by Zwi and colleagues (2007), three-quarters of those measuring anxiety-based reactions (e.g., increased dependency, fear of strangers, and aggression) found adverse effects for children in their intervention groups, suggesting that adverse effects are distinct possibilities, and should be measured routinely in outcome studies.

Tertiary Prevention

The currently accepted gold standard of treatment for children who are suffering the consequences of sexual abuse is trauma-focused cognitive-behavioral therapy (TF-CBT), which involves victimized children and, ideally, their nonoffending parent(s) (Cohen et al. 2006). Through TF-CBT, children and parents are informed of common reactions to and symptoms stemming from the abuse, and are taught to regulate negative affects and how feelings, thoughts, and behaviors are interrelated. The developers of TF-CBT suggest that one of the most important aspects of the treatment is the child's development of a trauma narrative (a story of what occurred during the abuse, how it felt, and what it meant to the child) in order to impose order on the abuse experience. Consistently, TF-CBT has been found to reduce traumatic symptoms in the child (Berliner and Elliott 2002).

Domestic Violence

Concerns about the prevalence of domestic violence or intimate partner violence in the United States are fairly recent. Thus, development, dissemination, and evaluation of universal prevention efforts are in the early stages. Tertiary prevention services are better established and available in most communities.

Primary Prevention

In 1994, The Family Violence Prevention and Services Act was passed to support the work of local prevention projects. Recognizing that domestic violence is a preventable public health problem, the Centers for Disease Control and Prevention launched Domestic Violence Prevention Enhancement and Leadership Through Alliances (DELTA) in 2002 (http://www.cdc.gov/ncipc/DELTA/DELTA_AAG.pdf). DELTA takes a systematic approach to reduction of first-time victimization and perpetration by funding demonstration projects and supporting domestic violence coalitions that target prevention-focused training, technical assistance, and interventions. One example is *Choose Respect.* This comprehensive, community-based, multimedia curriculum invites parents and schools to partner with youths ages 11–14 years to learn about healthy relationships and prevent future domestic violence (Martin et al. 2009).

Secondary Prevention

Screening for domestic violence in primary care and mental health clinics is a viable secondary prevention strategy to reach women and children who are at high risk for exposure to or who are already experiencing family violence and are in need of help to achieve safety. In primary care settings, screening and assessment for domestic violence and subsequent referrals can be effective in interrupting and preventing recurrence of domestic violence and associated trauma (McFarlane et al. 2006). Many professional medical organizations, including the American Academy of Pediatrics, the American Medical Association, and the American Academy of Family Physicians, recommend that physicians remain alert for the signs and symptoms of family violence in medical visits, though it is not mandatory to use screening tools to help identify victims of domestic violence. Many professionals feel reluctant to screen for domestic violence because they lack training in this area, feel concerned about offending families and discussing marital issues in front of children, and know of few screening tools to identify parents and children affected by domestic violence and community resources to refer them to (Nygren et al. 2004). Cultural and contextual variants impact providers' willingness to screen as well as patients' comfort with disclosing domestic violence. Children and parents report concerns that disclosure might escalate the violence and that child welfare authorities might be contacted and result in family separation along with loss of their home and established support systems, including neighbors, siblings, school contacts, and peer groups.

Tertiary Prevention

Hotlines, shelters, and advocacy services are vital resources for domestic violence victims. Hotlines offer crisis assistance, support, and information and are usually staffed by trained volunteers or paraprofessionals and supervised by professional staff. For example, the National Domestic Violence Hotline at (800) 799-7233 (the last four digits spell *SAFE*; there is also a TTY number, [800] 787-3224, for access via teletypewriters) provides 24-hour crisis assistance and referrals to local services, including shelters. Shelters provide temporary safe havens for families and, depending on funding, can offer an array of advocacy and mental health treatments. In a statewide evaluation of Illinois's domestic violence services, these resources were deemed effective in helping victims of domestic violence acquire safety, gain information about violence, increase social support, and improve decision-making, self-efficacy, and coping skills (Bennett et al. 2004). The Community Advocacy Project is an effective advocacy program that trains paraprofessionals to help families obtain needed community resources and social support. This empowerment-based intervention has been shown to improve quality of life and decrease the risk of repeated abuse in randomized clinical trials (Bybee and Sullivan 2002).

In addition to using these services, victims of domestic violence can apply for a protective order or restraining order. The perpetrator is ordered by the court to stay away from the victim's home or workplace; however, such orders often do not override court-ordered visitation or custody agreements. Court-ordered supervised visitations are another resource for parents and children affected by domestic violence. Supervised visitation programs may be effective in reducing further exposure to violence and minimizing the symptoms of trauma (Van Horn and Groves 2006).

Evidence-based mental health interventions designed to help parents and children recover from the impact of domestic violence (summarized in Table 9–5) include Kids' Club and Moms Empowerment, and Child-Parent Psychotherapy for Family Violence (CPP-FV). Kids' Club and Moms Empowerment are 10-week, concurrent programs for mothers and children exposed to domestic violence. In Kids' Club, children are taught about the attitudes and beliefs associated with family violence and the skills needed to support their emotional adjustment and social skills development. The program aims to enhance the child's sense of safety, to develop the therapeutic alliance, and to create a common vocabulary of emotions for making sense of violent experiences. Later sessions address responsibility for violence, managing feelings and family relationships, and conflict resolution. Moms Empowerment is a parenting program that supports mothers by empowering them to understand

Table 9–5. Practices to address the impact of domestic violence on children and parents: summary of outcomes

Practice	Outcomes
CPP-FV	Has been tested in two RCTs by the developer and by an independent researcher. Positive results were demonstrated in child symptom reduction, reduction of caregiver avoidance, and attachment.
Kids' Club and Moms Empowerment	A pseudo-RCT demonstrated that children's externalizing and internalizing behaviors decreased and that mothers' and children's knowledge and attitudes about violence improved.
AMEND	Meta-analyses and three urban batterer program evaluations of AMEND outcomes show tentative effects. Program completion reduced the probability of reassault during the 15-month follow-up by 33% for the full sample, and by nearly 50% for the court-ordered men.
DAIP	In an RCT, those assigned to the intervention showed significantly lower levels of reassault, based on official arrest and complaint records. However, during the 12-month follow-up, victims reported no significant differences in rates of overall abuse or severe abuse.

Note. AMEND = Abusive Men Exploring New Directions; CPP-FV = Child-Parent Psychotherapy for Family Violence; DAIP = Domestic Abuse Intervention Project; RCT = randomized, controlled trial.

the impact of violence on their child's development by increasing parental competence and safety skills (Graham-Bermann et al. 2007).

CPP-FV is a psychotherapy model that targets parents with children from infancy through the age of 8 years. It integrates psychodynamic, attachment, trauma, cognitive-behavioral, and social-learning theories into a dyadic treatment approach designed to restore the child-parent relationship and improve the child's developmental trajectory as well as to effect recovery from the traumatic experience of domestic violence (Lieberman et al. 2006; Toth et al. 2002). In addition to psychotherapy, the clinician offers "concrete assistance with problems in daily living" and works with the family in the home or in community settings. In two randomized clinical trials by the developer and an independent researcher, CPP-FV was found to reduce child and maternal

PTSD symptoms as well as improve attachment (Cicchetti et al. 2006; Lieberman et al. 2005, 2006; Toth et al. 2002).

In addition to these effective interventions, there are promising practices that engage in collaborative community partnerships to serve families affected by domestic violence. The Child Witness to Violence Project is a counseling, advocacy, and outreach project in Boston that focuses on helping families with young children exposed to domestic violence or community violence, by helping them gain access to comprehensive services including medical care, mental health care, and legal services (Groves and Gewirtz 2006). Domestic Violence Home Visit Intervention is a collaborative project between the Yale University Child Study Center and the New Haven (Connecticut) Police Department. The project provides training to and collaborates with members of law enforcement, community-based advocacy, and mental health agencies to increase child safety and decrease negative psychological effects of exposure to domestic violence (Berkman et al. 2004). The project conducts outreach home visits by teams of advocates and patrol officers who provide information on the judicial processes, available community resources, and children's responses to violence and trauma.

Lastly, two interventions targeting male abusers are Abusive Men Exploring New Directions (AMEND) and the Domestic Abuse Intervention Project (DAIP); results of these interventions are summarized in Table 9–5. AMEND is a 9-month, court-ordered or voluntary program with some degree of success in preventing repeated assault (Gondolf and Jones 2001). The program offers counseling aimed at improving skills (e.g., conflict resolution, anger management, communication) needed to reduce domestic violence, and advocacy services are offered to partners and children. DAIP is a collaborative model that brings together law enforcement, the criminal and civil courts, and human service providers to offer a 28-week curriculum-based educational program for offenders. DAIP also offers advocacy services, community resources, and educational programs to the female partners who were abused (Taylor et al. 2001). A systematic approach that supports families over time and offers assistance with the problems that contribute to high-stress situations (e.g., unemployment, substance abuse, unstable housing), is needed to sustain initial gains made in batterer programs.

Principles of the Prevention of Family Violence for Practicing Mental Health Professionals

Many influential organizations, including the American Medical Association, the American Academy of Child and Adolescent Psychiatry, and the American Academy of Pediatrics, call for physicians to take a major role in lessening the prevalence, scope, and severity of child maltreatment and domestic violence (as well as elder abuse, which is another important form of family violence). The prevalence of family violence is such that most physicians encounter individuals who are affected by violence in their practices. Additionally, family violence is more likely to be present in clinical, rather than nonclinical, populations; thus, psychiatrists are likely to have patients who are victims of, or perpetrators of, family violence. It is imperative that psychiatrists become aware of the antecedents of family violence, develop a system for identifying incidents of family violence, and have a means of referral and treatment once they are identified. Whereas psychiatrists sometimes use primary prevention strategies that address family violence as a public health issue, secondary or tertiary prevention to lessen the impact of early abuse and to prevent a pattern of escalating abuse is utilized with greater frequency in the clinical setting.

Primary Prevention

Individuals often view physicians as valuable sources of information about health-related topics. The Surgeon General's Workshop on Violence and Public Health, conducted in October 1985, represented a new beginning in how the medical system in the United States addresses the issue of violence and violence prevention. This public health approach encouraged all health professionals to respond constructively to family violence. Historically, when confronted by circumstances of violence, medical professionals have tacitly agreed that violence was the exclusive province of the legal system, leaving the matter to the police and courts. These agents of public safety and justice have served the public interest well, but are not equipped to address violence prevention.

Psychiatrists are uniquely positioned to educate the public about family violence. Psychiatrists have a good understanding of the antecedents of violence, including biological, psychological, and social factors. There are many venues available in which to share this information. These include small forums such as during individual meetings with patients, the public areas of one's office (with educational materials placed there), or small group educational settings in the community. Additionally, medical professionals are frequently invited to make presentations in community forums, in schools, at religious centers, and in the media (newspapers, television, magazines, etc.). These settings are beneficial in educating the public about family violence. Extending the message that family violence prevention is crucial to the development of healthy families and the overall well-being of individuals is an important advocacy role for psychiatrists.

Secondary Prevention

One of the critical tasks for psychiatrists is learning to identify family violence in the early stages. The psychiatrist should become proficient at screening for all forms of family violence. Unfortunately, many psychiatric residency training programs do an inadequate job of preparing physicians to recognize family violence, whether it is child abuse, spousal/intimate partner violence, or elder abuse. Moreover, it is often difficult for the psychiatrist to identify violence given that many victims will not acknowledge their own victimization. For example, many domestic partners develop alternative explanations for the abuser's behavior, especially when it is early in the course of the relationship. Many victims will not spontaneously discuss violence, even when it is recognized, because of embarrassment or fear of the consequences that may occur for a husband, father, wife, mother, daughter, or son. Furthermore, many victims will deny the presence of violence when asked in a busy clinical setting or in the presence of their spouse or domestic partner. Many children will not discuss violence in the presence of their parents, just as many elderly parents will not discuss violence in front of their adult children.

Therefore, the psychiatrist must be diligent in seeking this information in an empathic and caring manner. If there are suspicions of violence, the psychiatrist must ensure that the patient feels safe in discussing it. The interview should be conducted in a quiet location that is away from a busy emergency room or clinical setting. Delivery of supportive mental health services depends on early identification of victims and abusers through adequate screening processes. Adult clients should routinely be screened for domestic violence whenever any of the following occurs (New York State Office of the Prevention of Domestic Violence 2008):

- A woman requests services (regardless of her age, economic status, sexual orientation, or presenting problem).
- A couple requests couples counseling, family therapy, or mediation.
- A woman is referred because she is identified as a batterer.
- A male client shows physical, emotional, or behavioral signs of abuse.

Note that careful attention should be paid when a woman:

- Begins or ends a relationship
- Is in the middle of a struggle over child custody or visitation
- Has visible physical injuries
- Appears to have suffered from any type of accident
- Expresses concerns about her partner's alcoholism or drug use
- Complains about her partner's temper or mistreatment of children
- Shows any signs of posttraumatic stress disorder or depressive/anxiety symptoms
- Has a recent onset of or worsening in mental health symptoms
- Has a partner who insists on attending treatment sessions

Child clients should be screened for child abuse whenever any of the following occurs:

- A child presents with recurrent traumatic injuries.
- A child's behavior changes substantially.
- There are physical symptoms that are nonspecific and unexplained.
- A recent change in living arrangements has occurred.
- A child's school grades become worse.
- A youth becomes more aggressive toward adults or peers.
- There is an unexplained increase in the level of irritability, aggression, or anxiety.
- There are physical, emotional, or behavioral signs of abuse.

Tertiary Prevention

Family violence is an antecedent for a number of health problems, including stress-related disorders such as hypertension and frequent viral illness. Early detection and treatment are key to preventing health problems and/or decreasing the impact that disorders will have on the lives of clients. Once a psychiatrist has identified a case of family violence, it is important to act on this information. Although psychiatrists are not mandated to report domestic violence in all states, they are required to report cases of physical abuse, sexual abuse, or neglect of children and adolescents in all states. It is important that psychiatrists act to assist patients in developing a plan to attain safety and get treatment, because many victims may not have other support measures in place to assist them in dealing with the traumatic situation. There are three tasks that psychiatrists can undertake to assist victims in escaping chronic family violence:

1. *Help the victim develop a safety plan.* The mental health response in cases of family violence should be aimed at providing for the safety of the victim(s) and reinforcing accountability of the perpetrator. Special care must be given to victims who have preexisting mental health or physical health concerns because many of these individuals are more likely to be victimized than individuals who have no history of health concerns.

   Although most episodes of violence occur in the home, they have a significant impact on all aspects of the lives of family members. Many adult victims have experienced harassment from or threatening behaviors of their domestic partner at their worksites. This level of intrusion by their domestic partner can have a serious impact on their current employment as well as future employability. Many children become victims in a number of settings, including schools, sports activities, and other community settings. Many victims live under intense stress because the occurrences of violent behavior are unpredictable and unprovoked. Living with this degree of stress and daily anxiety may cause significant psychiatric impairment, which will have to be addressed in the context of psychiatric care. Although incidents do also occur outside the home, the most dangerous place for victims of family violence is in the home setting.

   The psychiatrist is often one of the first individuals who may hear about a family's lack of safety. Many victims are reluctant to disclose information and remain at continued risk of family violence while they de-velop the ability to move forward with protecting themselves. It is during this time period that it is critical for the psychiatrist to remain supportive. The following guidelines should be shared with victims of family violence when developing safety plans:

- Obtain a protection or restraining order to prevent physical contact with the perpetrator if there is a fear for personal or child safety.
- Obtain copies of any court orders and keep them in your (the victim's) possession at all times.
- Plan escape routes from the home and memorize emergency phone numbers.
- Avoid rooms in the home where family members may become trapped (e.g., bathrooms without windows, closets).
- Have a friend or neighbor available and a safe location to flee to in times of crisis.
- Teach the children to call 911 if they are old enough to do so.
- Have a cellular phone and keep it with you at all times.
- Keep money and a set of car keys in a safe place that is outside of the home but easily accessible.
- Rehearse these actions until everyone in the family knows what to do.

It is also often helpful to refer the family to a domestic violence or child maltreatment advocacy agency for assistance in putting into action a de-tailed safety plan beyond that which is being developed with the psychia-trist.

2. *Address the physical health care of the victim.* It is critical that victims' so-matic health be assessed quickly, as many victims may have unidentified internal injuries or head injuries. Furthermore, it is important to docu-ment the level of injuries experienced by the victim so that there will be an adequate record for any future legal proceedings. Although the psychia-trist may not be the primary physician addressing the somatic health care needs of an individual, it is important that the psychiatrist advocate for the victim and make sure that these issues are adequately addressed. Many victims may be reluctant to seek health care because of lack of insurance and a fear that the perpetrator may face legal repercussions as a result of the attacks. Many victims, or caregivers of victims, are also reluctant to

seek physical health care, as it becomes an admission that the injuries may have occurred as a result of domestic violence or child abuse. It is often important to confront the intense denial that may be present in the lives of many victims as they are encouraged and supported in seeking care.

3. *Provide mental health care for the victim.* A large number of people experience significant emotional distress as a result of family violence, but many psychiatrists feel ill-prepared to help these individuals. Many of the clinical interventions that psychiatrists use are for treating the consequences of violence (e.g., posttraumatic stress disorder, depression) rather than the violence itself. Psychiatrists may feel that it is not their duty to advocate or address the underlying issues directly. As a result, the clinician may refer the victim to an advocacy program or a shelter, which may be able to advocate for the victim but may not understand the clinical implications. Furthermore, some advocates may view "treatment" as implying that there is something wrong with the victim rather than understanding that there are larger sociological issues at play.

There are steps a treating psychiatrist can take to provide effective services to victims of family violence. First, create a safe, stable, and nurturing family environment so that all members of the family have a place to adequately recover from the traumatic events. It is important to work with the entire family to begin to address the issues involved and to help prevent future episodes of violence.

Second, identify mental health problems that may be experienced by the victims. Victims often have significant mental health problems that may go unnoticed. Unaddressed mental health problems make it more difficult for victims to identify appropriate services and may cause them to be more isolated from others than they would be otherwise. Although many women take steps to protect their children from an abusive partner, many do not take adequate steps to protect their own physical or emotional well-being. Be aware of the need to carefully consider caregivers' symptoms and the impact of these symptoms on family functioning. The reality is that a significant number of children of abused mothers are also abused, despite the protective caregiver's efforts. Furthermore, witnessing the abuse of one's caregiver is almost certainly experienced as traumatic by the dependent child. The most commonly used assessment technique is a focused clinical interview that explores the individual's experience with violence along with the associated symptoms. A clinical interview should be supplemented by standardized tools to measure trauma exposure and symptoms, as well as information to give the family on services including social service agencies and other community resources.

Third, reduce the number of symptoms that family members are experiencing. Make use of empirically supported treatments where available; treatment may involve individual therapy, group interventions, parental training, family therapy, or school consultation. Substance abuse is a common problem among families dealing with violence, so programs that provide both mental health care and substance abuse treatment are often necessary. Promote an open discussion of the family's experiences. Numerous studies have demonstrated that allowing victims to openly discuss their experiences promotes healing and the ability to integrate their experiences in a meaningful way (e.g., Brown and Kolko 1999; Kolko 1996). It also reduces the sense of isolation, which is likely to occur if the family is unable to share their experiences with others. Many victims become isolated from their support systems, including family members and friends. Without these supports in place, if psychiatric illness occurs in abuse victims they are much more likely to have a severe and protracted course of illness. Helping families connect with support systems is an important treatment strategy.

Key Points

- Family violence is a major public health concern. The prevalence is high and the negative consequences for all members of the family and for society are substantial, both short- and long-term.

- Violence within the family crosses biopsychosocial domains and is impacted by forces at work in the individual, as well as within the context of the family, community, and larger society. Additionally, stressors interact with protective factors to form a complex dynamic of risk and resilience.

- Primary and secondary prevention efforts, including mass media campaigns, reporting laws, and community practice standards regarding screening, appear to effectively raise awareness of the problem. However, evidence of their ability to reduce the prevalence of family violence has been limited.

- Evidence suggests that tertiary interventions can reduce adverse effects of child maltreatment and domestic violence.
- Although mental health professionals are most familiar and comfortable with tertiary prevention, the public health risks associated with family violence make it imperative that they become involved in primary and secondary prevention efforts.

References

Beckett C: The Swedish myth: the corporal punishment ban and child death statistics. Br J Soc Work 35:125–138, 2005

Belsky J: Etiology of child maltreatment: a developmental-ecological analysis. Psychol Bull 114:413–434, 1993

Bennett L, Riger S, Schewe P, et al: Effectiveness of hotline, advocacy, counseling, and shelter services for victims of domestic violence. J Interpers Violence 19:815–829, 2004

Berkman M, Casey R, Berkowitz S, et al: Police in the lives of children exposed to domestic violence: collaborative approaches to intervention, in Protecting Children from Domestic Violence: Strategies for Community Intervention. Edited by Jaffe PG, Baker LL, Cunningham AJ. New York, Guilford, 2004, pp 153–170

Berliner L, Elliott DM: Sexual abuse of children, in The APSAC Handbook on Child Maltreatment, 2nd Edition. Edited by Myers JEB, Berliner L, Briere J, et al. Thousand Oaks, CA, Sage, 2002, pp 55–78

Biederman J, Milberger S, Faraone SV, et al: Family-environment risk factors for attention-deficit hyperactivity disorder: a test of Rutter's indicators of adversity. Arch Gen Psychiatry 52:464–470, 1995

Bornstein RF: The complex relationship between dependency and domestic violence: converging psychological factors and social forces. Am Psychol 61:595–606, 2006

Brown EJ, Kolko DJ: Child victims' attributions about being physically abused: an examination of factors associated with symptom severity. J Abnorm Child Psychol 27:311–322, 1999

Bybee DI, Sullivan CM: The process through which a strengths-based intervention resulted in positive change for battered women over time. Am J Community Psychol 30:103–132, 2002

Campbell JC: Health consequences of intimate partner violence. Lancet 359:1331–1336, 2002

Chaffin M: Response to letters. Child Abuse Negl 29:241–249, 2005

Chaffin M, Silovsky JF, Funderburk B, et al: Parent-child interaction therapy with physically abusive parents: efficacy for reducing future abuse reports. J Consult Clin Psychol 72:500–510, 2004

Cicchetti D, Rogosch FA, Toth SL: Fostering secure attachment in infants in maltreating families through preventive interventions. Dev Psychopathol 18:623–650, 2006

Cohen JA, Mannarino AP, Deblinger E: Treating Trauma and Traumatic Grief in Children and Adolescents. New York, Guilford, 2006

Daro D, McCurdy KP: Interventions to prevent child maltreatment, in Handbook of Injury and Violence Prevention. Edited by Doll LS, Bonzo SE, Mercy JA, et al. New York, Springer, 2007, pp 137–155

DePanfilis D, Dubowitz H, Kunz J: Assessing the cost-effectiveness of Family Connections. Child Abuse Negl 32:335–351, 2008

Durrant JE, Janson S: Law reform, corporal punishment and child abuse: the case of Sweden. International Review of Victimology 12:139–158, 2005

Durrant JE, Olsen GM: Parenting and public policy: contextualizing the Swedish Corporal Punishment ban. Journal of Social Welfare and Family Law 19:443–461, 1997

Eckenrode J, Ganzel B, Henderson CR Jr, et al: Preventing child abuse and neglect with a program of nurse home visitation: the limiting effects of domestic violence. JAMA 284:1385–1391, 2000

Emery RE, Laumann-Billings L: An overview of the nature, causes, and consequences of abusive family relationships. Am Psychol 53:121–135, 1998

Fosco GM, DeBoard RL, Grych JH: Making sense of family violence: implications of children's appraisals of interparental aggression for their short- and long-term functioning. European Psychologist 12:6–16, 2007

Geeraert L, Van den Noortgate W, Grietens H, et al: The effects of early prevention programs for families with young children at risk for physical child abuse and neglect: a meta-analysis. Child Maltreat 9:277–291, 2004

Gelles RJ, Maynard PE: A structural family systems approach to intervention in cases of family violence. Fam Relat 38:270–275, 1987

Gondolf EW, Jones AS: The program effect of batterer programs in three cities. Violence Vict 16:693–704, 2001

Goodman PE: The relationship between intimate partner violence and other forms of family and societal violence. Emerg Med Clin N Am 24:889–903, 2006

Graham-Bermann SA, Seng J: Violence exposure and traumatic stress symptoms as additional predictors of health problems in high-risk children. J Pediatr 146:349–354, 2005

Graham-Bermann SA, Lynch S, Banyard V, et al: Community based intervention for children exposed to intimate partner violence: an efficacy trial. J Consult Clin Psych 75:199–209, 2007

Groves BM: Children Who See Too Much: Lessons from the Child Witness to Violence Project. Boston, Beacon Press, 2002

Groves BM, Gewirtz A: Interventions with children exposed to domestic violence: promising approaches, in Children Exposed to Violence: Research, Intervention and Policy. Edited by Feerick M, Silverman G. Baltimore, MD, Brookes Press, 2006, pp 106–136

Herron WG, Javier RA, McDonald-Gomez M, et al: Sources of family violence. Journal of Social Distress and the Homeless 3:213–227, 1994

Hill R: Generic features of families under stress. Soc Casework 49:139–150, 1958

Jaffe P, Wolfe D: Similarities in behavioral and social maladjustment among child victims and witnesses to family violence. Am J Orthopsychiatry 56:142–146, 1986

Kaufman J, Zigler E: Do abused children become abusive parents? Am J Orthopsychiatry 37:186–192, 1987

Kolko DS: Individual cognitive-behavioral treatment and family therapy for abused children and their attending parents: a comparison of child outcomes. Child Maltreat 1:322–342, 1996

Kolko D: Child physical abuse, in The APSAC Handbook on Child Maltreatment, 2nd Edition. Edited by Myers JEB, Berliner L, Briere J, et al. Thousand Oaks, CA, Sage, 2002, pp 21–54

Lieberman AF, Van Horn P, Ghosh Ippen C: Toward evidence-based treatment: child-parent psychotherapy with preschoolers exposed to marital violence. J Am Acad Child Adolesc Psychiatry 44:1241–1248, 2005

Lieberman AF, Van Horn P, Ghosh Ippen C: Child-parent psychotherapy: 6-month follow-up of a randomized controlled trial. J Am Acad Child Adolesc Psychiatry 45:913–918, 2006

MacMillan HL, Thomas BH, Jamieson E, et al: Effectiveness of home visitation by public-health nurses in prevention of the recurrence of child physical abuse and neglect: a randomized controlled trial. Lancet 365:1786–1793, 2005

Mahoney A, O'Donnelly WO, Boxer P, et al: Marital and severe parent-to-adolescent physical aggression in clinic-referred families: mother and adolescent reports on co-occurrence and links to child behavior problems. J Fam Psychol 17:3–19, 2003

Martin SL, Coyne-Beasley T, Hoehn M, et al: Primary prevention of violence against women: training needs of violence practitioners. Violence Against Women 15(1):44–56, 2009

McCloskey L, Figuerdo AJ, Koss MP: The effects of systematic family violence on children's mental health. Child Dev 66:1239–1261, 1995

McFarlane JM, Groff JY, O'Brien JA, et al: Secondary prevention of intimate partner violence: a randomized controlled trial. Nurs Res 55:52–61, 2006

New York State Office for the Prevention of Domestic Violence: Guidelines for Mental Health Professionals. 2008. Available at: http://www.opdv.state.ny.us/professionals/mental_health/index.html. Accessed November 3, 2008.

Nygren P, Nelson, HD, Klein J: Screening children for family violence: a review of the evidence for the US Preventive Services Task Force. Ann Fam Med 2:161–169, 2004

Olds DL, Eckenrode J, Henderson CR, et al: Long-term effects of home visitation on maternal life course and child abuse and neglect: fifteen-year follow-up of a randomized trial. JAMA 278:637–643, 1997

Peterson L, Tremblay G, Ewigman B, et al: Multilevel selected primary prevention of child maltreatment. J Consult Clin Psychol 71:601–612, 2003

Pianta R, Egeland B, Erickson MF: The antecedents of maltreatment: results of the mother-child interaction project, in Child Maltreatment: Theory and Research on the Causes and Consequences of Child Abuse and Neglect. Edited by Cicchetti D, Carlson V. Cambridge, MA, Cambridge University Press, 1997, pp 203–253

Statistiska Centralbyrån (SCB): Spanking and other forms of physical punishment: a study of adults' and middle school students' opinions, experience, and knowledge. Demografiska Rapporter 1.2 1996

Sweet MA, Appelbaum MI: Is home visiting an effective strategy?: a meta-analytic review of home visiting programs for families with young children. Child Dev 75:1435–1456, 2004

Taylor BG, Davis RC, Maxwell CD: The effects of a group batterer treatment program: a randomized experiment in Brooklyn. Justice Quarterly 18:171–201, 2001

Toth SL, Maughan A, Manly JT, et al: The relative efficacy of two interventions in altering maltreated preschool children's representational models: implications for attachment theory. Dev Psychopathol 14:877–908, 2002

U.S. Department of Justice, Bureau of Justice Statistics: Family violence statistics. June 2005. Available at: http://www.ojp.usdoj.gov/bjs/abstract/fvs.htm. Accessed October 27, 2008.

Van Horn P, Groves BM: Children exposed to domestic violence: making trauma-informed custody and visitation decisions. Juv Fam Court J 57:51–60, 2006

Wolfe D, Wekerle C, Reitzel D, et al: Strategies to address violence in the lives of high risk youth, in Ending the Cycle of Violence: Community Responses to Children of Battered Women. Edited by Peled E, Jaffee PG, Edleson JL. New York, Sage, 1995

Zellman GL, Fair CC: Preventing and reporting abuse, in The APSAC Handbook on Child Maltreatment, 2nd Edition. Edited by Myers JEB, Berliner L, Briere J, et al. Thousand Oaks, CA, Sage, 2002, pp 449–475

Zwi KJ, Woolfenden SR, Wheeler DM, et al: School-based education programmes for the prevention of child sexual abuse. Cochrane Database Syst Rev Issue 3, Art No CD004380. DOI: 10.1002/14651858.CD004380.pub2, 2007

10

Prevention Principles for Adolescents in Psychiatric Practice

Preventing Conduct Disorder and Other Behavioral Problems

Kareem Ghalib, M.D.

Gordon Harper, M.D.

Adolescence is a time of great growth, as well as great vulnerability. Biology, psychology, and environment are in flux. Many adolescents do not yet have the internal or external resources to successfully navigate the complex path toward adulthood. These characteristics make adolescents an important population for the prevention-minded psychiatrist.

Prior chapters have addressed adolescence in the context of identifying and preventing early onset of mood disorders, anxiety disorders, psychotic disorders, substance abuse, and suicide. Although it is important to keep in mind that these conditions may begin in adolescence, this chapter does not repeat those discussions. Rather, we focus on preventing and reducing the harm associated with behavioral problems that are specific to youth but commonly come to the attention of the general psychiatrist, either from an adolescent patient or from concerned parents. Examples include conduct disorder as well as violence, delinquency, and other problem behaviors not defined by DSM-IV-TR (American Psychiatric Association 2000).

In this chapter, first we briefly review normal (psychologically healthy) adolescent development. Second, we discuss the epidemiology and public health impact of conduct disorder in youth. Third, we summarize the risk factors for conduct and other behavioral problems and, fourth, describe interventions designed to prevent problem behaviors in youth. Fifth, protective factors and health promotion interventions, including resilience, are reviewed. Finally, we offer recommendations for preventing harm and promoting strength.

Normal Adolescence

Many general psychiatrists have adolescent patients. Although rushed schedules and force of habit may lead us to treat these patients like younger versions of their adult counterparts, important differences between adults and adolescents have implications for prevention. For example, adolescents are still developing. Table 10–1 lists cognitive, social, behavioral, and emotional features typical of normal (nonpathological) adolescent development. These do not always correspond to biological age, so it is important to assess each child individually. As the table indicates, an individual's developmental status informs our understanding of what is happening in the individual and in his or her family and peers, including how developed the person's capacity is for abstract thought and the person's vulnerability to risky behaviors. This information can be used in diagnosis, risk assessment, treatment planning, and building a therapeutic alliance.

Conduct Disorder: A Brief Overview

DSM-IV-TR defines conduct disorder as "a repetitive and persistent pattern of behavior in which the basic rights of others or major age-appropriate soci-

Table 10–1. Three stages of adolescent development across four domains: key features

	Cognitive	Social	Behavioral	Emotional
Early adolescence (ages 10–13)	Thought patterns are largely concrete	Primary reference group begins to change from family to peers	Experimentation with new behavior begins	Emotional separation from parents begins
Middle adolescence (ages 14–16)	Abstract thought begins, but sense of invulnerability remains	Enormous influence of peers/school environment	Health-risk behaviors peak	Sense of self begins to develop
Late adolescence (ages 17–19)	Abstract thought allows realistic assessments	Family and peer influence more balanced	Risky behaviors decline	Sense of self consolidates

Source. Adapted from Kantor 1999.

etal norms or rules are violated…" (American Psychiatric Association 2000). As noted in Table 10–2, youths meet DSM-IV-TR criteria for this disorder if they have exhibited at least three of the behaviors listed below in the past year, and at least one in the past 6 months:

- Aggression toward people and animals
- Destruction of property
- Deceitfulness or theft
- Serious violations of rules

The disorder is characterized as childhood- or adolescent-onset depending on whether criteria were met prior to age 10 years. Severity is classified as mild, moderate or severe, according to how many criteria are met and how much harm the youth causes other people.

Epidemiology and Public Health Impact

Conduct disorder is common. Disorders that co-occur with conduct disorder are also common, including learning disorders, internalizing disorders, and attention-deficit/hyperactivity disorder. Youths with conduct disorder are also at greater risk for dropping out of school than those without the disorder (Powell et al. 2007).

Conduct disorder is associated with substantial costs to society. According to an analysis of data from youths with conduct disorder in four poor U.S. communities, the conduct disorder–related public expenditures per child, including schooling, general health care, mental health care, and juvenile justice system costs, were $70,000 greater than public expenditures for nondiagnosed community youths (Foster and Jones 2005).

Risk Factors for Conduct Disorder and Other Behavioral Problems

Over the past three decades, risk factors for conduct disorder and other behavioral problems have been identified. These risk factors guide preventive interventions. Drawing on early work on delinquency (Hawkins et al. 1988) and a report by the Institute of Medicine (1989), Coie and colleagues (1993) grouped generic risk factors into the seven *conceptual clusters* listed below (examples are given in parentheses):

1. Family circumstances (family conflict, poor family bonding)
2. Emotional difficulties (emotional dyscontrol, low self-esteem)
3. School problems (academic failure, school dropout)
4. Adverse ecological contexts (victim of racial prejudice, extreme poverty)
5. Constitutional handicaps (complicated birth history, sensory deficits)
6. Interpersonal problems (peer rejection, alienation)
7. Skill development delays (mental retardation, learning disabilities)

As part of their Communities That Care initiative, Hawkins and Catalano (1992) categorized risk factors for adolescent problem behavior into four groups: those related to community, family, school, and peer group/the individual (Substance Abuse and Mental Health Services Administration 2003). Within these groups, they outlined 20 risk factors that predict vulnerability to two or more problem behaviors (Table 10–3).

Multiple risk factors make it more likely that a youth will develop multiple problem behaviors. Additional risk factors for problem behaviors include adverse childhood events and early entry into adult roles. Physical, sexual, or emotional abuse, and neglect, are risk factors for negative mental health outcomes. Given the stigma and shame associated with these experiences, the victim may not spontaneously reveal them. If they are identified, the risk of problem behaviors developing can be moderated by prompt intervention (Chapman et al. 2007). Regarding early entry into adult roles, teenage parenthood, living independently, and leaving school early increase the risk of unstable relationships, aggression, and exposure to violence (Roche et al. 2006).

Preventive Interventions

Multiple primary, secondary, and tertiary interventions have been tested with the goal of preventing conduct disorder (Powell et al. 2007). For example, Hill and colleagues (2004) reviewed the effectiveness of early screening for conduct problems. We summarize primary prevention first, including that aimed at young children.

Table 10–2.   DSM-IV-TR criteria for conduct disorder

A.   A repetitive and persistent pattern of behavior in which the basic rights of others or major age-appropriate societal norms or rules are violated, as manifested by the presence of three (or more) of the following criteria in the past 12 months, with at least one criterion present in the past 6 months:

Aggression to people and animals

(1)   often bullies, threatens, or intimidates others

(2)   often initiates physical fights

(3)   has used a weapon that can cause serious physical harm to others (e.g., a bat, brick, broken bottle, knife, gun)

(4)   has been physically cruel to people

(5)   has been physically cruel to animals

(6)   has stolen while confronting a victim (e.g., mugging, purse snatching, extortion, armed robbery)

(7)   has forced someone into sexual activity

Destruction of property

(8)   has deliberately engaged in fire setting with the intention of causing serious damage

(9)   has deliberately destroyed others' property (other than by fire setting)

Deceitfulness or theft

(10) has broken into someone else's house, building, or car

(11) often lies to obtain goods or favors or to avoid obligations (i.e., "cons" others)

(12) has stolen items of nontrivial value without confronting a victim (e.g., shoplifting, but without breaking and entering; forgery)

Serious violations of rules

(13) often stays out at night despite parental prohibitions, beginning before age 13 years

(14) has run away from home overnight at least twice while living in parental or parental surrogate home (or once without returning for a lengthy period)

(15) is often truant from school, beginning before age 13 years

B.   The disturbance in behavior causes clinically significant impairment in social, academic, or occupational functioning.

C.   If the individual is age 18 years or older, criteria are not met for Antisocial Personality Disorder.

Table 10–2.   DSM-IV-TR criteria for conduct disorder *(continued)*

Code based on age at onset:

312.81   **Conduct Disorder, Childhood-Onset Type:**   onset of at least one criterion characteristic of Conduct Disorder prior to age 10 years

312.82   **Conduct Disorder, Adolescent-Onset Type:**   absence of any criteria characteristic of Conduct Disorder prior to age 10 years

312.89   **Conduct Disorder, Unspecified Onset:**   age at onset is not known

Specify severity:

Mild: few if any conduct problems in excess of those required to make the diagnosis **and** conduct problems cause only minor harm to others

Moderate: number of conduct problems and effect on others intermediate between "mild" and "severe"

Severe: many conduct problems in excess of those required to make the diagnosis **or** conduct problems cause considerable harm to others

Source.   Reprinted from American Psychiatric Association: *Diagnostic and Statistical Manual of Mental Disorders,* 4th Edition, Revised. Washington, DC, American Psychiatric Association, 2000. Copyright 2000, American Psychiatric Association. Used with permission.

Primary Preventive Interventions

Conduct Disorder and Delinquency

Waddell and colleagues (2007) reviewed prevention of childhood mental disorders, including primary prevention of conduct disorder. Seven targeted and one universal intervention met inclusion criteria for their review; that is, interventions began before children met criteria for conduct disorder. Children were ages 0–8 years and displayed mild conduct symptoms, had a low IQ, were of a low socioeconomic status, or had a parent with a mental illness and/or other difficulties. Favorable outcomes, such as decreases in problem behaviors, were demonstrated for interventions using parental training, childhood social skills training, or their combination. These interventions, conducted by educators and clinicians, lasted 1–2 years and were delivered in homes or schools, not clinical settings.

Connor and colleagues (2006) evaluated interventions designed to prevent the onset of conduct problems, aggression, and antisocial behavior. They reviewed studies of young children, most no more than 12 years old. They found support for parent management training, a child-focused approach

Table 10–3. "Risk factor matrix" for selected adolescent problem behaviors (as described by Hawkins and Catalano for Communities That Care)

Environment and characteristics	Substance abuse	Delinquency	Teen pregnancy	School dropout	Violence
Community					
Availability of drugs	X				X
Availability of firearms		X			X
Community laws and norms favorable toward drug use, firearms, and crime	X	X			X
Transitions and mobility	X	X		X	
Low neighborhood attachment and community disorganization	X	X			X
Extreme economic deprivation	X	X	X	X	X
Family					
Family history of problem behaviors	X	X	X	X	X
Family management problems	X	X	X	X	X
Family conflict	X	X	X	X	X
Family attitude and involvement in problem behaviors	X	X			X
School					
Academic failure beginning in late elementary school	X	X	X	X	X
Lack of commitment to school	X	X	X	X	X
Peer and individual					
Early and persistent antisocial behavior	X	X	X	X	X
Rebelliousness	X	X		X	
Friends who engage in problem behaviors	X	X	X	X	X
Gang involvement	X	X			X
Favorable attitudes toward problem behaviors	X	X	X	X	X
Early initiation of problem behaviors	X	X	X	X	X
Constitutional factors	X				X

that draws on cognitive and behavioral principles to train parents to manage their child's behavioral problems.

Webster-Stratton and Taylor (2001) described multiple universal and selective interventions aimed at young children, their families, and communities, mostly school-based, that prevented later substance abuse, violence, and delinquency. Successful programs were broad-based, were developmentally informed, and focused on enhancing skills and strengths of both the parents and the children.

Hawkins and colleagues (2008) reported preliminary evidence of the effectiveness of a randomized community-level intervention to increase protective factors and reduce risk factors for delinquency and drug abuse in youths ages 10–14. As part of their Communities That Care prevention system, leaders from select communities in seven states were trained to choose and implement pretested prevention interventions. At initiation, more than 4,400 community elementary school students were being monitored for initiation of delinquent behavior or substance abuse. After less than 2 years, the children from communities that received the intervention were significantly less likely to exhibit delinquency. Positive results for substance abuse are expected to follow.

Other Behavioral Problems

Durlak and Wells (1997) conducted a meta-analysis of 177 primary prevention interventions focusing on behavioral and social problems in children and adolescents. Interventions occurred in a variety of settings and involved parents, teachers, undergraduate and graduate students, and/or mental health professionals. Effect sizes were largest for interventions that taught problem solving and emotional awareness to younger children (ages 2–7).

Beginning in the late 1970s, Olds and colleagues conducted home visits with 400 new mothers, approximately half of whom were impoverished and/or less than 19 years old. This program, which involved nurses teaching new mothers about healthy behaviors and promoting their personal development, improved maternal health and decreased rates of maternal problem behaviors (Olds et al. 1997). At long-term follow-up, adolescents born to visited mothers reported fewer arrests and less risky behavior involving sexual activity and drug use (Olds et al. 1998).

Secondary Preventive Interventions

In addition to their meta-analysis of studies on primary prevention, Durlak and Wells (1998) performed a meta-analysis of 130 secondary prevention interventions. Ten projects with children presenting early signs of externalizing disorders were clearly effective, as demonstrated by an effect size of 0.72. Here, as in primary preventive interventions, the interventions varied in effectiveness, but those that used cognitive or behavioral approaches and targeted younger children and their environments were most effective.

Oppositional defiant disorder (ODD), which DSM-IV-TR defines as "[a] pattern of negativistic, hostile and defiance behavior…" (American Psychiatric Association 2000), is often conceptualized as a precursor to conduct disorder (Moffitt 2007). For that reason, treatments for ODD can be considered secondary prevention interventions for conduct disorder. Best practices for the assessment and treatment of ODD have recently been summarized by the American Academy of Child and Adolescent Psychiatry (Steiner et al. 2007), and evidence-based reviews of treatment for ODD using medications (Turgay 2009) and psychosocial treatments (Eyberg et al. 2008) have also been conducted. A useful guide to discussing ODD with parents and family members, "ODD: A Guide for Families," is available for downloading from the American Academy of Child and Adolescent Psychiatry Web site (http://www.aacap.org/galleries/eAACAP.ResourceCenters/ODD_guide.pdf).

Natural Processes of Growth, Healing, and Adaptation

Secondary prevention should foster adaptation to the natural processes identified in the life of a teen and the family. Promoting adaptation is a strength-based, recovery-oriented complement to treating pathology. Adaptive processes are closer to a youth's experiences than are pathological diagnoses.

With adolescents, developmental milestones or other life events often necessitate adaptation. For instance, a family reforms after a period of separation. Remarriage triggers getting acquainted with a new stepparent and may trigger grieving for a lost closeness with the other. A child's entering a foster home or a child's return home triggers its own adjustments. For many children, disclosure of trauma or abuse initiates a period of recovery. Sometimes, a suspicion that trauma has occurred, though it sometimes cannot be confirmed, calls for something nearly as difficult—namely, living with ambiguity.

Asking about these processes (for instance, "Where do you see yourself in the process of adapting to…?") fosters reflection by the child or parent. It also acknowledges and validates an important part of their experience, often unstated.

Tertiary Preventive Interventions

Tertiary prevention has been directed at children and adolescents who meet criteria for conduct disorder or have had contact with the juvenile justice system. Given that youths with conduct disorder are often opposed to active participation in treatment, tertiary prevention is often directed at parents and other family members.

Several clinical trials have assessed intervening early with young children who have chronic conduct disorder and/or are chronically delinquent. Beauchaine and colleagues (2005) combined data from six interventions that involved a combination of parent training, teacher training, and/or social skills training for more than 500 children ages 3–8.5, They then used a latent growth curve analysis to investigate the mediators and moderators of 1-year response. Moderators of outcomes included comorbid anxiety or depression, paternal substance use, and maternal depression. Poorer outcome was predicted by a harsh, critical, or otherwise ineffective parenting style.

A meta-analysis of family and parenting interventions in children with conduct disorder and delinquency, defined by referral from juvenile justice or another legal system, examined eight randomized, controlled clinical trials involving almost 750 youths ages 10–17 (Woolfenden et al. 2002). Interventions with parents and families reduced the time the delinquent child spent in institutions, the risk of the juvenile being rearrested, and the rate of subsequent arrests 1–3 years later. Three of these interventions used multisystemic therapy (Borduin et al. 1995; Henggeler et al. 1992, 1997), which assumes that problem behaviors are multi-faceted and therefore require multiple home-based interventions.

For many, the standard in tertiary intervention for conduct disorder has become multisystemic therapy. Henggeler and colleagues have demonstrated, through program reports and randomized trials, reductions in criminal activity and violence with this method (Henggeler and Borduin 1990; Henggeler and Sheidow 2003; Henggeler et al. 1996, 2002).

In addition to reviewing the evidence pertaining to the primary prevention of conduct disorder, Connor and colleagues (2006) also described interventions designed to reduce the harm associated with established conduct disorder in adolescents age 12 and older with juvenile criminal records. This review again highlights the effectiveness of intensive, multi-faceted and community-based services, whether at home as part of multisystemic therapy, or as part of multidimensional treatment foster care.

Summary of Preventive Interventions

In summary, the literature contains evidence for primary and secondary prevention utilizing skills-based approaches for young children and their families and teachers. There is also evidence for the effectiveness of tertiary prevention in children and adolescents using multifaceted community-based interventions. A knowledge of risk factors can help determine which individuals may be the best targets for prevention. Successful prevention interventions aim to effect change not only in individuals but also in environments and institutions. Greenberg (2006) has both advocated for such programs and linked the individual skills to be attained (e.g., executive functioning) to recent findings in neuroscience research.

Protective Factors and Health Promotion Interventions

Knowledge of risk factors is only half the story. It is also important to identify and build on a patient's strengths. This can be done by identifying protective factors or assets, understanding resilience, and working toward positive development.

Protective Factors

The Search Institute is a nongovernmental organization that has developed a list of 40 *developmental assets* identified in prevention research (Search Institute 2009; Table 10–4). These assets, which can be categorized into one of several "internal" or "external" domains, describe a broad array of positive protective factors in adolescents' lives. They have been demonstrated to correlate with decreased risk behaviors and increased academic achievement (Scales and Roehlkepartain 2003; Roehlkepartain et al. 2003).

Table 10–4.   The Search Institute's 40 developmental assets for youths ages 12–18 years

	Asset Name	Definition
External assets		
Support	Family support	Family life provides high levels of love and support
	Positive family communication	Young person and his or her parent(s) communicate positively, and young person is willing to seek advice and counsel from parent(s)
	Other adult relationships	Young person receives support from ≥3 nonparent adults
	Caring neighborhood	Young person experiences caring neighbors
	Caring school climate	School provides a caring, encouraging environment
	Parental involvement in schooling	Parent(s) are actively involved in helping young person succeed in school
Empowerment	Community values youth	Young person perceives that adults in the community value youth
	Youth as resources	Young people are given useful roles in the community
	Service to others	Young person serves in the community ≥1 hour per week
	Safety	Young person feels safe at home, at school, and in the neighborhood
Boundaries and expectations	Family boundaries	Family has clear rules and consequences, and monitors the young person's whereabouts
	School boundaries	School provides clear rules and consequences
	Neighborhood boundaries	Neighbors take responsibility for monitoring young people's behavior
	Adult role models	Parent(s) and other adults model positive, responsible behavior
	Positive peer influence	Young person's best friends model responsible behavior
	High expectations	Both parent(s) and teachers encourage the young person to do well

Table 10–4. The Search Institute's 40 developmental assets for youths ages 12–18 years (continued)

	Asset Name	Definition
External assets (continued)		
Constructive use of time	Creative activities	Young person spends ≥3 hours per week in lessons or practice in music, theater, or other arts
	Youth programs	Young person spends ≥3 hours per week in sports, clubs, or organizations at school and/or in community organizations
	Religious community	Young person spends ≥1 hour per week in activities in a religious institution
	Time at home	Young person is out with friends "with nothing special to do" ≤2 nights per week
Internal assets		
Commitment to learning	Achievement motivation	Young person is motivated to do well in school
	School engagement	Young person is actively engaged in learning
	Homework	Young person reports doing ≥1 hour of homework every school day
	Bonding to school	Young person cares about her or his school
	Reading for pleasure	Young person reads for pleasure ≥3 hours per week
Positive values	Caring	Young person places high value on helping other people
	Equality and social justice	Young person places high value on promoting equality and reducing hunger/poverty
	Integrity	Young person acts on convictions and stands up for her or his beliefs
	Honesty	Young person "tells the truth even when it is not easy"
	Responsibility	Young person accepts and takes personal responsibility
	Restraint	Young person believes it is important not to be sexually active or to use alcohol or other drugs

Table 10–4. The Search Institute's 40 developmental assets for youths ages 12–18 years *(continued)*

	Asset Name	Definition
Internal assets *(continued)*		
Social competencies	Planning and decision making	Young person knows how to plan ahead and make choices
	Interpersonal competence	Young person has empathy, sensitivity, and friendship skills
	Cultural competence	Young person has knowledge of and comfort with people of different cultural/racial/ethnic backgrounds
	Resistance skills	Young person can resist negative peer pressure and dangerous situations
	Peaceful conflict resolution	Young person seeks to resolve conflict nonviolently
Positive identity	Personal power	Young person feels he or she has control over "things that happen to me"
	Self-esteem	Young person reports having a high self-esteem
	Sense of purpose	Young person reports that "my life has a purpose"
	Positive view of personal future	Young person is optimistic about his or her personal future

Pittman and colleagues (2003) have identified seven kinds of *basic inputs*, organized around services, supports, and opportunities, that provide the environment necessary for healthy development. These inputs, or protective factors, are as follows:

- *Services,* such as:
  - Stable places (e.g., a safe, permanent place to live)
  - Basic care and services (e.g., access to health care and education)
- *Supports,* such as:
  - Healthy relationships with peers and adults
  - High expectations and standards
  - Role models, resources, and networks
- *Opportunities,* such as:
  - Challenging experiences and opportunities to participate and contribute
  - High-quality instruction and training

Resilience and Positive Youth Development

Rutter defines *resilience* as the ability to remain competent when faced with stress, or the ability to overcome adversity (Rutter 1985, 1996, 2006, 2007). Masten and Obradovic (2006) discuss the importance of understanding resilience in a developmental context, where success or failure on one developmental test affect individuals ability to survive the next. Some building blocks for resilience, such as sound executive functioning and the ability to self-regulate (Dishion and Connel 2006; Greenberg 2006) may be innate (Rutter 2006). Other correlates of resilience, however, such as having social support (Ozbay et al. 2008), can be developed and nurtured.

The positive youth development movement provides prevention-minded psychiatrists with information regarding interventions that promote healthy development and resiliency (The Education Alliance 2007). Catalano and colleagues (2002) emphasized that positive youth development requires that programs do the following:

- Promote bonding, as well as social, emotional, cognitive, behavioral, and moral competence

- Foster belief in the future, clear and positive identity, prosocial norms (health standards for behavior), resilience, self-determination, self-efficacy, and spirituality
- Provide recognition for positive behavior and opportunities for prosocial involvement

Catalano and colleagues (2002) also described 25 health promotion programs that used a variety of methods, from mentoring to community organizing, to engage and promote the health of youths ages 6–20 years. All interventions aimed to increase a broad array of individual competencies, as well as to promote prosocial behavior with the youths' family and community. Improved outcomes included increased school attendance and performance; improved interpersonal interactions with adults and peers; and decreased aggression, violence, and high-risk behaviors.

Bauer and Webster-Stratton (2006) encourage pediatricians to incorporate principles of *positive parenting* into routine visits. These principles, which can be incorporated into evaluations or collateral work with adolescents, include:

- Using a collaborative, systems-based approach
- Emphasizing nonpunitive discipline
- Utilizing the power of parental attention
- Encouraging parents to model appropriate behaviors
- Teaching parents coping techniques

The Transition to Adulthood

The prevention minded psychiatrist should keep in mind that, just as adversity sometimes leads to a downward life trajectory, at other times it provides individuals with an opportunity to develop in more positive ways. Obradovic and colleagues (2006) describe the transition to adulthood as a developmental phase in which individuals are particularly vulnerable, but also have an opportunity for dramatic improvement in their life circumstance. For this reason psychiatrists treating older adolescents or young adults exhibiting problem behaviors should not succumb to fatalism, but rather hold onto the hope that their patients can change, and look to convert crises into opportunities for intervention (Masten et al. 2004).

Translating the Research: Recommendations for Preventing Harm and Promoting Strength in Youth

After reviewing risk and protective factors, the evidence-based interventions, and theories of resilience and health promotion, the prevention-minded general psychiatrist can consider the recommendations below when working with individuals and families affected by conduct disorder and other behavioral problems in adolescence:

1. Review adolescent development. In order to recognize deviance, it is important to know what is normal at different stages of development.
2. Discuss confidentiality with the adolescent and her or his parents or guardian. Having this conversation upfront can prevent subsequent misunderstanding.
3. Create and maintain an alliance with the parents and with the adolescent. The most effective interventions draw largely on parents, and the individual practitioner needs to do the same.
4. Review and recommend effective parenting principles, such as those distributed by the American Academy of Child and Adolescent Psychiatry (2001) or the American Academy of Pediatrics (Stein and Perrin 1998).
5. Ask about risk factors for behavioral problems. Identify, when possible, any impact they have had on the youth's life. Address them, either in the office or via a referral.
6. Review strengths and assets. Build on strengths and be mindful of how to promote developing more strengths.
7. If your patient is of child-bearing age, always keep in mind the next generation. As Olds and colleagues (1998) demonstrated, intervening with mothers can have significant protective effects for offspring.
8. Given that interpersonal problems are a risk factor (Coie et al. 1993), consider referring patients for individual and family therapy to decrease conflict and increase interpersonal connectedness.
9. Make your office a positive developmental setting, as suggested by Duncan and colleagues (2007) (Table 10–5).
10. Be an advocate in the community.

Table 10–5.   Positive youth developmental features and clinical applications

Positive youth developmental feature	Application in the clinical or office setting
Physical and psychological safety	Clarify confidentiality practices
Clear and appropriate structure	Explain organization of sessions
Supportive relationships	Show interest in the person's life, in addition to symptoms; encourage staff to be courteous
Opportunities to belong	Offer materials and an environment appropriate to adolescents
Positive social norms	Model respect; express nonjudgmental concern regarding risky behavior
Support for self-efficacy	Make direct recommendations to the adolescent first, then to his or her parents; acknowledge the adolescent's responsibility for his/her own health
Opportunities for skill building	Post or otherwise communicate appropriate volunteer opportunities
Integration of family, school, and community	Contact area schools to find out how they are implementing positive youth developmental concepts

Source.   Adapted from Duncan et al. 2007.

Key Points

- Adolescents are not simply young adults, and should not be treated as such. Approaches to prevention must begin with assessing an adolescent's cognitive, social, behavioral, and emotional developmental stage, and interventions must be targeted accordingly.

- Conduct disorder and other behavioral problems are common and exact a heavy economic and emotional cost. Risk factors for these problems are identifiable, and primary and secondary preventive interventions, particularly those that start early and endure, have proven to be effective.

- Factors that protect against conduct problems have also been identified. Through work with adolescents, their families, and communities, prevention-minded clinicians can develop and build on such protective factors, which will further foster positive development.

- Rather than giving up on older youths with conduct disorder or other behavioral problems, clinicians should know that research indicates the transition to adulthood provides opportunities to intervene and, quite possibly, alter a young person's life trajectory.

References

American Academy of Child and Adolescent Psychiatry: Facts for families: parenting: preparing for adolescence. June 2001. Available at: http://www.aacap.org/cs/root/facts_for_families/parenting_preparing_for_adolescence. Accessed November 9, 2008.

American Psychiatric Association: Diagnostic and Statistical Manual of Mental Disorders, 4th Edition, Text Revision. Washington, DC, American Psychiatric Association, 2000

Bauer NS, Webster-Stratton C: Prevention of behavioral disorders in primary care. Curr Opin Pediatr 18:654–660, 2006

Beauchaine TP, Webster-Stratton C, Reid MJ: Mediators, moderators, and predictors of 1-year outcomes among children treated for early onset conduct problems: a latent growth curve analysis. J Consult Clin Psychol 73:371–388, 2005

Borduin CM, Mann BJ, Cone LT, et al: Multisystemic treatment of serious juvenile offenders: long-term prevention of criminality and violence. J Consult Clin Psychol 63:569–578, 1995

Catalano RF, Hawkins JD, Berglund ML, et al: Prevention science and positive youth development: competitive or cooperative frameworks? J Adolesc Health 31 (suppl 6):230–239, 2002

Chapman DP, Dube SR, Anda RF: Adverse childhood events as risk factors for negative mental health outcomes. Psychiatr Ann 37:359–364, 2007

Coie JD, Watt NF, West SG, et al: The science of prevention: a conceptual framework and some directions for a national research program. Am Psychol 48:1013–1022, 1993

Connor DF, Carlson GA, Chang KD, et al: Juvenile maladaptive aggression: a review of prevention, treatment, and service configuration and a proposed research agenda. J Clin Psychiatry 67:808–820, 2006

Dishion TJ, Connell A: Adolescents' resilience as a self-regulatory process: promising themes for linking intervention with developmental science. Ann N Y Acad Sci 1094:125–138, 2006

Duncan PM, Garcia AC, Frankowski BL, et al: Inspiring healthy adolescent choices: a rationale for and guide to strength promotion in primary care. J Adolesc Health 41:525–535, 2007

Durlak JA, Wells AM: Primary prevention mental health programs for children and adolescents: a meta-analytic review. Am J Community Psychol 25:115–152, 1997

Durlak JA, Wells AM: Evaluation of indicated prevention intervention (secondary prevention) mental health programs for children and adolescents. Am J Community Psychol 26:775–802, 1998

The Education Alliance: Positive youth development: policy implications and best practices. 2007. Available at: http://www.educationalliance.org/Downloads/Research/PYDResearch.pdf. Accessed July 6, 2009.

Elliott DS: Serious violent offenders: onset, developmental course, and termination: the American Society of Criminology 1993 presidential address. Criminology 32:1–21, 1994

Eyberg SM, Nelson MM, Boggs SR: Evidence-based psychosocial treatments for children and adolescents with disruptive behavior. J Clin Child Adolesc Psychol 37:215–237, 2008

Foster EM, Jones DE: The high costs of aggression: public expenditures resulting from conduct disorder. Am J Public Health 95:1767–1772, 2005

Greenberg MT: Promoting resilience in children and youth: preventive interventions and their interface with neuroscience. Ann N Y Acad Sci 1094:139–150, 2006

Hawkins JD, Catalano RF: Communities That Care: Action for Drug Abuse Prevention. San Francisco, Jossey-Bass, 1992

Hawkins JD, Jenson JM, Catalano RF, et al: Delinquency and drug abuse: implications for social services. Soc Serv Rev 62:258–284, 1988

Hawkins JD, Brown EC, Oesterle S, et al: Early effects of communities that care on targeted risks and initiation of delinquent behavior and substance abuse. J Adolesc Health 43:15–22, 2008

Henggeler SW, Borduin CM: Family Therapy and Beyond: A Multisystemic Approach to Treating the Behavioral Problems of Children and Adolescents. Pacific Grove, CA, Brooks/Cole, 1990

Henggeler SW, Sheidow AJ: Conduct disorder and delinquency. J Marital Fam Ther 29:505–522, 2003

Henggeler SW, Cunningham PB, Pickrel SG, et al: Multisystemic therapy: an effective violence prevention approach for serious juvenile offenders. J Adolesc 19:47–61, 1996

Henggeler SW, Melton GB, Smith LA: Family preservation using multisystemic therapy: an effective alternative to incarcerating serious juvenile offenders. J Consult Clin Psychol 60:953–961, 1992

Henggeler SW, Melton GB, Brondino MJ, et al: Multisystemic therapy with violent and chronic juvenile offenders and their families: the roles of treatment fidelity in successful dissemination. J Consult Clin Psychol 65:821–833, 1997

Henggeler SW, Clingempeel WG, Brondino MJ, et al: Four-year follow-up of multisystemic therapy with substance-abusing and substance-dependent juvenile offenders. J Am Acad Child Adolesc Psychiatry 41:868–874, 2002

Hill LG, Coie JD, Lochman JE, et al: Effectiveness of early screening for externalizing problems: issues of screening accuracy and utility. J Consult Clin Psychol 72:809–820, 2004

Institute of Medicine: Research on Children and Adolescents with Mental, Behavioral, and Developmental Disorders: Mobilizing a National Initiative. Washington, DC, National Academy Press, 1989

Kantor L: Tailoring pregnancy prevention programs to stages of adolescent development, in Get Organized: A Guide to Preventing Teen Pregnancy. National Campaign to Prevent Teen Pregnancy. Washington, DC, U.S. Department of Health and Human Services, 1999. Available at: http://aspe.hhs.gov/hsp/get-organized99/ch2.pdf. Accessed July 7, 2009.

Masten AS, Obradovic J: Competence and resilience in development. Ann N Y Acad Sci 1094:13–27, 2006

Masten AS, Burt KB, Roisman GI, et al: Resources and resilience in the transition to adulthood: continuity and change. Dev Psychopathol 16:1071–1094, 2004

Moffitt TE, Arseneault L, Jaffee SR, et al: Research review: DSM-V conduct disorder: research needs for an evidence base. J Child Psychol Psychiatry 49:3–33, 2008

Obradovic J, Burt KB, Masten AS: Pathways of adaptation from adolescence to young adulthood: antecedents and correlates. Ann N Y Acad Sci 1094:340–344, 2006

Olds DL, Eckenrode J, Henderson CR Jr, et al: Long-term effects of home visitation on maternal life course and child abuse and neglect: 15-year follow-up of a randomized trial. JAMA 278:637–643, 1997

Olds D, Henderson CR Jr, Cole R, et al: Long-term effects of nurse home visitation on children's criminal and antisocial behavior: 15-year follow-up of a randomized controlled trial. JAMA 280:1238–1244, 1998

Ozbay F, Fitterling H, Charney D, et al: Social support and resilience to stress across the life span: a neurobiologic framework. Curr Psychiatry Rep 10:304–310, 2008

Pittman K, Irby M, Tolman J, et al: Preventing problems, promoting development, encouraging engagement: competing priorities or inseparable goals? Washington, DC, The Forum for Youth Investment, Impact Strategies, 2003. Available at: www.forumfyi.org/node/105. Accessed July 7, 2008.

Powell NR, Lochman JE, Boxmeyer CL: The prevention of conduct problems. Int Rev Psychiatry 19:597–605, 2007

Roche KM, Ensminger ME, Ialongo N, et al: Early entries into adult roles: associations with aggressive behavior from early adolescence into young adulthood. Youth Soc 38:236–261, 2006

Roehlkepartain EC, Benson PL, Sesma A: Signs of progress in putting children first: developmental assets among youth in St Louis Park, 1997–2001. Minneapolis, MN, Search Institute, 2003. Available at: http://www.search-institute.org/research/assets. Accessed July 7, 2009.

Rutter M: Resilience in the face of adversity: protective factors and resistance to psychiatric disorder. BMJ 147:598–611, 1985

Rutter M: Transitions and turning points in developmental psychopathology: as applied to the age span between childhood and mid-adulthood. Int J Behav Dev 19:603–626, 1996

Rutter M: Implications of resilience concepts for scientific understanding. Ann N Y Acad Sci 1094:1–12, 2006

Rutter M: Resilience, competence, and coping. Child Abuse Negl 31:205–209, 2007

Scales PC Roehlkepartain EC: Boosting student achievement: new research on the power of developmental assets. Search Institute Insights and Evidence 1:1–10, 2003

Search Institute: What kids need: developmental assets. 2007. Available at: http://www.search-institute.org/developmental-assets. Accessed May 27, 2009.

Stein MT, Perrin EL: American Academy of Pediatrics Committee on Psychosocial Aspects of Child and Family Health: Guidance for effective discipline. Pediatrics 101:723–728, 1998

Steiner H, Remsing L, AACAP Work Group on Quality Issues: Practice parameter for the assessment and treatment of children and adolescents with oppositional defiant disorder. J Am Acad Child Adolesc Psychiatry 46:126–141, 2007

Substance Abuse and Mental Health Services Administration (SAMHSA): Communities that care: key leader orientation: The Research Foundation: Trainer's Guide: Module 2. 2003. Available at: http://download.ncadi.samhsa.gov/Prevline/pdfs/ctc/KLO_TG_MOD2.pdf; "Risk Factors Matrix" available at http://ncadi.samhsa.gov/features/ctc/resources.aspx. Accessed July 7, 2009.

Turgay A: Psychopharmacological treatment of oppositional defiant disorder. CNS Drugs 23:1–17, 2009

Waddell C, Hua JM, Garland OM, et al: Preventing mental disorders in children: a systematic review to inform policy-making. Can J Public Health 98:166–173, 2007

Webster-Stratton C, Taylor T: Nipping early risk factors in the bud: preventing substance abuse, delinquency, and violence in adolescence through interventions targeted at young children (0–8 years). Prev Sci 2:165–192, 2001

Woolfenden SR, Williams K, Peat JK: Family and parenting interventions for conduct disorder and delinquency: a meta-analysis of randomized controlled trials. Arch Dis Child 86:251–256, 2002

11

Prevention Principles for Older Adults

Preventing Late-Life Depression, Dementia, and Mild Cognitive Impairment

Joanne A. McGriff, M.D., M.P.H.

William M. McDonald, M.D.

Paul R. Duberstein, Ph.D.

Jeffrey M. Lyness, M.D.

Across several disciplines, the definition of *prevention* has shifted over the past 40 years. In the 1960s, the concept of prevention narrowly referred to averting "the development of a pathological state and all measures—definitive therapy among them—that limit the progression of disease at any stage of its course" (Clark and MacMahon 1967). Steadily, however, the notions of risk factor identification and disease-specific prevention have replaced the generic,

297

population-based approach to achieving improved health and well-being. The 1998 World Health Organization's emphasis on risk factor reduction and the publication of clinical prevention studies focusing on identifying premorbid and morbid states, isolating relevant risk factors, and determining thresholds for appropriate intervention ushered in an era of considering prevention an integral part of disease management (Starfield et al. 2008). Whether this shift in the ideology of prevention is justified or appropriate is certainly debatable (e.g., Starfield et al. 2008).

In this chapter, we emphasize the principles of psychiatric (clinical) disease prevention and its focus on individual risk factors as they relate to late-life depression, dementia, and mild cognitive impairment (MCI). The complexities of diagnosing geriatric psychiatric illnesses and the relatively ubiquitous nature of clinically significant symptoms in the general older adult population warrant a narrower view toward (individual) case identification as a point of departure for understanding population-level intervention and prevention. In geriatric psychiatry, risk factor analysis and emphasis on improving case identification have led to the conceptualization and development of several innovative models of interventions for those afflicted with debilitating mental and emotional disorders. This perspective does not diminish the necessity of good mental health and well-being in the overall population.

As the global health sector focuses on trying to find effective methods to prevent disease and improve quality of life for an aging population, the issue of prevention in geriatric psychiatry has gained prominence, but its importance has not yet become paramount. Innovative prevention studies are underway for some of the most prevalent diseases affecting older adults, such as depression and dementia. These studies focus not only on traditional risk factor identification but also on determining high-risk profiles for particular subgroups of older adults, which convey implications for effective intervention (Schoevers et al. 2006; Smits [sic] et al. 2008).

Definition of Terms

In this chapter, we discuss prevention principles pertaining to late-life depression, dementia, and MCI. Our definitions are consistent with the classifications and conceptual framework of prevention outlined by the Institute of Medicine report on prevention of mental disorders (Mrazek and Haggerty

1994; Whyte and Rovner 2006). We subdivide the section on primary prevention of late-life depression into three categories: universal, selective, and indicated preventive interventions. *Universal preventive interventions* focus on the general population, which includes many individuals who have only minimal risk of developing a particular disorder. Examples include educating the general older adult population about the benefits of exercise for overall physical and mental well-being. *Selective preventive interventions* target specific groups at elevated risk due to the presence of certain risk factors. In late-life depression, selective preventive interventions may include enrolling recently bereaved older adults into a mutual help program for the widowed. *Indicated preventive interventions* focus on individuals with subsyndromal symptoms, in whom the likelihood of developing the syndromic disorder is highly probable. An example would be older adults with subthreshold symptoms of major depression being referred to a behavioral treatment program, which may help ameliorate or eliminate depressive symptoms and prevent the development of a full depressive disorder. In principle, secondary and tertiary prevention are the mainstays of current clinical prevention strategies in geriatric mental health.

Late-Life Depression

Depression is the second most debilitating psychiatric syndrome in older adults, after cognitive impairment (Blazer 2008; Charney et al. 2003). The effects of this chronic, recurrent disorder extend beyond affective and somatic disturbances into complications with chronic medical illnesses, cognitive impairment, functional disability, and reduced psychosocial capacity (Blazer 2003). Moreover, the cumulative effects of depressive symptoms that do not meet criteria for major depression also pose significant challenges to overall geriatric health and have important implications for treatment and prevention.

Clinical Characteristics

Most of the clinical characteristics of geriatric depression can be captured by the DSM-IV-TR criteria for major depression (Alexopoulos et al. 2002; American Psychiatric Association 2000). However, many diagnostic features and issues distinctive to older adults are not emphasized within this framework (Blazer 2008). For instance, Lyness and colleagues (1995) found that depressed older adults in an inpatient hospital setting tended to underreport depressive symptoms, especially ideational/affective dysfunction, compared with their reporting of somatic and cognitive symptoms. Further, older patients in primary care rarely spontaneously report feelings of sadness, worthlessness, or guilt but tend to emphasize a lack of feeling or general anhedonia (Alexopoulos et al. 2002; Blazer 2008). Gallo and Rabins (1999) propose the concept of "depression without sadness" to describe the tendency of primary care older adults to report feelings of apathy, loss of interest, fatigue, difficulty sleeping, and other somatic symptoms.

In addition to the challenges posed by the underreporting of particular symptoms, primary care practitioners often have difficulty disentangling the common complaints of aging and symptoms of chronic diseases from possible symptoms of major depression (e.g., insomnia, fatigue, loneliness) (Alexopoulos et al. 2002; Lawhorne 2005). This could lead to the underdiagnosis of mood disorders. In addition, the competing demands within busy primary care offices often undermine the careful attention required in monitoring changes in mood and physical capacity that may indicate a psychiatric illness in those with one or more comorbid chronic diseases (Klinkman 1997).

Epidemiology

The incidence and prevalence of major depression in older adults in the United States depend on the segment of population under study: community members, primary care patients, hospitalized patients, or older adults in long-term care facilities (Lawhorne 2005). In general, rates tend to be higher in medical settings than in the community.

Among community-dwelling older adults, the prevalence of major depression ranges from 1%–4%, with the incidence estimated at 0.15% per year (Alexopoulos 2005; Blazer 2003). Rates of depressive *symptoms* are significantly higher, with a prevalence of 8%–16% in older adults (Blazer 2003). The prevalence of major depression is higher in women (Alexopoulos 2005), but evidence for racial or ethnic differences is scant. However, a recent psychiatric epidemiological study documented a higher prevalence of major depressive disorder among African American and Caribbean blacks in the United States and a higher risk of persistence of major depressive disorder in black persons compared with white persons (Williams et al. 2007).

As noted above, major depression is more prevalent in primary care clinics, hospitals, and long-term care settings than in community settings. Some 5%–10% of older adults seen in primary care settings have major depression and up to one-third may have depressive symptoms (Blazer 2003). In studies of older adults hospitalized for medical and surgical services, 10%–12% had major depression and an additional 23% had significant symptoms of depression (Alexopoulos 2005; Blazer 2003; Lyness et al. 2007).

Patients in long-term care facilities tend to have higher rates of both major depression and depressive symptoms compared with patients seen in primary care settings and individuals in the community. Among those living in long-term care facilities, the incidence of major depression ranges from 6% to 17% per year, prevalence ranges from 12% to 14%, and 17%–35% of patients exhibit clinically significant depressive symptoms (Alexopoulos 2005; Lawhorne 2005).

Risk Factors

A systematic review of 20 longitudinal studies conducted in community settings highlighted a number of important risk factors (Cole 2008). Other important considerations for risk of late-life depression can be classified as biological or psychosocial.

Biological

The presence of a comorbid medical illness is a common risk factor for major depression. A comprehensive list prioritizes cardiovascular conditions such as cardiovascular disease, post–myocardial infarction, and post–coronary artery bypass surgery as special contributors to the incidence of depression (Krishnan 2002). Other medical illnesses include cancer, neurological conditions (such as stroke, Parkinson disease, and Alzheimer disease), endocrine disorders (e.g., thyroid dysfunction, diabetes) and nutritional deficiencies (e.g., B vitamin deficiency) (Krishnan 2002; Lawhorne 2005). Notably, vascular depression and the pattern of hyperintensities viewed on magnetic resonance imaging secondary to cerebrovascular changes have been associated with older-age depression (Alexopoulos 2005; Krishnan 2002). One recent study suggests that overall medical illness burden may be more important than disease of any specific organ system (Lyness et al. 2006).

Psychosocial

Psychosocial risk factors thought to be related to late-life depression have been studied prospectively and include stressful life events such as relational stress during late adulthood, bereavement, certain personality characteristics, caregiver burden, social isolation, and loss of meaningful social roles (Blazer 2003; Lawhorne 2005; Mrazek and Haggerty 1994). A meta-analysis of 25 studies documented significant associations of depression in older adults with financial strain and relationship difficulties (Kraaij et al. 2002). Neuroticism, the dispositional tendency to experience moodiness and distress, has been shown prospectively to amplify risk of depression, even into the ninth decade of life (Duberstein et al. 2008).

Of note, bereavement is a particular life event that requires considerable attention when considering the mental health of older adults. Older widows and widowers frequently experience sadness, anger, guilt, and despair immediately after, and 1 year or more following, the death of a spouse and are often at risk for developing a depressive episode (Holley and Mast 2007; Ott et al. 2007). In addition, the multiple life transitions and disruptions that occur after the loss of a spouse often leave widows and widowers alone to cope with a new, single lifestyle that may not provide the meaningful social interaction that they were accustomed to (Mrazek and Haggerty 1994).

Treatment

In general, management of late-life depression should begin with the identification of any drug or medical illness that may underlie changes in mood (Alexopoulos 2005). Once the putative causal element is removed or the illness resolves, then more proactive forms of therapy may begin if depressive symptoms persist. Treatment studies for late-life depression confirm the efficacy of pharmacological therapy, psychotherapy, and electroconvulsive therapy (ECT) (Cole 2008). The preferred treatment option is a combination of both pharmacotherapy and psychotherapy (Alexopoulos 2005), particularly for complex, refractory, or recurrent depressive illness.

In terms of antidepressants, selective serotonin reuptake inhibitors and dual serotonin and norepinephrine reuptake inhibitors appear to be effective and better tolerated than tricyclic antidepressants (Charney et al. 2003). These classes of antidepressants also do not require blood concentration level monitoring or electrocardiography analysis prior to initiation of therapy (Reynolds et al. 2001).

Evidence supports the need for providers to target full remission in the treatment of elderly patients (Charney et al. 2003; Reynolds et al. 2001). Partially treated patients are subject to increased risk of relapse and continued disability. In 1997, the U.S. National Institutes of Health consensus panel on the diagnosis and treatment of late-life depression recommended that depressed geriatric patients experiencing their first episode of depression continue taking antidepressant medications for at least 6 months after the resolution of symptoms (Lebowitz et al. 1997).

Most psychotherapies are designed to help older adults respond effectively to life events and chronic stress. Cognitive-behavioral therapy, supportive psychotherapy, problem-solving therapy, interpersonal therapy, and reminiscence therapy (the latter involves the review of the past in order to help find meaning in the present, as well as an exploration of coping responses to reduce fear and guilt) are suggested psychotherapies for late-life depression (Pinquart et al. 2006); there is some evidence that cognitive-behavioral therapy and reminiscence therapy may be more efficacious than the other approaches (Pinquart et al. 2006). A meta-analysis points to the potential superiority of psychotherapies versus pharmacological interventions in older adults with minor depression or dysthymia (Pinquart et al. 2007), but further research specifically focused on this issue is still needed.

ECT has been shown to be a very effective and safe treatment for geriatric depression (O'Connor et al. 2001). ECT is usually reserved for the more treatment-resistant patients but should be considered earlier in the treatment plan for patients who are psychotic, have severe depression and are at risk for suicide, or are physically compromised due to a lack of nutrition and fluids and need more immediate treatment (Alexopoulos 2005).

Adherence needs to be addressed at every stage with patients and their families. Education should be provided about the potential for relapse and recurrence due to nonadherence to treatment regimens (Reynolds et al. 2001).

Prevention of Late-Life Depression

A survey of the literature on prevention of late-life depression since 2000 shows a significant shift in focus from tertiary prevention approaches (i.e., methods to reduce the occurrence of relapse and chronic disability) to primary prevention (reducing the emergence of new cases) (Reynolds 2008; Smits [sic] et al. 2008; Sriwattanakomen et al. 2008). Much of this shift can be attributed to the acknowledgment by practitioners and caretakers that depression is not a part of the normal aging process. With this perspective, recognition of sub-threshold depressive symptoms that may progress to full syndromic depression, and research into assessment tools and techniques to help identify new cases, have gained greater importance. Another contribution to the shift in prevention focus came from the sheer volume of incident cases of late-life depression and its relationship to the quickly expanding cohort of older adults throughout the world (Smits [sic] et al. 2008). Recent studies of this phenomenon show that one in every five cases of late-life depression is a new condition (Smit et al. 2006; Smits [sic] et al. 2008), such that attention must now turn to prevention at stages that precede disease inception or shortly thereafter (as in secondary prevention). Lastly, as the older birth cohort grows and the number of incident cases increases, recognition and treatment (tertiary prevention) must progress to prevent the negative consequences of untreated or undertreated depression, such as excess morbidity and mortality (Reynolds et al. 2001; Schoevers et al. 2006), high medical service utilization (Luber et al. 2001), high health care costs (Katon et al. 2003), and increased demands on caregivers (Charney et al. 2003).

Primary Prevention

Universal preventive interventions.   Currently, there is little evidence in the psychiatric literature of any late-life depression interventions targeting older adults in general, regardless of the presence of known risk factors. A recent meta-analysis of psychological interventions for depression found only two randomized, controlled trials of universal preventive interventions and concluded that they were less effective than selective or indicated interventions (Cuijpers et al. 2008). One possible explanation for the lack of research on universal preventive interventions may be the risk of negative consequences of interventions directed toward low-risk older adults and the ethical and financial implications of such an approach (Schoevers et al. 2006).

Selective preventive interventions.   Intervention research studies have targeted groups known to be at risk (Rovner et al. 2007) and observational studies have indicated that focusing the design of late-life depression prevention on older adults with specific risk indicators could potentially yield higher overall health gains compared with universal interventions (Schoevers et al. 2006; Smits [sic] et al. 2008).

Smit and colleagues (2006) looked at known risk factors for late-life depression in an analysis to estimate the potential cost-effectiveness of primary prevention programs aimed at reducing incident cases. Using two waves of population-based data from a 3-year longitudinal study in The Netherlands, the researchers reported a depression incidence of 2.8 cases per 100 person-years among community residents ages 55–85 years. Next, distilling a comprehensive list of putative risk factors for depression, the authors devised a model consisting of only six statistically significant risk factors that predicted 83% of the incident cases:

1. Female sex
2. Low educational level (elementary school)
3. Having two or more chronic diseases
4. The presence of functional limitations
5. Having an above-average number of depressive symptoms (Center of Epidemiologic Studies Depression Scale [CES-D] scores of >5 and <16)
6. Having a small social network (<13 persons)

In their discussion, the authors identified an even smaller risk profile that could allow for the greatest health benefits to be achieved and the smallest number of people needed to treat to reduce the rate of new cases of late-life depression. This profile comprises people who 1) have depressive symptoms, 2) have functional limitations, 3) have a small social network, and 4) have one of the first three items listed above (are female or have a low level of education (elementary school) or have two or more chronic diseases).

In a later study, this same research group (Smits [*sic*] et al. 2008) found three additional risk profiles for predicting new cases of chronic or recurrent depression, defined as persons with CES-D scores of greater than 16 at baseline and at 3-year follow-up. The profiles are:

1. People who have anxiety or a score of 8 or higher on the Hospital Anxiety and Depression Scale

2. People who do not have anxiety but do have functional impairments, two or more chronic diseases, and low educational attainment (elementary education vs. high school and higher)

3. People who do not have anxiety or chronic illnesses, but do have functional impairments, have a below-average sense of mastery (locus of control), and live without a partner

The implication of this research lies in its ability to narrow the focus of potentially costly interventions to smaller populations of at-risk older adults.

Although actual intervention programs have not yet been tested based on the risk indicators identified in the Dutch studies, Rovner and colleagues (2007) attempted to prevent depression in older adults (>64 years of age) who have age-related macular degeneration (AMD). Research has shown that these individuals are at particular risk for depression given the functional challenges that come with loss of vision (Rovner et al. 2007). In a selective preventive intervention trial (known as the *Preventing Depression in AMD Trial*), Rovner and colleagues (2007) demonstrated the short-term effectiveness of using problem-solving treatment (a skills-enhancing behavioral treatment strategy that assumes that problems of daily life cause and maintain depressive symptoms and that by systematically identifying and addressing these problems, patients can reduce depressive symptoms) to prevent the onset of a depressive disorder in older adults recently diagnosed with AMD. Although the prevention benefit was not maintained throughout 6 months of follow-up, the authors suggest the use of booster or rescue treatments as a possible key to sustaining the effects of this behavioral treatment (Rovner et al. 2007).

Indicated preventive interventions.   Schoevers and colleagues (2006) demonstrated the potential benefit of using an indicated preventive intervention in older adults ages 65–84 years in primary care settings. Using data from the Amsterdam Study of the Elderly, the authors found seven significant risk indicators for the development of late-life depression: medical illness, disability, a personal history of depression, recent loss of a spouse, sleep disturbance, generalized anxiety disorder, and subsyndromal depression (defined as a level of 1–2 at baseline on the Geriatric Mental State AGECAT [Automated Geriatric Examination for Computer Assisted Taxonomy] system). In fact, subjects with subsyndromal depressive symptoms accounted for nearly one-fourth of the new cases of depression at follow-up 3 years later (Schoevers et al. 2006). The study suggested that using an indicated preventive intervention strategy that identifies individuals with subsyndromal depression might be the preferred strategy for efficiently identifying high-risk groups for intervention.

Secondary Prevention

Perhaps the greatest attention and effort in the prevention of late-life depression has been placed on secondary prevention strategies. Improvement in case identification for late-life depression has clarified the need to enhance the knowledge base of general practitioners, engage family members and friends in assessments, and reorganize systems of care. Key issues such as consensus on a validated screening tool for older adults, especially for ethnic and low-income subpopulations, remain unresolved. In addition, cultural sensitivity and the need for alternative diagnostic approaches for ethnic minorities have broad implications for increasing case identification and the prevention of late-life depression. For instance, black older adults often struggle with mistrust of physicians and hospitals and feel significant stigma is attached to mental disorders and their treatments (Sriwattanakomen et al. 2008). Although most older adults are reluctant to disclose psychological symptoms, older black patients have even greater challenges when dealing with an untrusted health care provider. Further, a number of studies have shown that depressed black patients tend to cope differently with the emotional distress of depression and often seek spiritual and social support from informal (or community) networks before or instead of traditional clinical care (Cooper-Patrick et al. 1997). Hence, the challenges of secondary prevention or early case identification for some groups require approaches that expand beyond primary care clinics into families and communities. It is imperative that new methods of case identification be developed that are well suited to the circumstances of particular subgroups.

Below, we highlight two examples of secondary prevention programs that demonstrate the intervention strategies being developed on the primary care system level and the home-based, community level.

Depression care management.   The depression care management (DCM) model has emerged as an alternative team approach to treating depressed older

adults in primary care (Unutzer et al. 2002). Features of the model include diagnosing depression using a validated screening instrument, administering
antidepressant treatments using an algorithmic approach, and conducting
observer-based assessments to monitor and guide treatment (Snowden et al.
2008). This is a collaborative effort, with a trained social worker, nurse, or
other practitioner working together with a consulting psychiatrist to educate,
monitor, track the progress of, and adjust the treatment regimen for each patient (Unutzer et al. 2002). One randomized, controlled trial has demonstrated a reduction of depressive symptoms in those assigned to DCM versus
usual care (Unutzer et al. 2002).

Program to Encourage Active, Rewarding Lives for Seniors.   The Program to
Encourage Active, Rewarding Lives for Seniors (PEARLS) is a home-based
treatment intervention to help manage minor depression and dysthymia in
older community-dwelling adults. The older adult participants were randomized to either receive usual care or participate in the PEARLS program, in
which they received problem-solving therapy, social and physical activation
(including activities to increase patients' social interactions outside the home
and help patients develop a regular physical activity program), and possible
referral to the participant's physician for antidepressant medications (Ciechanowski et al. 2004). Results showed that at 1 year the home-based program
had reduced depressive symptoms by 50% from baseline and improved quality of life measures, such as functional and emotional well-being (Ciechanowski et al. 2004).

Tertiary Prevention

Reynolds and colleagues (2001) note that keeping patients well after the acute
phase of a depressive episode subsides is a vital component of care. A common
error in clinical practice is the premature discontinuation of treatment before
full remission and recovery, and some practitioners are reluctant to use more
than one drug or adjunctive treatment such as psychotherapy (Reynolds et al.
2001). In fact, one study found that one in five elderly patients required the
use of antidepressants or adjunctive medication to achieve remission and to
avoid relapse (Reynolds et al. 2001, 2006).

Dementia

Clinical Characteristics

The DSM-IV-TR describes dementia as a clinical syndrome characterized by the development of multiple cognitive deficits that include memory impairment and at least one other cognitive disturbance, such as aphasia, apraxia, agnosia, or a disturbance in executive function, that impairs social or occupational functioning. Diagnostic criteria for Alzheimer disease—the most common cause of dementia, accounting for 60%–70% of all cases (Fratiglioni et al. 2007)—are shown in Table 11–1.

Dementia patients often present with impaired ability to learn new material or to recall previously learned material (such as misplacing valuables or getting lost in a familiar neighborhood). Other features include deterioration of language or difficulty with speech (aphasia), inability to recall the names of objects or persons (agnosia), inability to carry out motor activities despite intact motor function (apraxia), and impairment in planning or abstract thinking (deficits in executive function).

The dementias are further classified in DSM-IV-TR according to presumed etiology and include dementia of the Alzheimer's type, vascular dementia, dementia due to other general medical conditions, substance-induced persisting dementia, dementia due to multiple etiologies, and dementia not otherwise specified.

Epidemiology

The global prevalence of dementia in people more than 60 years old has been estimated at 3.9% (Qiu et al. 2007). The prevalence of dementia is generally lower in developing countries, though this likely reflects methodological artifacts and may not account for regional variation within developing countries. North America has a regional estimate of 6.4% (Ferri et al. 2005; see also Zhang et al. 2006).

The incidence of dementia worldwide is estimated to be 7.5 per 1,000 population with rates increasing exponentially with age (Ferri et al. 2005; Qiu et al. 2007). In the United States, major population-based studies have reported higher estimates of incidence, ranging from 19.3 to 25.5 per 1,000 person-years in adults more than 65 years old (Haan and Wallace 2004; Miech

Table 11–1. DSM-IV-TR diagnostic criteria for dementia of the Alzheimer's type

A.   The development of multiple cognitive deficits manifested by both

  (1)   memory impairment (impaired ability to learn new information or to recall previously learned information)

  (2)   one (or more) of the following cognitive disturbances:

    (a)   aphasia (language disturbance)

    (b)   apraxia (impaired ability to carry out motor activities despite intact motor function)

    (c)   agnosia (failure to recognize or identify objects despite intact sensory function)

    (d)   disturbance in executive functioning (i.e., planning, organizing, sequencing, abstracting)

B.   The cognitive deficits in Criteria A1 and A2 each cause significant impairment in social or occupational functioning and represent a significant decline from a previous level of functioning.

C.   The course is characterized by gradual onset and continuing cognitive decline.

D.   The cognitive deficits in Criteria A1 and A2 are not due to any of the following:

  (1)   other central nervous system conditions that cause progressive deficits in memory and cognition (e.g., cerebrovascular disease, Parkinson's disease, Huntington's disease, subdural hematoma, normal-pressure hydrocephalus, brain tumor)

  (2)   systemic conditions that are known to cause dementia (e.g., hypothyroidism, vitamin B_{12} or folic acid deficiency, niacin deficiency, hypercalcemia, neurosyphilis, HIV infection)

  (3)   substance-induced conditions

E.   The deficits do not occur exclusively during the course of a delirium.

F.   The disturbance is not better accounted for by another Axis I disorder (e.g., Major Depressive Disorder, Schizophrenia).

  Code based on presence or absence of a clinically significant behavioral disturbance:

    294.10   Without Behavioral Disturbance: if the cognitive disturbance is not accompanied by any clinically significant behavioral disturbance

    294.11   With Behavioral Disturbance: if the cognitive disturbance is accompanied by a clinically significant behavioral disturbance (e.g., wandering, agitation)

Table 11–1. DSM-IV-TR diagnostic criteria for dementia of the Alzheimer's type *(continued)*

Specify subtype:

      With Early Onset: if onset is at age 65 years or below

      With Late Onset: if onset is after age 65 years

Coding note: Also code 331.0 Alzheimer's disease on Axis III. Indicate other prominent clinical features related to the Alzheimer's disease on Axis I (e.g., 293.83 Mood Disorder Due to Alzheimer's Disease, With Depressive Features, and 310.1 Personality Change Due to Alzheimer's Disease, Aggressive Type).

Source. Reprinted from American Psychiatric Association: *Diagnostic and Statistical Manual of Mental Disorders,* 4th Edition, Revised. Washington, DC, American Psychiatric Association, 2000. Copyright 2000, American Psychiatric Association. Used with permission.

et al. 2002). Moreover, a separate study examined the incidence of dementia among African Americans older than 65 years and reported a rate of 32.4 per 1,000 person-years (Haan and Wallace 2004; Hendrie et al. 2001).

The two most common subtypes of dementia are Alzheimer disease and vascular dementia. Both have similar patterns of incidence and prevalence across regions, with Alzheimer disease and vascular dementia accounting for the majority of all cases (Haan and Wallace 2004; Qiu et al. 2007).

Risk Factors

Age

Age is the principal risk factor for dementia. As individuals age, their chances of developing progressive memory loss and dementia increase. Although few cases of dementia occur before age 60, meta-analyses show prevalence rates that increase as individuals surpass age 65 and double every 4 years to about 30% by age 80 (Ritchie and Lovestone 2002).

Presence of Mild Cognitive Impairment

Individuals with MCI are essentially normally functioning adults who do not have dementia but who present with a cognitive complaint (e.g., memory impairment) (Winblad et al. 2004). Often referred to as a transitional zone between normal cognition and dementia, MCI progresses to Alzheimer dementia at a rate of 10%–15% per year (Cummings et al. 2007). Although the delineation of the relationship between MCI and dementia continues, there is growing evidence that the relationship between these cognitive states offers important opportunities for prevention research.

Genetic Factors

The most recognized genetic risk for the occurrence of dementia is the APOE gene, which is responsible for encoding the cholesterol transport protein apolipoprotein E (ApoE). In particular, the allele producing the ε4 type of ApoE (the APOE*E4 allele) has a well-established relationship with an increased risk of both Alzheimer disease and vascular dementia (Breitner 2007; Haan and Wallace 2004). Individuals who have a family history of Alzheimer disease and who carry at least one copy of the APOE*E4 allele are more likely to experience neurocognitive changes by the fifth and sixth decades of life and to have the cognitive changes progress to full-blown dementia (Breitner 2007; Winblad et al. 2004). Those carrying homozygous pairs of the APOE*E4 allele have an even stronger risk of dementia than those with a heterozygous profile (Haan and Wallace 2004). APOE*E4 accounts for up to 40% of the genetic risk of developing late-onset Alzheimer disease, with variations across age, gender, and ethnicity (Haan and Wallace 2004). In one U.S. study, Evans and colleagues (2000) estimated that about 13% of dementia cases would be eliminated if the APOE*E4 allele did not exist.

Vascular Risk Factors and Disorders

The contribution of ApoE to the onset and progression of dementia is facilitated through its relationship to higher low-density lipoprotein (LDL) levels and secondary coronary heart or artery disease. Haan and Wallace (2004) suggest that cumulative effects of elevated LDL levels combined with amyloid deposition and oxidative stress increase the risk of both Alzheimer disease and vascular dementia, but perhaps especially the risk of vascular dementia. Hence, prevention approaches may need to encompass strategies to change dietary lifestyles, increase exercise, and make other changes to improve cardiac health and reduce high cholesterol levels. These modifications may have considerable protective significance for genetically vulnerable populations such as those carrying the APOE*E4 allele.

In addition, there is significant evidence suggesting that vascular factors and disorders are directly involved in the occurrence and progression of dementia (Qiu et al. 2007). Obesity, infrequent exercise, hypertension, stroke, and type 2 diabetes have been linked to both subtypes of dementia (Haan and Wallace 2004).

Dietary and Nutritional Factors

Nutritional considerations for dementia include the possible link between increased dietary antioxidants (e.g., vitamins C and E) and B vitamins (e.g., B_6 and B_{12}) and decreased risk of Alzheimer disease (Haan and Wilson 2004). However, clinical trials have failed to find any effect of vitamin E supplementation on cognitive decline (Qiu et al. 2007). In addition, a review of clinical trials found no evidence of an effect of folate or B vitamins (B_6 or B_{12}) intake on cognition (Balk et al. 2007). Debate is ongoing about the effects of vitamin supplementation in memory loss and overall health, and the issue remains unresolved.

Systemic Inflammation

The role of inflammation in the atherosclerotic process had led to hopes that anti-inflammatory agents might delay the onset of or prevent dementia. Epidemiological studies have suggested that the use of nonsteroidal anti-inflammatory drugs (NSAIDs) could be associated with a lower risk of Alzheimer disease; clinical trials, however, have found no such protective quality (as reviewed in Qiu et al. 2007; see also "Prevention of Dementia" section).

Physical Inactivity

At least six longitudinal studies have found that physical activity is associated with a lower risk of dementia (Qiu et al. 2007), and a meta-analysis has affirmed that fitness training increases general cognitive performance (Colcombe and Kramer 2003). What remains unclear is the delineation of exactly how cardiovascular exercise prevents neuronal damage and whether these changes are affected by baseline cognitive and fitness levels of older adults participating in exercise programs (Colcombe and Kramer 2003).

Social Network/Leisure Activities

Population-based cohort studies reveal a strong relationship between nonphysical leisure activity and cognitive performance (Fratiglioni et al. 2004). Older adults who are more engaged in social, mentally stimulating activities have a reduced risk of cognitive decline (Fratiglioni et al. 2004, 2007).

Educational Level

The *cognitive reserve hypothesis* (Stern 2006) suggests that individuals who attained higher levels of education have greater levels of cognitive reserve, and thus express clinical changes in response to normal brain aging and atrophy at a comparatively slower rate. A *larger brain reserve*, defined as larger brain mass or greater neuronal count due to increased stimulation, presumably protects against brain atrophy. It thus takes a greater amount of brain damage before reaching the threshold for clinical expression. This theory is largely based on several clinical case studies in which individuals without dementia, who at death showed advanced Alzheimer disease pathology, evidenced no or little expression of cognitive decline (Stern 2006).

Though this biological hypothesis may help explain some of the observed relationship between low educational level and risk of dementia, other issues that remain untested are the implications of education as an indicator for early life circumstances and socioeconomic status, and its effect on symptom recognition and early detection of dementia (Qiu et al. 2007).

Treatment of Dementia

The treatment of dementia is a multimodal, dynamic process that follows the progressive nature of the disease. Treatment strategies are characterized by ongoing assessments to monitor the evolution of cognitive and noncognitive deficits and their response to intervention (APA Work Group 2007). In addition, concomitant psychiatric symptoms such as psychosis, agitation, insomnia, and depressed mood also are evaluated and treated to provide maximum functional status.

Currently, three main pharmacological agents exist for the treatment of mild to moderate Alzheimer dementia—donepezil, rivastigmine, and galantamine (Blazer 2008). These drugs have been found to have modest benefits in clinical trial testing (APA Work Group 2007). Memantine, an agent in a new class of drugs known as noncompetitive N-methyl-D-aspartate antagonists, has been approved by the U.S. Food and Drug Administration to treat moderate and severe Alzheimer disease. It has been shown to provide modest benefits and have few side effects (APA Work Group 2007; Blazer 2008).

Additional considerations in treatment include the evaluation and management of co-occurring medical disorders, safety recommendations, and psychosocial support (APA Work Group 2007). Strong alliances with family members and other caregivers are also important to help in assessing changes in cognition and compliance with treatment regimens (Blazer 2008).

Prevention of Dementia

Direct application of the principles of prevention, as stated by the Institute of Medicine, to dementia poses a number of challenges. At the heart of preventive intervention research and application is the proper identification and prioritization of risk factors. In the prevention literature on dementia, conflicting views exist on the actual predictive value of risk factors in the development of dementia. Observational studies that have led the way in identifying presumably modifiable risk factors have not always been replicated by experimental (clinical trial) testing. For instance, the use of NSAIDs to slow or reduce the risk of developing Alzheimer disease remains controversial (Etminan et al. 2003; Qui et al. 2007; Szekely et al. 2008; Vlad et al. 2008). Longitudinal and twin studies have reported the possibility of a protective effect of NSAID use, but several clinical trials have not found the same benefit (Aisen et al. 2000, 2003; Van Gool et al. 2001) (see Etminan and colleagues 2003 for a meta-analysis).

Another challenge is that the appropriate points of intervention are unclear with a disease that is progressive in nature and manifests with a wide spectrum of cognitive and noncognitive symptoms that change over time. As discussed in the "Mild Cognitive Impairment" section, the boundaries between normal cognition, MCI, and dementia are not always clear and therefore pose a challenge in prevention research. Below we provide a brief discussion of key issues for consideration as the field of dementia prevention advances.

Primary Prevention

Cummings and colleagues (2007) have proposed a number of strategies for approaching the issue of primary prevention in dementia and Alzheimer disease research. For example, for universal preventive interventions, they suggest the possible use of age as the primary risk factor in clinical trials. They speculate that giving preventive pharmacotherapy to large samples of asymptomatic older adults (>80 years of age) without dementia may give us important information about the progression of cognitive decline and whether the medications in fact slow the development of dementia (Cummings et al. 2007).

Other primary prevention approaches include the use of risk factor research to identify groups of older adults at risk for dementia and targeting specific interventions to delay or prevent the development of cognitive dysfunction (selective and indicated preventive interventions) (Breitner 2007). The most important risk factors would probably include the presence of MCI and the APOE*E4 allele (Cummings et al. 2007). In addition, selection criteria related to cardiovascular risk factors (e.g., diabetes, hypertension, or a history of stroke) could also identify potentially useful subgroups for intervention.

Secondary Prevention

The most promising secondary prevention strategy is to use therapeutic agents that may slow the progression of dementia symptoms in individuals with MCI. Although a reversal of symptoms is not always expected, a delay in the onset of dementia is an acceptable outcome (Breitner 2007). Randomized clinical trials using cholinesterase inhibitors, antioxidants, and anti-inflammatory agents have shown variable reductions in the progression of MCI to dementia and Alzheimer disease, ranging from 4% or 5% to 16% per year (Breitner 2007; Cummings et al. 2007).

Tertiary Prevention

Tertiary prevention strategies include the long-term care of individuals with dementia and treatment strategies that optimize quality of life and minimize suffering (Fratiglioni et al. 2007). Ongoing assessment of cognitive and noncognitive symptoms, as well as treating co-occurring psychiatric symptoms (such as agitation and insomnia), is vital for the comfort and safety of those with dementia. Evaluation of the patient's living conditions, the adequacy of their supervision and support, and any evidence of neglect or abuse should also be part of maintenance care and treatment (APA Work Group 2007).

Mild Cognitive Impairment

MCI generally refers to cognitive deficits that do not meet diagnostic criteria for dementia and have not yet adversely affected daily functioning. As mentioned earlier in the context of dementia (see subsection "Risk Factors"), MCI represents a transitional state between normal functioning and dementia (Petersen 2004; Winblad et al. 2004). Currently there is very little agreement about the boundaries between normal cognition, MCI, and dementia. Furthermore, the heterogeneous nature of MCI and its nonspecific course blur the prognostic value of cognitive testing to confirm the diagnosis. More research is needed to elucidate the continuum of cognitive decline and determine whether MCI could be justifiably categorized as a disorder.

Clinical Characteristics

Petersen and colleagues (1999) identified five major features of MCI:

1. A memory complaint usually corroborated by an observer
2. Objective memory impairment for the person's age
3. Relatively preserved general cognitive function
4. Largely intact functional activities of daily living
5. Not meeting diagnostic criteria for dementia

In 2004, the definition of MCI was modified to include two clinical subtypes of MCI, amnestic and nonamnestic, given that the definition of MCI includes those who demonstrate impairment in cognitive domains other than memory (e.g., language, executive function, visuospatial skills; Petersen 2004). The definition of MCI was also modified to delineate impairment in single versus multiple cognitive domains (Petersen 2004).

Epidemiology

To date, estimates of the prevalence and incidence of MCI are highly variable, largely because studies vary considerably in methodology, including diagnostic criteria, classification, sampling, assessment measures, testing procedures, and follow-up periods. In a review of clinical and epidemiological studies of preclinical or "predementia" states between 1986 and 2004, the authors found several studies that offer disparate and even contradictory results (Panza et al. 2005). According to the report of the International Working Group on Mild Cognitive Impairment, more research is needed to establish both the prevalence and incidence of MCI in different populations and age groups (Winblad et al. 2004).

Risk Factors

Given the progressive nature of dementia, risk factors identified for dementia may also apply to MCI. However, both growing knowledge of biomarkers and genetic research may offer a divergent etiology for MCI.

Biomarkers

There is limited research on biomarkers for MCI. Research into the role of the cerebrospinal fluid biomarkers total tau protein and the 42-amino-acid form of β-amyloid protein have focused on the relationships between biomarker levels and the risk of Alzheimer disease (Rockwood et al. 2007; Winblad et al. 2004). It is not known how the levels of these markers may or may not affect MCI. In addition, studies of biomarkers of cognitive decline still must address the effect of baseline concentration levels of these markers in the cerebrospinal fluid of older adults, as well as the impact of medications (Winblad et al. 2004).

Genetics

The APOE gene, particularly the APOE*E4 allele, has been associated with the progression of MCI to dementia (Albert and Blacker 2006; Winblad et al. 2004), but research is needed to understand the predictive and prognostic value of the APOE*E4 allele as well as the dynamics of gene-environment interactions among older adults (Winblad et al. 2004).

Treatment

Primary treatment strategies for MCI center on appropriate recognition of cognitive deficits. Subjective cognitive complaints from older patients warrant verification by objective cognitive or neuropsychological testing (Petersen 2004; Winblad et al. 2004). Persistent or worsening cognitive impairment should be referred to a specialist's care.

Although there is some evidence of efficacy in studies of pharmacological treatments in Alzheimer disease (Cummings et al. 2007), the design of the clinical trials, including methodological decisions about diagnostic criteria and the selection of memory tests and study populations, remains controversial (Albert and Blacker 2006; APA Work Group 2007). Most clinical trials have used the rate of conversion from MCI to Alzheimer disease or another form of dementia as the primary outcome measure. Given the methodological differences across studies, the rates of conversion from MCI to Alzheimer disease are variable, ranging from 6% to 16% per year (Albert and Blacker 2006). More studies are needed to evaluate the efficacy of pharmacological treatment of MCI.

Prevention of Mild Cognitive Impairment

As the global population of older adults expands, the potential increase in cognitive deficits and dementia becomes inevitable and creates the need for a committed focus on prevention. With greater understanding of MCI and the prodromal stages of cognitive deterioration, opportunities for primary prevention have surfaced.

Primary Prevention

On a population level, there is little evidence that screening for MCI would yield great public health benefit. There is still disagreement about the validity of MCI related to the sensitivity and specificity of the diagnostic criteria and appropriateness of specific tools for identifying potential cases of MCI (e.g., cognitive tests, imaging studies, and cerebrospinal fluid collection) (Winblad et al. 2004). More research is needed to delineate which instruments will yield accurate information while minimizing cost and personal distress to the older adult. Meanwhile, management of treatable causes of cognitive impairment (e.g., hypothyroidism, polypharmacy, medication side effects, modifiable cerebrovascular risk factors, depression, and vitamin deficiencies, to name a few) and long-term monitoring and assessment of cognitive symptoms are well advised.

Additionally, memory training programs to improve basic memory skills may prevent MCI. For example, Small (2002) and colleagues at the UCLA (University of California, Los Angeles) Center on Aging have developed a simple memory loss prevention program that offers a series of memory exercises, diet plans for a healthy brain, and in-depth psychoeducational discussions to help educate the general public about cognitive deficits and the small steps that can be taken to decrease the risk of sustained memory loss (e.g., Alzheimer dementia).

Randomized, controlled trials of cognitive training interventions have also shown promise. Willis and colleagues (2006) conducted a 5-year, single-blind

Advanced Cognitive Training for Independent and Vital Elderly (ACTIVE) trial with 2,832 seniors (>65 years of age) recruited from the community, hospitals, and clinics to investigate the effect of cognitive training on daily functioning. The interventions consisted of 10 sessions of training in memory, reasoning, or speed of processing, with four booster sessions approximately 1 and 3 years later. The authors found that subjects who participated in the reasoning training reported less difficulty in performing instrumental activities of daily living at year 5. Also, improvement in the cognitive ability that training targeted occurred across the intervention groups and was sustained for up to 5 years (Willis et al. 2006). Though this study did not show specific effects on individuals with cognitive decline, it does indicate great potential for the development of primary prevention strategies in the future.

Secondary Prevention

Current research has not established the absolute efficacy of pharmacological treatments for MCI. Though clinical trials have shown moderate benefits of some agents in treating mild Alzheimer disease, there is not yet a consensus regarding the use of these drugs for patients with MCI. Presumably, strategies to slow the progression of disease in identified cases would begin with a thorough assessment to eliminate the possibility of general medical causes and to treat co-occurring psychiatric symptoms (e.g., depression). Few controlled studies exist on the efficacy of cognitive training programs in those with symptomatic cognitive decline.

Tertiary Prevention

As noted above, there is little evidence for the efficacy of current agents in the treatment and maintenance of individuals with MCI. As clinical trials continue, there is still debate about whether MCI should be viewed as a predementia state or as a separate psychiatric syndrome that has a variable course. One study found that 58.5% of participants ages 55 years and older with one cognitive impairment at baseline did not progress to dementia and 17% actually reverted back to an unimpaired cognitive state by 3–5 years after initial assessment (Alexopoulos et al. 2006). Researchers question whether or not this challenges the paradigm of MCI as a prodromal stage of dementia and whether it is a valid target for prevention strategies (Alexopoulos et al. 2006; Rockwood et al. 2007).

Key Points

- Prevention of late-life depression has shifted in focus from tertiary prevention (the reduction of relapse and chronic disability) and secondary prevention (early case identification) to primary prevention (reducing the emergence of new cases). Epidemiological studies demonstrate that focusing on older adults with selective risk indicators or risk profiles could potentially yield higher overall health gains.

- Secondary prevention strategies in late-life depression have revealed the need to enhance the knowledge base of general practitioners, engage family members and friends in assessments, and reorganize systems of care. Issues such as consensus on a validated screening tool and alternative diagnostic approaches for ethnic and low-income subpopulations remain unresolved.

- Tertiary prevention of late-life depression includes avoiding the premature discontinuation of treatment before full remission and recovery. Also, practitioners should consider the use of more than one antidepressant or adjunctive treatment, such as psychotherapy.

- Prevention of dementia faces the challenge that conflicting views exist on the value of risk factors for predicting the development of dementia. Although observational studies have led the way in identifying risk factors, they have not always been replicated by experimental (clinical trial) testing.

- The most promising secondary prevention strategy for dementia involves the use of therapeutic agents that may help slow the progression of dementia symptoms in individuals with mild cognitive impairment (MCI). Tertiary prevention strategies emphasize optimizing quality of life and minimizing suffering.

- There is still disagreement about the validity of MCI related to the sensitivity and specificity of the diagnostic criteria and appropriateness of specific tools for identifying potential cases of MCI.

- Management of treatable causes of cognitive impairment (e.g., hypothyroidism, polypharmacy, medication side effects, modifiable cerebrovascular risk factors, depression, vitamin deficiencies) and long-term monitoring and assessment of cognitive symptoms are well advised. Current research has not established the absolute efficacy of pharmacological treatments for MCI.

References

Aisen PS, Davis KL, Berg JD, et al: A randomized controlled trial of prednisone in Alzheimer's disease. Neurology 54:588–593, 2000

Aisen PS, Schafer KA, Grundman M, et al: Effects of rofecoxib or naproxen vs placebo on Alzheimer disease progression: a randomized controlled trial. JAMA 289:2819–2826, 2003

Albert MS, Blacker D: Mild cognitive impairment and dementia. Annu Rev Clin Psychol 2:379–388, 2006

Alexopoulos GS: Depression in the elderly. Lancet 365:1961–1970, 2005

Alexopoulos GS, Borson S, Cuthbert DP, et al: Assessment of late life depression. Biol Psychiatry 52:164–174, 2002

Alexopoulos P, Grimmer T, Perneczky R, et al: Do all patients with mild cognitive impairment progress to dementia? J Am Geriatr Soc 54:1008–1010, 2006

American Psychiatric Association: Diagnostic and Statistical Manual of Mental Disorders, 4th Edition, Text Revision. Washington, DC, American Psychiatric Association, 2000

APA Work Group on Alzheimer's Disease and other Dementias; Rabins PV, Blacker D, Rovner BW, et al: American Psychiatric Association practice guideline for the treatment of patients with Alzheimer's disease and other dementias: second edition. Am J Psychiatry 164 (suppl 12):5–56, 2007

Balk EM, Raman G, Tatsioni A, et al: Vitamin B_6, B_{12}, and folic acid supplementation and cognitive function: a systematic review of randomized trials. Arch Intern Med 167:21–30, 2007

Blazer DG: Depression in late life: review and commentary. J Gerontol A Biol Sci Med Sci 58:249–265, 2003

Blazer DG: Treatment of seniors, in The American Psychiatric Publishing Textbook of Psychiatry, 5th Edition. Edited by Hales RE, Yudofsky SC, Gabbard GO. Arlington, VA, American Psychiatric Publishing, 2008, pp 1449–1470

Breitner JCS: Prevention of Alzheimer's disease: principles and prospects, in The Recognition and Prevention of Major Mental and Substance Use Disorders. Edited by Tsuang MT, Stone WS, Lyons MJ. Washington, DC, American Psychiatric Publishing, 2007, pp 319–328

Charney DS, Reynolds CF 3rd, Lewis L, et al; Depression and Bipolar Support Alliance: Depression and Bipolar Support Alliance consensus statement on the unmet needs in diagnosis and treatment of mood disorders in late life. Arch Gen Psychiatry 60:664–672, 2003

Ciechanowski P, Wagner E, Schmaling K, et al: Community integrated home-based depression treatment in older adults: a randomized controlled trial. JAMA 291:1569–1577, 2004

Clark DW, MacMahon B: Preventive Medicine. Boston, MA, Little, Brown, 1967

Colcombe S, Kramer AF: Fitness effects on the cognitive function of older adults: a meta-analytic study. Psychol Sci 14:125–130, 2003

Cole MG: Brief interventions to prevent depression in older subjects: a systematic review of feasibility and effectiveness. Am J Geriatr Psychiatry 16:435–443, 2008

Cooper-Patrick L, Powe NR, Jenckes MW, et al: Identification of patient attitudes and preferences regarding treatment of depression. J Gen Intern Med 12:431–438, 1997

Cuijpers P, Van Straten A, Smit F, et al: Preventing the onset of depressive disorders: a meta-analytic review of psychological interventions. Am J Psychiatry 165:1272–1280, 2008

Cummings JL, Doody R, Clark C: Disease-modifying therapies for Alzheimer disease: challenges to early intervention. Neurology 69:1622–1634, 2007

Duberstein PR, Pálsson S, Waern M, et al: Personality and risk for depression in a birth cohort of 70-year-olds followed for 15 years. Psychol Med 38:663–671, 2008

Etminan M, Gil S, Samii A: Effect of non-steroidal anti-inflammatory drugs on risk of Alzheimer's disease: systematic review and meta-analysis of observational studies. BMJ 327:1–5, 2003

Evans RM, Emsley CL, Gao S, et al: Serum cholesterol, APOE genotype, and the risk of Alzheimer's disease: a population based study of African Americans. Neurology 54:240–242, 2000

Ferri CP, Prince M, Brayne C, et al: Global prevalence of dementia: a Delphi consensus study. Lancet 366:2112–2117, 2005

Fratiglioni L, Palliard-Borg S, Winblad B: An active and socially integrated lifestyle in late life might protect against dementia. Lancet Neurol 3:343–353, 2004

Fratiglioni L, Winblad B, von Strauss E: Prevention of Alzheimer's disease and dementia: major findings from the Kungsholmen Project. Physiol Behav 92:98–104, 2007

Gallo JJ, Rabins PV: Depression without sadness: alternative presentations of depression in late life. Am Fam Physician 60:820–826, 1999

Haan MN, Wallace R: Can dementia be prevented?: brain aging in a population-based context. Annu Rev Public Health 25:1–24, 2004

Hendrie HC, Ogunniyi A, Hall KS, et al: Incidence of dementia and Alzheimer disease in 2 communities: Yoruba residing in Ibadan, Nigeria, and African Americans residing in Indianapolis, Indiana. JAMA 285:739–747, 2001

Holley CK, Mast BT: The effects of widowhood and vascular risk factors on late-life depression. Am J Geriatr Psychiatry 15:690–698, 2007

Katon WJ, Lin E, Russo J, et al: Increased medical costs of a population-based sample of depressed elderly patients. Arch Gen Psychiatry 60:897–903, 2003

Klinkman MS: Competing demands in psychosocial care: a model for the identification and treatment of depressive disorders in primary care. Gen Hosp Psychiatry 19:98–111, 1997

Kraaij V, Arensman E, Spinhoven P: Negative life events and depression in elderly persons: a meta-analysis. J Gerontol B Psychol Sci Soc Sci 57:87–94, 2002

Krishnan KR: Biological risk factors in late life depression. Biol Psychiatry 52:185–192, 2002

Lawhorne L: Depression in the older adult. Prim Care 32:777–792, 2005

Lebowitz BD, Pearson JL, Schneider LS: Diagnosis and treatment of depression in late life: consensus statement update. JAMA 278:1186–1190, 1997

Luber MP, Meyers BS, Williams-Russo PG: Depression and service utilization in elderly primary care patients. Am J Geriatr Psychiatry 9:169–174, 2001

Lyness JM, Cox C, Curry J, et al: Older age and the underreporting of depressive symptoms. J Am Geriatr Soc 43:216–221, 1995

Lyness JM, Niculescu A, Tu X, et al: The relationship of medical comorbidity and depression in older, primary care patients. Psychosomatics 47:435–439, 2006

Lyness JM, Kim J, Tang W, et al: The clinical significance of subsyndromal depression in older primary care patients. Am J Geriatr Psychiatry 15:214–223, 2007

Miech RA, Breitner JC, Zandi PP, et al: Incidence of AD may decline in the early 90s for men, later for women: the Cache County study. Neurology 58:209–218, 2002

Mrazek P, Haggerty R (eds): Reducing Risks for Mental Disorders: Frontiers for Preventive Intervention Research. Washington, DC, National Academy Press, 1994

O'Connor MK, Knapp R, Husain M, et al: The influence of age on the response of major depression to electroconvulsive therapy: a C.O.R.E. report. Am J Geriatr Psychiatry 9:382–290, 2001

Ott CH, Lueger RJ, Kelber ST, et al: Spousal bereavement in older adults: common, resilient, and chronic grief with defining characteristics. J Nerv Ment Dis 195:332–341, 2007

Panza F, D'Introno A, Colacicco A, et al: Current epidemiology of mild cognitive impairment and other pre-dementia syndromes. Am J Geriatr Psychiatry 13:633–644, 2005

Petersen RC: Mild cognitive impairment as a diagnostic entity. J Intern Med 256:183–194, 2004

Petersen R, Smith G, Waring S, et al: Mild cognitive impairment: clinical characterization and outcome. Arch Neurol 56:303–308, 1999

Pinquart M, Duberstein PR, Lyness JM: Treatments for later-life depressive conditions: a meta-analytic comparison of pharmacotherapy and psychotherapy. Am J Psychiatry 163:1493–1501, 2006

Pinquart M, Duberstein PR, Lyness JM: Effects of psychotherapy and behavioral interventions on clinically depressed older adults: a meta-analysis. Aging and Mental Health 11:645–657, 2007

Qiu C, De Ronchi D, Fratiglioni L: The epidemiology of the dementias: an update. Curr Opin Psychiatry 20:380–385, 2007

Reynolds CF: Preventing depression in old age: it's time. Am J Geriatr Psychiatry 16:433–434, 2008

Reynolds CF, Alexopoulos GS, Katz IR, et al: Chronic depression in the elderly: approaches for prevention. Drugs Aging 18:507–514, 2001

Reynolds CF, Dew M, Pollock BG, et al: Maintenance treatment of depression in old age. N Engl J Med 354:1130–1138, 2006

Ritchie K, Lovestone S: The dementias. Lancet 360:1759–1766, 2002

Rockwood K, Chertkow H, Feldman HH: Is mild cognitive impairment a valid target of therapy. Can J Neurol Sci 34 (suppl 1):S90–S96, 2007

Rovner BW, Casten RJ, Hegel MT, et al: Preventing depression in age-related macular degeneration. Arch Gen Psychiatry 64:886–892, 2007

Schoevers RA, Smit F, Deeg DJH, et al: Prevention of late-life depression in primary care: do we know where to begin? Am J Psychiatry 163:1611–1621, 2006

Small G: The Memory Bible. New York, Hyperion, 2002

Smit F, Ederveen A, Cuijpers P, et al: Opportunities for cost-effective prevention of late-life depression: an epidemiological approach. Arch Gen Psychiatry 63:290–296, 2006

Smits [sic] F, Smits N, Schoevers R, et al: An epidemiological approach to depression prevention in old age. Am J Geriatr Psychiatry 16:444–453, 2008

Snowden M, Steinman L, Frederick J: Treating depression in older adults: challenges to implementing the recommendations of an expert panel. Prev Chronic Dis 5:1–7, 2008

Sriwattanakomen R, Ford AF, Thomas SB, et al: Preventing depression in later life: translation from concept to experimental design and implementation. Am J Geriatr Psychiatry 16:460–468, 2008

Starfield B, Hyde J, Gérvas J, et al: The concept of prevention: a good idea gone astray? J Epidemiol Community Health 62:580–583, 2008

Stern Y: Cognitive reserve and Alzheimer disease. Alzheimer Dis Assoc Disord 20:112–117, 2006

Szekely CA, Green RC, Breitner JC, et al: No advantage of A beta 42-lowering NSAIDs for prevention of Alzheimer dementia in six pooled cohort studies. Neurology 70:2291–2298, 2008

Unutzer J, Katon W, Callahan CM, et al: Collaborative care management of late life depression in primary care setting: a randomized controlled trial. JAMA 288:2836–2845, 2002

Van Gool WA, Weinstein HC, Scheltens P, et al: Effect of hydroxychloroquine on progression of dementia in early Alzheimer's disease: an 18-month randomised, double-blind, placebo-controlled study. Lancet 358:455–460, 2001

Vlad SC, Miller DR, Kowall NW, et al: Protective effects of NSAIDs on the development of Alzheimer disease. Neurology 70:1672–1677, 2008

Whyte EM, Rovner B: Depression in late-life: shifting the paradigm from treatment to prevention. Int J Geriatr Psychiatry 21:746–751, 2006

Williams DR, González HM, Neighbors H, et al: Prevalence and distribution of major depressive disorder in African Americans, Caribbean blacks, and non-Hispanic whites: results from the National Survey of American Life. Arch Gen Psychiatry 64:305–315, 2007

Willis SL, Tennstedt SL, Marsiske M, et al: Long-term effects of cognitive training on everyday functional outcomes in older adults. JAMA 296:2805–2814, 2006

Winblad B, Palmer K, Kivipelto M, et al: Mild cognitive impairment—beyond controversies, towards a consensus: report of the International Working Group on Mild Cognitive Impairment. J Intern Med 256:240–246, 2004

Zhang ZX, Zahner GE, Román GC, et al: Socio-demographic variation of dementia subtypes in China: methodology and results of a prevalence study in Beijing, Chengdu, Shanghai, and Xian. Neuroepidemiology 27:177–187, 2006

12

Health Promotion and Prevention of Somatic Illnesses in Psychiatric Settings

Ann L. Hackman, M.D.

Eric B. Hekler, Ph.D.

Lisa Dixon, M.D., M.P.H.

T his chapter addresses the role of physical health promotion and prevention of medical illnesses in psychiatric settings. We primarily focus on people with severe and persistent mental illnesses, such as schizophrenia and severe mood disorders who are receiving outpatient treatment in settings such as community mental health centers. However, we also touch on these issues in private practice, inpatient settings, and psychiatric emergency rooms. We first describe the scope of the problem of somatic illnesses in people with severe and persistent mental illnesses and review some definitions related to health promotion and disease prevention. We then explore some of the interventions that have been used to promote good physical health and prevent disease in nonpsychiatric settings, and consider current efforts to apply some of these approaches in routine psychiatric practice. Finally, we propose future directions for study and implementation.

Scope of the Problem

The challenges of health promotion and disease prevention have long been considered in the general population. Reasons to focus on preventive medicine and health promotion in mental health settings include:

1. Death rates are elevated in people with serious mental illnesses compared with rates in the general population.
2. Somatic illnesses occur frequently in people with serious mental illnesses.
3. Some problematic health behaviors (such as smoking) are prevalent in people with serious mental illnesses, and other factors increase the occurrence of somatic illness in psychiatric patients.
4. Health care disparities exist for psychiatric patients.
5. People with serious mental illnesses experience barriers to medical care.

Each of these is briefly reviewed below.

Death Rates

One essential reason for considering somatic health in people with serious mental illnesses is that these individuals have substantially elevated death rates compared with the general population (Dembling et al. 1999; Jones et al. 2004). Research published more than three decades ago revealed that mortality in people with schizophrenia was significantly greater than in the general population (Tsuang 1975); however, recent work (Capasso et al. 2008) suggests that the survival gap is increasing, perhaps because people with serious mental illnesses are not experiencing the continued lengthening of average lifespan seen in the general population. Death rates for public mental health clients in eight states throughout the country are 1.2–4.9 times higher than expected based on rates in the general population, resulting in an average of 13–30 years of potential life lost per person (Colton and Manderscheid

2006). Further, an Ohio study of more than 20,000 psychiatric patients in public mental health hospitals over a 4-year period, from 1998 through 2002, found that the number of deaths was three times higher than expected, with an average of 32 years of potential life lost per person. Although these numbers did include suicides, heart disease was the leading cause of death for these individuals (Miller et al. 2006).

Somatic Illnesses

The elevated death rates observed among people with serious mental illnesses result in part from elevated rates of somatic diseases. In the general U.S. population, chronic diseases account for 10 of the 15 leading causes of death (Kung et al. 2008). Although people with serious mental illnesses do have higher rates of suicide and death due to accidental injury than do those in the general population (Dalmau et al. 1997; Dickey et al. 2004; Prior et al. 1996; Wan et al. 2006), most deaths in people with serious mental illnesses are attributable to co-occurring and often chronic medical conditions (Lambert et al. 2003; Miller et al. 2006; Prior et al. 1996). We have known for some time that medical illnesses co-occur in three-quarters (Jones et al. 2004) or more (Maricle et al. 1987) of people with serious mental illnesses. The 2005 Clinical Antipsychotic Trials of Intervention Effectiveness (CATIE) study that involved schizophrenia patients found significantly elevated rates of diabetes, hypertension, and cardiac disease (Goff et al. 2005). Other studies have indicated elevated rates of hepatic diseases (Sokal et al. 2004), pulmonary disease including chronic bronchitis and emphysema (Himelhoch et al. 2004; Keyes 2004; Sokal et al. 2004), and infectious diseases such as hepatitis (Goldberg et al. 2005) and human immunodeficiency virus (HIV) infection (Blank et al. 2002; Cournos et al. 1994). The problem of co-occurring medical conditions in people with serious mental illnesses is further complicated because it is common for medical problems to go undiagnosed in this population (Felker et al. 1996; Koran et al. 2002).

Health Behaviors and Other Illness- and Medication-Related Factors

It is likely that several factors—including adverse health behaviors, the impact of a chronic mental illness, and the side effects of medications used to treat chronic mental illnesses—act synergistically to determine health status and mortality risk (Berrigan et al. 2003). Despite the apparent interaction between these factors, study of multiple health indicators to assess overall health status of people with serious mental illnesses has been limited (Dickerson et al. 2006).

Compared with the general population, people with serious mental illnesses engage in fewer health-promoting behaviors. In one study using five selected indicators of good health (the first four of which relate directly to health behaviors), only 1% of people with serious mental illnesses (N=200) met criteria for all five indicators, compared with 10% of the general population (Dickerson et al. 2006). In individuals with serious mental illnesses the rate of smoking is 2–4 times higher than in the general population (Compton et al. 2006; Lasser et al. 2000; Rohde et al. 2003), with higher rates of smoking correlated with more co-occurring medical disorders, greater perceived stress, and poorer quality of life (Dixon et al. 2007). One startling estimate is that 44% of the cigarettes sold in the United States are sold to individuals with a mental illness (Lasser et al. 2000). Individuals with serious mental illnesses are less physically active than the general population (Brown et al. 1999; Daumit et al. 2005) and are more likely to have walking as their sole form of exercise (Daumit et al. 2005). This population also has poor dental care; more than one-third of people with serious mental illness in a large sample of those receiving care through the U.S. Department of Veterans Affairs health care system reported oral health problems severe enough to make eating difficult (Kilbourne et al. 2007). Further, people with serious mental illnesses are at least 50% more likely to be overweight (Compton et al. 2006) and have diets higher in fat and lower in fiber than the general population (Brown et al. 1999). Health behaviors also lead to increased risk of some infectious diseases such as hepatitis (Goldberg et al. 2005) and HIV (Blank et al. 2002; Cournos et al. 1994), with substance abuse explaining much of the increased risk (Himelhoch et al. 2007).

High rates of somatic illness are thought to be multifactorial and derive from shared vulnerability and genetic factors (Mitchell and Malone 2006). Psychiatric illness itself may predispose people to glucose intolerance (Ryan et al. 2003) and nicotine dependence (Tidey et al. 2005). Depressive or deficit symptoms can lead to decreased motivation, rendering individuals less likely to engage in positive health behaviors and proactively address health problems (Dickerson et al. 2006).

In addition to the effects of the psychiatric illness, psychiatric medications also cause some somatic problems. Many antipsychotic and mood-stabilizing medications, especially olanzapine and clozapine, produce weight gain (Allison et al. 1999; Bustillo et al. 1996; Conley and Mahmoud 2001). The issue has become so problematic that it inspired a consensus report from the American Diabetes Association, American Psychiatric Association, American Association of Clinical Endocrinologists, and North American Association for the Study of Obesity (American Diabetes Association et al. 2004) to address treating emergent hyperglycemia and diabetes related to the use of second-generation antipsychotics, with particular focus on olanzapine and clozapine because they may induce insulin resistance independent of weight gain (Melkersson et al. 1999, 2000). Medications, particularly second-generation antipsychotics, can also induce elevated cholesterol levels, resulting in the metabolic syndrome (Meyer 2001; Meyer and Koro 2004). Some antipsychotic medications also cause elevation of the prolactin level, leading to galactorrhea in 14% of patients (Windgassen et al. 1996); this can lead to further complications such as sexual dysfunction and possibly an increased risk of breast cancer (Schyve et al. 1978; Wang et al. 2002).

Health Care Disparities

The medical care received by individuals with serious mental illnesses is often of lower quality than that received by the general population, despite the fact that people with serious mental illnesses are seen regularly in medical settings (Hellerstein et al. 2007; Uebelacker et al. 2006) and may be even more likely to receive certain types of general medical care, such as regular physical examinations (Dickerson et al. 2003). Several medical quality deficits have been noted in the literature, including overuse of some services, underuse of evidence-based general medical services, and misuse or medical errors (Druss and Newcomer 2007).

People with serious mental illnesses often access emergency room services for medical care needs and receive poorer quality care over the long term. Among Medicaid patients, one study found that people with serious mental illnesses received less health care overall than their counterparts without mental illnesses and were more likely to receive their care in emergency room settings than nonemergency settings (Berren et al. 1999). Also, people with serious mental illnesses tend to receive their general medical care in the emergency department at higher rates than the general population (Dickerson et al. 2003; Goldberg and Gmyrek 2007; Hackman et al. 2006). The quality of emergency care for people with psychiatric illnesses is problematic given that evidence suggests that misdiagnosis of urgent medical problems within an emergency room has occurred due to issues including: co-occurring substance use/intoxication, inadequate physical examination, lack of mental status examination, failure to obtain laboratory studies, and failure to obtain an available medical history (Reeves et al. 2000).

Nonemergency settings also present quality of care concerns, though the data are not completely consistent. On one hand, veterans with and without mental illnesses have been found to receive equivalent care (Krein et al. 2006). However, in a study of diabetic patients, Goldberg and colleagues (2007) showed that patients receiving services in community mental health centers were less likely than patients without mental illnesses to receive the full complement of services recommended by the Diabetes Improvement Project (Fleming et al. 2001). Such psychiatric patients also receive less education about diabetes (Goldberg et al. 2007) and have more gaps in their diabetes knowledge (Dickerson et al. 2005).

Individuals with mental illnesses and co-occurring cardiovascular disease also experience quality of care deficits. Druss and colleagues (2000) found that patients with a psychiatric illness who had a myocardial infarction were less likely to undergo cardiac revascularization procedures than those without a psychiatric illness. Studies in nonacute settings have also revealed problems, in that patients with schizophrenia and elevated cholesterol levels were less likely to receive a statin and may also have received less rigorous monitoring of cholesterol levels (Hippisley-Cox et al. 2007) than the general population. The CATIE study (Nasrallah et al. 2006) found that 88% of patients with elevated fasting lipid levels were not receiving statins and 62% of individuals who met criteria for hypertension were not receiving medication for that condition. Such deficits have also been found in people with a mental illness and multiple general medical conditions; compared with mentally healthy individuals with diabetes, community mental health care consumers with diabetes received less aggressive treatment to reduce their cardiac risk: they were less likely to have their lipid levels checked (Goldberg et al. 2007) and were less likely to be treated with cardioprotective medications, such as statins (Dixon et al. 2004; Kreyenbuhl et al. 2008).

Cancer rates among people with serious mental illnesses are not necessarily higher (Lawrence et al. 2000) and may even be lower than among those without a mental illness for some types of cancer, such as prostate cancer (Torrey 2006). Interestingly, however, an Australian study found that people with a mental illness are more likely to die of cancer than those without a mental illness, a phenomenon possibly explained by deficiencies in patient screening and treatment (Lawrence et al. 2000). For instance, in a community mental health center sample, older women with a mental illness were less likely to have mammograms and to perform breast self-examinations than older women in the general population (Dickerson et al. 2002). In a group of patients treated through the U.S. Department of Veterans Affairs health care system, cancer screening was less likely to occur in individuals with a mental illness, including screening for colorectal cancer (fecal occult blood, sigmoidoscopy, colonoscopy) and prostate cancer, even if they had more medical visits than individuals without a mental illness (Druss et al. 2002). For people with a mental illness, more complex or multistep cancer screenings may be less likely to occur than simpler screenings, and individuals who are dually diagnosed (i.e., those with psychiatric illness and a co-occurring substance use disorder) are less likely to receive cancer screenings than those with a mental illness alone (Druss et al. 2002). Lack of screening among peoples with mental illness can lead to the detection of cancers at a later pathological stage than those without a mental illness, thus resulting in higher mortality rates.

Barriers to Health Care

Barriers to health care for people with serious mental illnesses can be related to the patient (the health care consumer) and/or his or her illness, to the provider, or to the system:

- Some consumer-related factors include the socioeconomic status of persons with serious mental illnesses (Farnam et al. 1999), limited knowledge (Farnam et al. 1999), and limited social networks and emotional supports (Barreira 1999).
- Provider-related barriers to prompt and appropriate general medical care include lack of understanding by health care professionals of the issues faced by mental health care consumers and their challenges in navigating

the health care system (Muir-Cochrane 2006), lack of knowledge about psychiatric illnesses and medications on the part of primary care providers (O'Day et al. 2005), and limited ability of psychiatrists to access general medical care services, including referrals, hospital admissions, and imaging studies (Fang and Rizzo 2007).

- Systems barriers involve geographic, financial, and organizational and cultural separation between medical and mental health care as well as other issues, including lack of integrated care and inadequate collaboration between psychiatric and general medical care providers (Druss and Newcomer 2007).

Inadequate insurance coverage and denial of health insurance claims also create barriers to health care (Druss and Rosenheck 1998; Fang and Rizzo 2007).

Somatic illnesses can carry large financial costs and detrimentally impact quality of life, which further drives the need to provide preventive somatic medicine and health promotion services to patients with serious mental illnesses (American Heart Association 2008; Dixon et al. 2000; National Heart Lung and Blood Institute 2007). These costs may be even higher in those with a co-occurring mental illness than in those without mental illness (Kuriyama et al. 2004), in part because of the high utilization of certain services such as hospital emergency departments (Hackman et al. 2006) and in part because medical problems exacerbate psychiatric symptoms (Dixon et al. 2000). For these reasons, over the past several decades interest in improving general medical care services, including disease prevention and health promotion services, to people with serious mental illnesses has increased substantially (Dickerson et al. 2006; McCarrick et al. 1986).

Health Promotion and Illness Prevention: Definitions

As defined by the Canadian Best Practices Portal for Health Promotion and Chronic Disease Prevention (World Health Organization 2004), illness prevention includes 1) interventions aimed at decreasing the likelihood of a disease affecting an individual and 2) interventions designed to interrupt or impede the progress of a disorder. *Health promotion* is defined in a variety of ways. Green and Kreuter (1990) suggest that health promotion includes both educational and environmental factors. O'Donnell (1989) describes health promotion as both a science and an art focused on facilitating lifestyle change with the goal of helping the individual achieve optimal health. Essential components of health promotion include enhancing awareness of healthy behaviors and the impact of unhealthy behaviors, effecting behavioral change, and creating environments that support good health practices. The World Health Organization (WHO) Ottawa Charter for Health Promotion (1986) places some focus on the individual, describing health promotion not only as a process whereby people may improve their health but also as a process of enabling them to increase control over determinants of their health. As described in the WHO Health Promotion Glossary (World Health Organization 1998), health promotion involves a complex social and political process encompassing both actions that are aimed at enhancing the skills and abilities of individuals and actions that are aimed at changing social, environmental, and economic conditions to alleviate their negative impact on public health. Strategies for health promotion described in the Ottawa Charter (World Health Organization 1986) include advocating for health (in the political, economic, social, cultural, and environmental arenas), enabling people to fulfill their full health potential, and mediating between different interests in society in the pursuit of health.

WHO (1986, 1998) advocates a comprehensive approach that includes using settings that offer a practical opportunity to implement comprehensive strategies, including increasing patients' health literacy and knowledge. Community mental health centers and other psychiatric treatment settings provide an accessible and appropriate venue for both preventive somatic medicine and physical health promotion in people with serious mental illnesses.

Health Promotion Within the General Population

Before considering disease prevention and physical health promotion among individuals with serious mental illnesses, we describe some of the ways in which preventive medicine and physical health promotion have been applied in the general population. The reasons for employing health-promoting and preventive medical strategies—including reducing mortality, improving quality of life, and decreasing costs (American Heart Association 2008; National Heart Lung and Blood Institute 2007)—are the same in persons with or without a mental illness. Cardiovascular disease is the leading cause of death in the United States (American Heart Association 2008) and cardiovascular disease and its risk factors are significantly impacted by health behaviors. Our focus in this section is on cardiovascular disease because it provides a good model for discussing prevention and health promotion and allows us to outline specific health promotion recommendations. It is important to note, however, that many of the lifestyle recommendations for patients with cardiovascular disease are also effective for patients with other chronic diseases, including cancer (Thomas and Davies 2007).

Cardiovascular disease is an umbrella term that encompasses several conditions including coronary heart disease, myocardial infarction, cerebrovascular disease, and heart failure (American Heart Association 2008). Several chronic medical problems are risk factors for cardiovascular disease, including high cholesterol and lipid levels, hypertension, being overweight or obese, and diabetes. Cholesterol and lipid levels are evaluated by measuring blood levels of low-density lipoprotein (LDL) and high-density lipoprotein (HDL) (Lichtenstein et al. 2006); the American Heart Association (AHA) recommends that LDL levels remain below 100 mg/dL and that HDL levels be greater than 50 mg/dL in women and greater than 40 mg/dL in men (Lichtenstein et al. 2006). *Hypertension* is currently defined as systolic blood pressure greater than 140 and diastolic blood pressure greater than 80 (Chobanian et al. 2003). Overweight/obesity is most commonly assessed using the body mass index (BMI), with ideal weight defined as a BMI between 18.5 and 24.9 kg/m; being *overweight* is defined as having a BMI between 25 and 29.9 kg/m^2 and *obese* as a BMI of 30 kg/m^2 or greater (Wadden et al. 2002). Diabetes is defined by elevated blood glucose levels, including fasting glucose levels of 126 mg/dL or higher (American Diabetes Association 2005) and includes type 1 diabetes, a usually juvenile-onset condition characterized by a lack of insulin production; gestational diabetes; and type 2 diabetes, a usually adult-onset condition in which individuals produce insulin but either have some resistance to it or do not produce enough (American Diabetes Association 2008). Obesity plays an important role in increasing a person's risk of type 2 diabetes, given that approximately three-quarters of all individuals with type 2 diabetes are or have been obese (American Diabetes Association 2005). Therefore, weight management and other lifestyle factors play an important role in diabetes prevention and management.

The AHA offers guidelines for living with a healthy lifestyle. Recommended behaviors fall broadly into four domains: exercising regularly, managing weight, maintaining a nutritious diet, and quitting smoking if one smokes (Lichtenstein et al. 2006). Managing weight is largely controlled by a balance between physical activity and diet.

Physical Activity

For individuals ages 18–65 years, the American College of Sports Medicine and AHA recommend, at minimum, moderate-intensity aerobic physical activity for 30 minutes per day, 5 days per week, or vigorous aerobic activity 20 minutes per day on at least 3 days per week, as well as strength training twice weekly (Haskell et al. 2007). Because there appears to be a dose-response relationship between physical activity and reduction in cardiovascular disease risk (Kesaniemi et al. 2001), the Institute of Medicine (2002) recommends additional exercise for those who are prone to being overweight or obese (45–60 minutes of moderate intensity activity per day) and those who are already overweight or obese (60–90 minutes daily). Aerobic physical activity has been linked with positive health outcomes including improved lipid levels and lipoprotein profiles (Donnelly et al. 2000), blood pressure (Moreau et al. 2001), fasting plasma insulin levels (Donnelly et al. 2000), cardiorespiratory fitness (Donnelly et al. 2000; Jackicic et al. 1999; Moreau et al. 2001; Murphy et al. 2002), and weight control (Jackicic et al. 1999). Additionally, there may be an inverse association between strength training and all-cause mortality (Fitzgerald et al. 2004). Further, in the general population, regular exercise is also beneficial for the prevention and treatment of depression (Warburton et al. 2006) and possibly for the prevention of dementia (Solfrizzi et al. 2008).

Extensive research has addressed interventions that are aimed at promoting physical activity in the general population (for a review, see Marcus et al. 2006). Research has examined physical activity promotion in a variety of settings, including at home, school, and work, within hospitals and other health care agencies, and through larger public health initiatives (Marcus et al. 2006). Regarding interventions employed in health care settings, brief advice or educational interventions (of ≤10 minutes) appear to be more effective if advice is delivered by members of the health care team other than a physician, such as a nurse, and include both written and verbal advice (Eakin et al. 2000; Simons-Morton et al. 1998). More intensive interventions such as self-monitoring, setting goals, and supervised exercise are generally, although not consistently, more effective than education alone (Simons-Morton et al. 1998). Finally, physical activity promotion at a hospital or other health care center appears to be effective in promoting physical activity in the short term, but a home-based approach appears to be more effective in promoting long-term adherence to a physical activity plan (Ashworth et al. 2005).

Diet

A healthy diet is another key lifestyle recommendation. AHA recommendations include the following (Lichtenstein et al. 2006):

- Balancing caloric intake and physical activity to maintaining a healthy body weight
- Eating fruits and vegetables as well as whole-grain and high-fiber foods
- Eating fish twice weekly
- Eating lean meats and consuming low-fat dairy products, thereby limiting one's intake of saturated fats, *trans* fats, and cholesterol
- Limiting the use of added sugars and salt

These recommendations take into consideration the impact of an entire balanced diet, not simply separate components, because evidence supports the advantage of focusing on overall diet for reducing the risk of cardiovascular disease and reducing risk factors for cardiovascular disease (Appel et al. 1997, 2005; Knoops et al. 2004). Effective interventions for promoting a healthy diet are generally theoretically based (usually grounded in social cognitive theory); include the family when appropriate; involve goal setting and other behavioral planning; and have clear definitions of and messages about a healthy diet (Sahay et al. 2006).

Tobacco Use

Tobacco use is the leading cause of preventable death in the United States; it is linked with approximately 440,000 deaths per year and causes damage to "nearly every organ of the body" (U.S. Department of Health and Human

Services 2004) (see also Chapter 13, "The Prevention of Cigarette Smoking: Principles for Psychiatric Practice," this volume). Considerable progress has been made in reducing smoking in the United States, with the number of current smokers reduced to half of what it was in 1964 when the first U.S. Surgeon General's report about the negative effects of smoking was published (U.S. Department of Health and Human Services 2004). Nonetheless, prevalence rates are still troublingly high in several groups—including people with serious mental illnesses, some racial and ethnic minority groups, and individuals with low levels of education (U.S. Department of Health and Human Services 2004). Research indicates that a number of interventions are effective at promoting smoking cessation (U.S. Department of Health and Human Services 2000), and the U.S. Department of Health and Human Services recommends that health care professionals offer treatment for tobacco dependence to all individuals who smoke. For those who are currently smoking and unwilling to stop, motivational enhancement techniques are recommended. For those who are willing to quit, there are various recommended treatment approaches. Although brief treatments have been shown to be effective, there appears to be a dose-response relationship between the intensity of treatment and outcomes (see Chapter 13, this volume). Key aspects of effective behavioral therapies include motivational enhancement techniques, problem-solving skills training, within-treatment social support, and facilitation of securing social support beyond treatment (U.S. Department of Health and Human Services 2000). Finally, there are several effective pharmacotherapies including nicotine replacement strategies (gum, inhaler, nasal spray, or patch), sustained-release bupropion, and varenicline.

Although interventions aimed at a single aspect of health promotion do provide benefits, a review of well-controlled studies indicates that comprehensive efforts to promote a healthy lifestyle, including regular exercise and a healthy diet, lead to more beneficial changes in physical activity, eating habits, and physiological outcomes (Blue and Black 2005). These interventions generally use a combination of behavior-changing strategies (e.g., goal setting, self-monitoring) and education, and outcomes have persisted for the duration of the intervention trials, up to 5 years. Studies attempting to promote both smoking cessation and physical activity suggest that vigorous physical activity improves the overall efficacy of a cognitive-behavioral treatment for smoking cessation (Marcus et al. 1999), although findings have differed when moderate-intensity exercise has been used (Ussher et al. 2000). It is unclear how best to facilitate change in multiple health behaviors (Marcus et al. 2006), but there is some indication that a person's readiness to change one behavior may not match her or his degree of readiness to change another behavior, so a sequential intervention may be more effective than an integrated approach (Taylor et al. 2004).

In considering the health-promoting behaviors that can reduce morbidity and mortality from cardiovascular disease, another concern is that even in the general population long-term adherence to health behaviors after interventions are completed is troublingly low (Appel et al. 2006; Marcus et al. 2006). As such, new theories are being developed that focus specifically on understanding maintenance of health behaviors (e.g., Rothman et al. 2004). In addition, societal and other environmental factors (e.g., the design of cities that are conducive to physical activity, the availability of healthy food, or bans on smoking in public areas) are all being examined as areas of intervention to promote a healthy lifestyle (Marcus et al. 2006). These broader factors apply to health promotion in people with serious mental illnesses as well as in the general population.

Prevention and Health Maintenance in People With Serious Mental Illnesses

A variety of research programs and techniques have been implemented to promote somatic health maintenance and disease prevention among individuals with serious mental illnesses, but they have not received as much research attention and are not as broadly employed as programs and techniques used in the general population. For example, evidence suggests that patients with a regular source of health care are more likely to receive recommended prevention services (Bindman and Grumbach 1992). In addition, mental health practitioners often serve as the only regular source of health care for people with serious mental illnesses. Therefore interventions that take advantage of the opportunity this regular contact provides have been explored. Such programs can be organized loosely as interventions targeted to 1) the mental health consumer (including behaviors and knowledge base), 2) the mental health care provider and her or his practice, and 3) the system of care and its structure. These distinctions are somewhat artificial in that many of the evaluated approaches involve more than one of these aspects of care, and a significant system-based change (such as an integrated psychiatry–primary care program) would be expected to change both providers' practices and consumers' health behaviors. Nonetheless, this distinction is valuable because it allows us to organize consideration of the primary target of interventions.

The Consumer

For the purposes of this discussion we will consider *consumer-based interventions* to be those that target changes in the patient's behavior and enhancement of his or her knowledge base, such as community mental health center–based wellness programs. As noted for the general population, changing behavior is a challenging proposition given that fewer than half of participants remain within a program aimed at behavioral change, such as an exercise program, for more than 6 months (Richardson et al. 2005). Therefore it seems unreasonable to expect more from people with serious mental illnesses. However, some research indicates that adherence is enhanced in these individuals when such programs are made available as part of psychiatric services (Martinsen 1990). Further, interventions used in the general population can often be adapted for use in people with serious mental illnesses (see Goff et al. 2005). Many programs developed to promote somatic health and well-being in people with serious mental illnesses involve enhancing health-promoting behaviors and increasing the consumer's knowledge base through health education.

Engaging in regular exercise often requires a significant change in behavior, particularly for people with serious mental illnesses. Strategies that have been employed to promote physical activity among individuals with serious mental illnesses include structured activities and lifestyle interventions; individually tailored programs including ones that incorporate computer-generated motivational messages; and self-monitoring interventions (including ones that use Web-based logs, objective monitoring devices such as pedometers, and one-on-one sessions) (Richardson et al. 2005). Flexibility is necessary with exercise programs offered in the context of mental health treatment. For example, evidence suggests that it is important to encourage patients to attend regularly but to allow them to miss some sessions without this resulting in expulsion from the program (Richardson et al. 2005). Unfortunately, programs for mental health care providers to use to address physical activity in patients with serious mental illnesses often have been fragmented and inadequate (Eden et al. 2002).

Community mental health center–based wellness programs focusing on both exercise and diet have received some research attention, particularly those that are administered by psychiatric nurses. Some evidence does suggest that lifestyle interventions involving diet and exercise can reduce weight gain in patients with serious mental illnesses (Faulkner et al. 2003; Menza et al. 2004). One nurse-administered program based in community mental health centers in Brisbane, Australia (O'Sullivan et al. 2006), involving three teaching modules on nutrition and healthy eating, physical health, and community-based activities, resulted in high consumer satisfaction.

Smoking cessation is another area of health behavior that can be addressed with people with serious mental illnesses in mental health settings. Current evidence generally supports the use of group therapy, nicotine replacement, and bupropion to promote smoking cessation. The American Psychiatric Association (1996) recommends that psychiatrists assess the patient's readiness to quit and quitting history and, when indicated, provide advice to motivate quitting and integrate smoking cessation efforts into psychiatric care. Mental health center–based interventions that have been explored include:

- Psychotherapeutic interventions alone, such as group programs for social skills training and motivational enhancement (Ziedonis et al. 1997)
- Pharmacological interventions alone such as bupropion and nicotine replacement treatment (Evins et al. 2007)
- Combined behavior modification and nicotine replacement (Addington et al. 1998)
- Combined group psychotherapy, nicotine replacement, and bupropion (Gershon Grand et al. 2007).

However, as with the general population, studies suggest that long-term maintenance of smoking cessation remains low. Research indicates quitting rates of 36% (Gershon Grand et al. 2007) to 42% (Addington et al. 1998) for individuals completing the studies; however, 6 months after study completion, only 12% (Addington et al. 1998) to 13% (Ziedonis et al. 1997) remained abstinent—although one study did indicate that at 6 months 40% of individuals completing the study had decreased their smoking by half (Ziedonis et al. 1997).

Mental health center–based interventions incorporating education, cognitive-behavioral principles, and/or social skills training have been studied as ways to reduce high-risk behaviors associated with the transmission of HIV and hepatitis in people with serious mental illnesses. Programs to reduce HIV risk utilizing brief behavioral interventions and education (Kalichman et al. 1995; Katz et al. 1995), interactive groups (Susser et al. 1998), and cognitive-behavioral group intervention with advocacy training (Kelly et al. 1997) had significant impact on enhancing AIDS-related knowledge (Kalichman et al. 1995; Katz et al. 1995) and improving self-reported safe sex practices (Kalichman et al. 1995; Kelly et al. 1997), including reductions in rates of unprotected sex (Kelly et al. 1997; Susser et al. 1998) and a decrease in the number of sexual partners (Kelly et al. 1997).

In summary, consumer-based interventions employed in mental health care settings and designed to change patient behavior and enhance knowledge have been studied with diet and exercise, cigarette smoking, and high-risk sexual behaviors. However, these studies have generally been small and their results unreplicated.

The Provider

For the purposes of this chapter, *provider-* or *practice-based interventions* include those primarily involving a change in what the mental health practitioner does to facilitate health promotion or prevention of somatic disease. We know that psychiatrists believe prevention services are important and have reasonably good baseline knowledge about guidelines for preventive medical services, and even may be more likely than internists to ask and counsel about some aspects of prevention such as substance use and possession of weapons (Carney et al. 1998). In addition, many psychiatrists are currently providing some prevention services. According to National Ambulatory Medical Care Survey data from 1992 through 1999, some sort of clinical preventive medical services (most commonly blood pressure measurements) were provided at 11% of routine, office-based psychiatry visits (Daumit et al. 2002). One community mental health center–based study found that psychiatrists offered smoking cessation counseling at 12.4% of visits for patients who smoke (Himelhoch and Daumit 2003), and other research indicates that psychiatrists in a community mental health center discuss issues related to diabetes with almost half of patients with diabetes (Goldberg et al. 2007) and do some screening and counseling for hepatitis and HIV (Goldberg et al. 2005). Further, mental health care providers may be targeting patients at greater risk. Daumit and colleagues (2002) found that psychiatrists were more likely to offer prevention services to people with chronic medical conditions such as diabetes, hypertension, and obesity. Another study indicated that psychiatrists were more likely to provide smoking cessation counseling to patients older than 50 years and those with co-occurring medical problems (Himelhoch and Daumit 2003). Mental health care consumers find education from mental health care providers helpful; these consumers may be more likely than the general population to rely on health information received from health care providers, including mental health care providers such as nurses and psychiatrists, and are less likely to rely on information from media and print sources (MacHaffie 2002).

Extensive practice recommendations exist for mental health care providers about general medical monitoring of people with serious mental illnesses. A decade ago, Carney and colleagues (1998) recommended treatment guidelines that included the following:

- Assessment of cigarette smoking and treatment of nicotine dependence by psychiatrists
- Screening at an initial psychiatric visit to determine whether the patient has a primary care provider
- Use of both inpatient and outpatient psychiatric settings for preventive medical care
- Administration of certain clinical prevention services in high-risk settings (e.g., counseling for individuals at high risk for HIV; pneumococcal vaccination for appropriate populations; tetanus boosters for homeless persons with serious mental illnesses; and vaccination against hepatitis B virus for individuals who use intravenous drugs or engage in high-risk sexual behaviors)

More recently, the 2002 Mount Sinai Conference consensus guidelines (Marder et al. 2004) addressed regular health monitoring for schizophrenia patients who are taking antipsychotic medications; these interventions dealt with screening for problems related to antipsychotic medications, which are prescribed in the vast majority of psychiatric settings. These recommendations include the following:

- Monitor patients' weights (initially and at subsequent visits), BMI, and waist circumference, and provide weight gain interventions including education, engagement in weight management, or medication changes.
- Monitor for diabetes according to American Diabetes Association recommendations (Expert Committee on the Diagnosis and Classification of Diabetes Mellitus 2003), including baseline measurements and checks of fasting plasma glucose or hemoglobin A_{1c} levels every 4 months, particularly when using the second-generation antipsychotics clozapine and olanzapine. Assess the patient for and provide consumer education about diabetes symptoms such as polyuria and polydipsia, and ensure follow-up with a knowledgeable medical care provider when results indicate possible diabetes.
- Recommendations on hyperlipidemia and hypercholesterolemia include routine lipid screening at baseline and, at minimum, biannually when LDL levels are normal; screen once every 6 months if LDL levels are greater than 130 mg/dL, and refer patients to a medical care provider when LDL levels are greater than 130 (although the guidelines note that treatment for hyperlipidemia may be implemented by mental health care providers).
- Obtain a baseline electrocardiogram (ECG) for patients taking antipsychotics associated with prolongation of the QT interval.
- Inquire about visual changes suggestive of cataracts and perform yearly ocular evaluation of patients more than 40 years old who are taking quetiapine.
- Monitor for signs and symptoms of myocarditis in patients taking clozapine.
- Monitor for extrapyramidal symptoms, akathisia, and tardive dyskinesia every 6 months in patients taking conventional antipsychotics, every 12 months in patients taking second-generation antipsychotics, and every 3 months in patients at high risk.

Although the Mount Sinai consensus guidelines are part of the psychiatric literature, it is not clear what percentage of clinicians follow these recommendations. Other recommendations for psychiatrists include the American Psychiatric Association (1996) guidelines directing psychiatrists to assess smoking status including readiness to quit and quitting history, to provide advice to motivate quitting, and to integrate smoking cessation efforts within psychiatric care.

Recommendations from the nursing literature are similar to the Mount Sinai consensus guidelines. Nursing recommendations (Lumby 2007) for people with schizophrenia who are taking medications include a baseline work-up consisting of taking the patient's medical history, including smoking history; assessing current smoking status; assessing and counseling the patient regarding nutrition and physical activity; and determining BMI, waist circumference, blood pressure, fasting plasma glucose level, and fasting lipids profile. Lumby (2007) recommends that for people with schizophrenia who are taking medications a baseline workup include regular assessment of smoking status (and counseling when appropriate); annual evaluation including fasting glucose level, lipid levels, blood pressure, nutrition and physical activity assessment, and an ECG; and focused evaluation 12 weeks after initiation or switching of antipsychotics (including BMI, waist circumference, blood pressure, fasting plasma glucose level, fasting lipid levels, and an ECG).

Approaches designed to facilitate implementation of these and other guidelines in mental health settings include specialized nursing case management for medical issues in people with serious mental illnesses, and targeting specific components of care such as client identification and outreach, assessment, service planning, monitoring of service delivery, and advocacy (Worley et al. 1990). Psychiatric nursing has also been proactive with wellness programs designed to identify, treat, and monitor somatic issues, with referral to appropriate specialist services, and introducing and implementing consumer self-monitoring and self-regulation tools such as health diaries (Ohlsen et al. 2005).

Many mental health care providers are implementing some aspects of somatic preventive medicine and health promotion into their practices. And there are recommendations in the literature for doing so, such as the Mount Sinai consensus guidelines noted above. Still, more research is necessary and should consider current strategies for implementing preventive medical interventions in mental health treatment; further assess how often and to what extent guidelines are being implemented; and assess how implementation impacts consumer outcomes.

The System

System-based interventions are those involving significant restructuring of the approach to treatment, including changes in the treatment setting and practitioners; they may also involve substantial innovations in usual practice. Such interventions include integrated care (either through colocation of programs or medical management by physician extenders embedded in a psychiatric treatment program) (Kilbourne et al. 2008), changes in training of mental health care providers to allow for delivery of primary care services, and other significant institutional changes aimed at health promotion and disease prevention.

The U.S. Department of Veterans Affairs has employed innovative approaches to integrated care for people with serious mental illnesses, including colocation of services (i.e., psychiatric and somatic services at the same location) and shared medical records (Druss et al. 2001). One such program emphasized preventive care, patient education, and close collaboration between medical and psychiatric providers. Mental health consumers receiving integrated care had enhanced outcomes, including the following (Druss et al. 2001):

1. Being more likely to visit a primary care provider
2. Being more likely to have received preventive interventions (e.g., assessment of weight and blood pressure; a rectal exam and sigmoidoscopy; screening for hepatitis, diabetes, hypercholesterolemia, and tuberculosis; education about exercise, nutrition, smoking, and advance directives)
3. Showing improvement in general health

The authors noted that the integrated program used additional staff resources to improve access and adherence, and required some basic reintegration of services including one site/common chart (Druss et al. 2001). Factors found to be helpful in integrated programs included case management services and a shared medical record, especially an electronic medical record (Kilbourne et al. 2008).

General medical care providers embedded in mental health clinics constitute another significant system-based innovation for providing health-promoting services and preventing somatic illnesses. One excellent example of such an intervention was designed to address viral hepatitis and other blood-borne diseases, including HIV. This project, STIRR (screen, test, immunize, reduce risk, and refer), is a model public health intervention designed to provide best-practice services, as specified by the Centers for Disease Control and Prevention, to people with co-occurring psychiatric and substance use disorders (Rosenberg et al. 2004). This is a brief intervention that screens individuals for risk factors, tests for HIV and hepatitis, immunizes against the hepatitis A and B viruses, provides risk reduction counseling, and refers individuals for further treatment when appropriate. The intervention is delivered at mental health care sites by a mobile team of specialists including an advanced practice nurse. Initial study results show that more than two-thirds of appropriate consumers were tested and immunized with an average cost per client of less than $220. Mental health care providers, who may be reluctant to master and deliver the infectious disease–related services, recognize the value of such services and are able to support such interventions when they are provided on-site by an outside team of experts. The STIRR approach to preventing blood-borne diseases is currently being further evaluated in other community mental health settings.

The *primary care psychiatrist*—a psychiatrist with additional training in primary care who is supervised by an internist in treating common conditions and providing preventive care—is another treatment innovation being explored (Golomb et al. 2000). One such program is PsyCE, a Veterans Affairs program in Portland, Oregon, in which psychiatry residents provide primary care to patients with mental illnesses in a medical clinic (Dobscha and Ganzini 2001). A pilot program assessed this model compared with treatment as usual and found that psychiatry residents involved in this intervention were able to provide important health screening and preventive care, and that the care provided was equivalent to standard care and yielded very high patient satisfaction (Snyder et al. 2007).

Some other system-related interventions require less dramatic changes than extensive restructuring of services or the retraining of psychiatrists. Such changes necessitate the reevaluation of treatment as usual based on what is known about the disease prevention and health promotion needs of people with serious mental illnesses. For example, a wellness program implemented in 16 Norwegian inpatient psychiatric hospitals involved modifying the patients' diets, from the standard diet provided in general hospitals to a diet specifically formulated to address the special needs of an inpatient population with serious mental illnesses, with resulting diminution in the severity of weight problems for these consumers (Thommessen et al. 2005).

In summary, system-based interventions, particularly those that involve integrated care, have been subject to some of the most rigorous research and have shown strong evidence of their effectiveness in providing preventive care and promoting physical health in mental health care settings. However, these interventions are complex to implement and require additional funding.

Conclusion and Future Directions

The approach to physical health promotion and disease prevention for people with serious mental illnesses in psychiatric settings continues to evolve. In 2006, the National Association of State Mental Health Program Directors issued a technical report underscoring the excess morbidity and mortality of people with serious mental illnesses and calling for national and local efforts to implement established standards of care for prevention, screening, assessment, and treatment of people with serious mental illnesses, including improved access to medical care and integration of psychiatric and medical care. However, there remains a lack of clarity regarding how much responsibility the mental health care system should take for the physical health of individuals receiving psychiatric services (Dixon et al. 2007; Hutchinson et al. 2006). One compelling point of view is that optimal health is more than simply the absence of disease; it is a basic human right, so those involved in mental health care systems have a responsibility to promote this aspect of recovery (Hutchinson et al. 2006). This approach supports the use of public health models proven within the general population but adapted for diverse groups of people; it includes focus on health literacy, access to health education and health promotion services, consideration of communication and social support, and development of practice guidelines (Hutchinson et al. 2006).

It is imperative that mental health systems and care providers take a more active role in the primary care of people with serious mental illnesses, particularly in issues of health promotion and disease prevention. We discovered some years ago that treatment of patients who are dually diagnosed with both a psychiatric illness and an addictive disorder is most effective when mental health care providers assume significant responsibility for treatment and when we take an integrated approach (Minkoff 1989). The same would seem to apply to patients with co-occurring psychiatric and somatic illnesses. In describing reasons to address exercise and promote physical activity in psychiatric settings, Richardson and colleagues (2005) note the following:

1. People with serious mental illnesses already have regular contact with the mental health system, so these practitioners are in a good position to provide the frequent reinforcement that is important to bringing about change in behavior.
2. Barriers specific to mental illnesses may best be addressed by mental health treatment providers.
3. Health-promoting behaviors (such as physical activity) can play a role in mental health recovery.

Mental health care providers must address the issues of mortality, morbidity, and inadequate general medical care in people with serious mental illnesses, including prevention of medical illness and health promotion. Further training is needed for both psychiatrists and primary care physicians, for the former to do more in treating somatic illnesses and for the latter to develop skills to work with people with serious mental illnesses (McCarrick et al. 1986). It is essential that behavioral health systems adopt protocols pertaining to medical monitoring, including ensuring that people in psychiatric treatment have a primary care provider and that there is an adequate mechanism for communication between psychiatrists and general medical care providers (Lester 2006; Miller et al. 2006; Vreeland 2007). Further, the role of psychiatry in addressing somatic concerns must be clarified (Dixon et al. 2007). Additional development and financing of services to promote healthy behaviors in persons with serious mental illnesses is required (Dickerson et al. 2006). More research is essential because there have been relatively few comprehensive studies designed to improve medical care, particularly preventive medical care, in people with serious mental illnesses (Druss and von Esenwein 2006) and because studies of health promotion in this population often lack the methodological rigor to provide what can be called evidence-based results (Hutchinson et al. 2006).

We must look specifically at recovery-based approaches that empower mental health care consumers to be active and informed participants in their own general medical care. This is particularly true regarding the development of evidence-based approaches to health promotion and disease prevention that involve educating consumers about and supporting them in making behavioral changes, especially as related to diet, exercise, and smoking. Further, there is evidence that interventions including education and social skills training can help mental health consumers to be better advocates for themselves with medical care providers (Heinssen et al. 2000). Interventions need to be tailored to the specific mental health consumer, designed, for example, to meet the needs of certain psychiatric populations such as persons who are homeless or have dual diagnoses (Carney et al. 1998). We also need to consider specialized, culturally sensitive interventions that are appropriate to the patient's racial and ethnic group (Hellerstein et al. 2007). In some instances it is also necessary to address challenging situations such as dealing with medical advance directives and end-of-life planning for people with serious mental illness, in ways that support recovery and affirm autonomy, choice, and self-determination (Foti et al. 2005).

It is vital that we educate providers and adapt standard practices to address issues of health promotion and disease prevention in psychiatric settings. The same prevention approaches developed for general populations are likely to be effective for individuals with serious mental illnesses, but some adaptation may be needed and mental health practitioners often lack the training and expertise to employ these services (Compton et al. 2006; Lambert et al. 2003). A decade ago, investigators evaluating differences in prevention services provided by general medical and psychiatric physicians recommended more training of psychiatrists in clinical preventive medical services and clearly defined educational guidelines for delivery of clinical preventive medical services in psychiatric settings (Carney et al. 1998). Certainly, there are other extensive recommendations such as the Mount Sinai consensus guidelines for treatment of persons with schizophrenia who are receiving antipsychotic medications (Marder et al. 2004). However, it is not clear to what extent mental health care providers are aware of, feel competent with, or are following these recommendations. Further, additional research is needed on how implementation of such guidelines impacts consumers' health outcomes. Although the American Psychiatric Association began to address preventive medicine and health promotion with its 1996 practice guideline regarding assessment and treatment of cigarette smoking, there is a need for additional directives to provide a comprehensive framework for mental health care providers.

Systems must undergo substantial changes to facilitate preventive somatic care and health promotion in psychiatric settings. These include adaptation of financing and reimbursement systems (Dickerson et al. 2005) to allow mental health care providers to implement recommendations such as the administration of certain immunizations, as well as funding to develop and implement additional training for mental health care providers. Use of available technology must increase, including using shared electronic medical records (Kilbourne et al. 2008) and automated systems with computerized prompts or reminders for mental health care providers regarding preventive medical screenings or interventions (Carney et al. 1998). We need to expand and further evaluate innovative pilot programs to provide truly integrated care such as colocated clinics (Druss et al. 2001) and incorporation of a general medical care provider into mental health teams (Rosenberg et al. 2004). Integrated care interventions present implementation challenges but hold real promise for reducing barriers to medical care, decreasing morbidity and mortality, and improving health behaviors in people with serious mental illnesses.

There is increasing recognition of the impact that co-occurring medical illnesses and problematic health behaviors have in people with serious mental illnesses, and growing awareness of the potential to make positive interventions focused on health promotion and disease prevention in mental health care settings. With further research and a recovery-based approach to collaboration with consumers—in terms of promoting healthy behaviors, providing appropriate training and guidelines for mental health care providers, and implementing well-thought-out system adaptations—health promotion and preventive medical interventions in mental health care settings can be expected to lead to significant improvement in the lives of people with serious mental illnesses.

Key Points

- On average, people with serious mental illnesses die at ages much younger than in the general population. They have more medical illnesses than those without mental illnesses. Increased morbidity and mortality appear to result from a variety of factors, including adverse health behaviors, illness- and medication-related influences, and often-inadequate general medical care.

- Because of increased morbidity and mortality associated with serious psychiatric illnesses, we need to provide preventive medical services and health promotion services for people with such disorders. For example, health promotion in the prevention of cardiovascular disease includes monitoring of parameters such as weight, blood pressure, serum glucose levels, and serum lipid levels, as well as employing techniques to change adverse health behaviors such as poor diet, physical inactivity, and cigarette smoking.

- Preventive medicine and health promotion for people with serious mental illnesses can be implemented in mental health settings. Interventions may be directed toward the consumer (e.g., smoking cessation programs based in community mental health centers), the provider (e.g., practice changes such as incorporation of the Mount Sinai consensus guidelines into usual care), or the system (e.g., colocation of mental health and general medical clinics, or primary care training for psychiatric care providers).

- Although some mental health–based programs for health promotion and disease prevention have been successful, further research, expanded guidelines, appropriate training for mental health practitioners, and funding to support such efforts are needed. The area of health promotion and disease prevention presents an excellent opportunity for mental health care providers and consumers to take a holistic and recovery-based approach to treatment.

References

Addington J, el-Guebaly N, Campbell W, et al: Smoking cessation treatment for patients with schizophrenia. Am J Psychiatry 155:974–976, 1998

Allison DB, Mentore JL, Heo M, et al: Antipsychotic-induced weight gain: a comprehensive research synthesis. Am J Psychiatry 156:1686–1696, 1999

American Diabetes Association; American Psychiatric Association; American Association of Clinical Endocrinologists; North American Association for the Study of Obesity: Consensus development conference on antipsychotic drugs and obesity and diabetes. Diabetes Care 27:596–601, 2004

American Diabetes Association: American Diabetes Association Complete Guide to Diabetes. New York, McGraw Hill, 2005

American Diabetes Association: Diagnosis and classification of diabetes mellitus. Diabetes Care 31:S55–S60, 2008

American Heart Association: Heart Disease and Stroke Statistics—2008 Update. Dallas, TX, American Heart Association, 2008

American Psychiatric Association: Practice guideline for the treatment of patients with nicotine dependence. Am J Psychiatry 153 (suppl 10):1–31, 1996

Appel LJ, Moore TJ, Obarzanek E, et al: Clinical trials of the effects of dietary patterns on blood pressure: Dash Collaborative Research Group. N Engl J Med 336:1117–1124, 1997

Appel LJ, Sacks FM, Carey VJ, et al; Omniheart Collaborative Research Group: The effects of protein, monounsaturated fat, and carbohydrate intake on blood pressure and serum lipids: results of the Omniheart Randomized Trial. JAMA 294:2455–2464, 2005

Appel LJ, Brands MW, Daniels SR, et al: Dietary approaches to prevent and treat hypertension: a scientific statement from the American Heart Association. Hypertension 47:296–308, 2006

Ashworth NL, Chad KE, Harrison EL, et al: Home versus center based physical activity programs in older adults. Cochrane Database Syst Rev Issue 1, Art No: CD004017. DOI: 10.1002/14651858.CD004017.pub2, 2005

Barreira P: Reduced life expectancy and serious mental illness. Psychiatr Serv 50:995, 1999

Berren MR, Santiago JM, Zent MR, et al: Health care utilization by persons with severe and persistent mental illness. Psychiatr Serv 50:559–561, 1999

Berrigan D, Dodd K, Troiano RP, et al: Patterns of health behavior in U.S. adults. Prev Med 36:615–623, 2003

Bindman AB, Grumbach K: America's safety net: the wrong place at the wrong time? JAMA 268:2426–2427, 1992

Blank MB, Mandell DS, Aiken L, et al: Co-occurrence of HIV and serious mental illness among Medicaid recipients. Psychiatr Serv 53:868–873, 2002

Blue CL, Black DR: Synthesis of intervention research to modify physical activity and dietary behaviors. Res Theory Nurs Pract 19: 25–61, 2005

Brown S, Birtwistle J, Roe L, et al: The unhealthy lifestyle of people with schizophrenia. Psychol Med 29:697–701, 1999

Bustillo JR, Buchanan RW, Irish D, et al: Differential effects of clozapine on weight: a controlled study. Am J Psychiatry 153:817–819, 1996

Capasso RM, Lineberry TW, Bostwick JM, et al: Mortality in schizophrenia and schizoaffective disorder: an Olmsted County, Minnesota cohort: 1950–2005. Schizophr Res 98:287–294, 2008

Carney C, Yates WR, Goerdt CJ, et al: Psychiatrists' and internists' knowledge and attitudes about delivery of clinical preventive medical services. Psychiatr Serv 49:1594–1600, 1998

Chobanian AV, Bakris GL, Black HR, et al; National Heart, Lung, and Blood Institute Joint National Committee on Prevention, Detection, Evaluation, and Treatment of High Blood Pressure; National High Blood Pressure Education Program Coordinating Committee: The Seventh Report of the Joint National Committee on Prevention, Detection, Evaluation, and Treatment of High Blood Pressure: the JNC 7 report. JAMA 289:1479–1485, 2003

Colton CW, Manderscheid RW: Congruencies in increased mortality rates, years of potential life lost, and causes of death among public mental health clients in eight states. Prev Chronic Dis 3(2):A42, 2006. Available at: http://www.cdc.gov/pcd/issues/2006/apr/05_0180.htm. Accessed October 29, 2008.

Compton MT, Daumit GL, Druss BG: Cigarette smoking and overweight/obesity among individuals with serious mental illnesses: a preventive perspective. Harv Rev Psychiatry 14:212–222, 2006

Conley RR, Mahmoud R: A randomized double-blind study of risperidone and olanzapine in the treatment of schizophrenia or schizoaffective disorder. Am J Psychiatry 158:765–774, 2001

Cournos F, Horwath E, Guido JR, et al: HIV-1 infection at two public psychiatric hospitals in New York City. AIDS Care 6:443–452, 1994

Dalmau A, Bergman B, Brismar B: Somatic morbidity in schizophrenia—a case control study. Public Health 111:393–397, 1997

Daumit GL, Crum RM, Guallar E, et al: Receipt of preventive medical services at psychiatric visits by patients with severe mental illness. Psychiatr Serv 55:884–887, 2002

Daumit GL, Goldberg RW, Anthony C, et al: Physical activity patterns in adults with severe mental illness. J Nerv Ment Dis 193:641–646, 2005

Dembling BP, Chen DT, Vachon L: Life expectancy and causes of death in a population treated for serious mental illness. Psychiatr Serv 50:1036–1042, 1999

Dickerson FB, Pater A, Origoni A: Health behaviors and health status of older women with schizophrenia. Psychiatr Serv 55:882–884, 2002

Dickerson FB, McNary SW, Brown CH, et al: Somatic healthcare utilization among adults with serious mental illness who are receiving community psychiatric services. Med Care 41:560–570, 2003

Dickerson FB, Goldberg RW, Brown CH, et al: Diabetes knowledge among persons with serious mental illness and type 2 diabetes. Psychosomatics 46:418–424, 2005

Dickerson FB, Brown CH, Daumit GL, et al: Health status of individuals with serious mental illness. Schizophr Bull 32:584–589, 2006

Dickey B, Dembling B, Azeni H, et al: Externally caused deaths for adults with substance use and mental disorders. J Behav Health Serv Res 31:75–85, 2004

Dixon L, Weiden P, Delehanty J, et al: Prevalence and correlates of diabetes in national schizophrenia samples. Schizophr Bull 26:903–912, 2000

Dixon LB, Kreyenbuhl JA, Dickerson FB, et al: A comparison of type 2 diabetes outcomes among persons with and without severe mental illnesses. Psychiatr Serv 55:892–900, 2004

Dixon LB, Adler DA, Berlant JL, et al: Psychiatrists and primary caring: what are our boundaries of responsibility? Psychiatr Serv 58:600–602, 2007

Dobscha SK, Ganzini L: A program for teaching psychiatric residents to provide integrated psychiatric and primary medical care. Psychiatr Serv 52:1651–1653, 2001

Donnelly JE, Jacobsen DJ, Heelan KS, et al: The effects of 18 months of intermittent vs. continuous exercise on aerobic capacity, body weight and composition, and metabolic fitness in previously sedentary, moderately obese females. Int J Obes Relat Metab Disord 24:566–572, 2000

Druss BG, Newcomer JW: Challenges and solutions to integrating mental and physical health care. J Clin Psychiatry 68:e09, 2007

Druss BG, Rosenheck RA: Mental disorders and access to medical care in the United States. Am J Psychiatry 155:1775–1777, 1998

Druss BG, von Esenwein SA: Improving general medical care for persons with mental and addictive disorders: systematic review. Gen Hosp Psychiatry 28:145–153, 2006

Druss BG, Bradford DW, Rosenheck RA, et al: Mental disorders and use of cardiovascular procedures after myocardial infarction. JAMA 283:506–511, 2000

Druss BG, Rohrbaugh RM, Levinson CM, et al: Integrated medical care for patients with serious psychiatric illness. Arch Gen Psychiatry 58:861–868, 2001

Druss BG, Rosenheck R, Desai MM, et al: Quality of preventive medical care for patients with mental disorders. Med Care 40:129–136, 2002

Eakin EG, Glasgow RE, Riley KM: Review of primary care-based physical activity intervention studies: effectiveness and implications for practice and future research. J Fam Pract 49:158–168, 2000

Eden KB, Orleans CT, Mulrow CD, et al: Does counseling by clinicians improve physical activity?: a summary of the evidence for the U.S. Preventive Services Task Force. Ann Intern Med 137:208–215, 2002

Evins AE, Cather C, Culhane MA, et al: A 12-week double-blind, placebo-controlled study of bupropion sr added to high-dose dual nicotine replacement therapy for smoking cessation or reduction in schizophrenia. J Clin Psychopharmacol 27:380–386, 2007

Expert Committee on the Diagnosis and Classification of Diabetes Mellitus: Report of the Expert Committee on the Diagnosis and Classification of Diabetes Mellitus. Diabetes Care 26 (suppl 1):S5–S20, 2003

Fang H, Rizzo JA: Do psychiatrists have less access to medical services for their patients? J Ment Health Policy Econ 10:63–71, 2007

Farnam CR, Zipple AM, Tyrrell W, et al: Health status risk factors of people with severe and persistent mental illness. J Psychosoc Nurs Ment Health Serv 37:16–21, 1999

Faulkner G, Soundy AA, Lloyd K: Schizophrenia and weight management: a systematic review of interventions to control weight. Acta Psychiatr Scand 108:324–332, 2003

Felker B, Yazell JJ, Short D: Mortality and medical comorbidity among psychiatric patients: a review. Psychiatr Serv 47:1356–1363, 1996

Fitzgerald SJ, Barlow CE, Kampert JB, et al: Muscular fitness and all-cause mortality: prospective observations. J Phys Act Health 1:7–18, 2004

Fleming BB, Greenfield S, Engelgau MM, et al: The Diabetes Quality Improvement Project: moving science into health policy to gain an edge on the diabetes epidemic. Diabetes Care 24:1815–1820, 2001

Foti ME, Bartels BJ, Merriman MP, et al: Medical advance care planning for persons with serious mental illness. Psychiatr Serv 56:576–584, 2005

Gershon Grand RB, Hwang S, Han J, et al: Short-term naturalistic treatment outcomes in cigarette smokers with substance abuse and/or mental illness. J Clin Psychiatry 68:892–898, 2007

Goff DC, Cather C, Evins AE, et al: Medical morbidity and mortality in schizophrenia: guidelines for psychiatrists. J Clin Psychiatry 66:183–194, 2005

Goldberg RW, Gmyrek AL: Use of medical emergency departments by veterans with schizophrenia. Psychiatr Serv 58:566–567, 2007

Goldberg RW, Himelhoch S, Kreyenbuhl J, et al: Predictors of HIV and hepatitis testing and related service utilization among individuals with serious mental illness. Psychosomatics 46:573–577, 2005

Goldberg RW, Cooke B, Hackman A: Mental health providers' involvement in diabetes management. Psychiatr Serv 58:1501–1502, 2007

Golomb BA, Pyne JM, Wright B, et al: The role of psychiatrists in primary care of patients with severe mental illness. Psychiatr Serv 51:766–773, 2000

Green L, Kreuter MW: Health promotion as a public health strategy for the 1990s. Annu Rev Public Health 11:319–334, 1990

Hackman AL, Goldberg RW, Brown CH, et al: Use of emergency department services for somatic reasons by people with serious mental illness. Psychiatr Serv 57:563–566, 2006

Haskell WL, Lee IM, Pate RR, et al: Physical activity and public health: updated recommendations for adults from the American College of Sports Medicine and the American Heart Association. Circulation 116:1081–1093, 2007

Heinssen RK, Liberman RP, Kopelowicz A: Psychosocial skills training for schizophrenia: lessons from the laboratory. Schizophr Bull 26:21–46, 2000

Hellerstein DJ, Almeida G, Devlin MJ, et al: Assessing obesity and other related health problems of mentally ill Hispanic patients in an urban outpatient setting. Psychiatr Q 78:171–181, 2007

Himelhoch S, Daumit G: To whom do psychiatrists offer smoking-cessation counseling? Am J Psychiatry 160:2228–2230, 2003

Himelhoch S, Lehman A, Kreyenbuhl J, et al: Prevalence of chronic obstructive pulmonary disease among those with serious mental illness. Am J Psychiatry 161:2317–2319, 2004

Himelhoch S, McCarthy JF, Ganoczy D, et al: Understanding associations between serious mental illness and HIV among patients in the VA Health System. Psychiatr Serv 58:1165–1172, 2007

Hippisley-Cox J, Parker C, Coupland C, et al: Inequalities in the primary care of patients with coronary heart disease and serious mental health problems: a cross-sectional study. Heart 93:1256–1262, 2007

Hutchinson DS, Gange C, Bowers A, et al: A framework for health promotion services for people with psychiatric disabilities. Psychiatr Rehabil J 29:241–250, 2006

Institute of Medicine of the National Academies, Food and Nutrition Board: Dietary Reference Intakes for Energy, Carbohydrate, Fiber, Fat, Fatty Acids, Cholesterol, Protein, and Amino Acids. Washington, DC, National Academies Press, 2002

Jackicic JM, Winters C, Lang W, et al: Effects of intermittent exercise and use of home exercise equipment on adherence, weight loss, and fitness in overweight women: a randomized trial. JAMA 282:1554–1560, 1999

Jones DR, Macias C, Barreira PJ, et al: Prevalence, severity, and co-occurrence of chronic physical health problems of persons with serious mental illness. Psychiatr Serv 55:1250–1257, 2004

Kalichman SC, Sikkema KJ, Kelly JA, et al: Use of a brief behavioral skills intervention to prevent HIV infection among chronic mentally ill adults. Psychiatr Serv 46:275–280, 1995

Katz RC, Westerman C, Beauchamp K, et al: Effects of AIDS counseling and risk reduction training on the chronic mentally ill. AIDS Educ Prev 8:457–463, 1995

Kelly JA, McAuliffe TL, Sikkema KJ, et al: Reduction in risk behavior among adults with severe mental illness who learned to advocate for HIV prevention. Psychiatr Serv 48:1283–1288, 1997

Kesaniemi YA, Danforth E Jr, Jensen MD, et al: Dose-response issues concerning physical activity and health: an evidence-based symposium. Med Sci Sports Exerc 33:S531–S538, 2001

Keyes CL: The nexus of cardiovascular disease and depression revisited: the complete mental health perspective and the moderating role of age and gender. Aging Ment Health 8:266–274, 2004

Kilbourne AM, Horvitz-Lennon M, Post EP, et al: Oral health in Veterans Affairs patients diagnosed with serious mental illness. J Public Health Dent 67:42–48, 2007

Kilbourne AM, Irmiter C, Capobiance J, et al: Improving integrated general medical and mental health services in community-based practices. Adm Policy Ment Health 35:337–345, 2008

Knoops KT, de Groot LC, Kromhout D, et al: Mediterranean diet, lifestyle factors, and 10-year mortality in elderly European men and women: the HALE project. JAMA 292:1433–1439, 2004

Koran LM, Sheline Y, Imai K, et al: Medical disorders among patients admitted to a public-sector psychiatric inpatient unit. Psychiatr Serv 53:1623–1625, 2002

Krein SL, Bingham CR, McCarthy JF, et al: Diabetes treatment among VA patients with comorbid serious mental illness. Psychiatr Serv 57:1016–1021, 2006

Kreyenbuhl J, Medoff DR, Seliger SL, et al: Use of medications to reduce cardiovascular risk among individuals with psychotic disorders and Type 2 diabetes. Schizophr Res 101:256–265, 2008

Kung HC, Hoyert DL, Xu J, et al: Deaths: final data for 2005. Natl Vital Stat Rep 56:1–120, 2008

Kuriyama S, Ohmori K, Miura C, et al: Body mass index and mortality in Japan: the Miyagi Cohort Study. J Epidemiol 14 (suppl 1):S33–S38, 2004

Lambert TJ, Velakoulis D, Pantelis C: Medical comorbidity in schizophrenia. Med J Aust 178 (suppl 9):S67–S70, 2003

Lasser K, Boyd JW, Woolhandler S, et al: Smoking and mental illness: a population-based prevalence study. JAMA 284:2606–2610, 2000

Lawrence D, Holman CD, Jablensky AV, et al: Excess cancer mortality in Western Australian psychiatric patients due to higher case fatality rates. Acta Psychiatr Scand 101:382–388, 2000

Lester H: Current issues in providing primary medical care to people with serious mental illness. Int J Psychiatry Med 36:1–12, 2006

Lichtenstein AH, Appel LJ, Brands M, et al: Diet and lifestyle recommendations revision 2006: a scientific statement from the American Heart Association Nutrition Committee. Circulation 114:82–96, 2006

Lumby B: Guide schizophrenia patients to better physical health. Nurse Pract 32:30–37, 2007

MacHaffie S: Health promotion information: sources and significance for those with serious and persistent mental illness. Arch Psychiatr Nurs 16:263–274, 2002

Marcus BH, Albrecht AE, King TK, et al: The efficacy of exercise as an aid for smoking cessation in women: a randomized controlled trial. Arch Intern Med 159:1229–1234, 1999

Marcus BH, Williams DM, Dubbert PM, et al: Physical activity intervention studies: what we know and what we need to know: a scientific statement from the American Heart Association Council on Nutrition, Physical Activity, and Metabolism (Subcommittee on Physical Activity); Council on Cardiovascular Disease in the Young; and the Interdisciplinary Working Group on Quality of Care and Outcomes Research. Circulation 114:2739–2752, 2006

Marder SR, Essock SM, Miller AL, et al: Physical health monitoring of patients with schizophrenia. Am J Psychiatry 161:1334–1349, 2004

Maricle RA, Hoffman WF, Bloom JD, et al: The prevalence and significance of medical illness among chronically mentally ill outpatients. Community Ment Health J 23:81–90, 1987

Martinsen EW: Physical fitness, anxiety and depression. Br J Hosp Med 43:194, 196, 199, 1990

McCarrick AK, Manderscheid RW, Bertolucci DE, et al: Chronic medical problems in the chronic mentally ill. Hosp Community Psychiatry 37:289–291, 1986

Melkersson KI, Hulting AL, Brismar KE, et al: Different influences of classical antipsychotics and clozapine on glucose-insulin homeostasis in patients with schizophrenia or related psychoses. J Clin Psychiatry 60:783–791, 1999

Melkersson KI, Hulting AL, Brismar KE: Elevated levels of insulin, leptin, and blood lipids in olanzapine-treated patients with schizophrenia or related psychoses. J Clin Psychiatry 61:742–749, 2000

Menza M, Vreeland B, Minsky S, et al: Managing atypical antipsychotic-associated weight gain: 12-month data on a multimodal weight control program. J Clin Psychiatry 65:471–477, 2004

Meyer JM: Effects of atypical antipsychotics on weight and serum lipid levels. J Clin Psychiatry 62 (suppl 27):27–34, 2001

Meyer JM, Koro CE: The effects of antipsychotic therapy on serum lipids: a comprehensive review. Schizophr Res 70:1–17, 2004

Miller BJ, Paschall CB 3rd, Svendsen DP: Mortality and medical comorbidity among patients with serious mental illness. Psychiatr Serv 57:1482–1487, 2006

Minkoff K: An integrated treatment model for dual diagnosis of psychosis and addiction. Hosp Community Psychiatry 40:1031–1036, 1989

Mitchell AJ, Malone D: Physical health and schizophrenia. Curr Opin Psychiatry 19:432–437, 2006

Moreau KL, Degarmo R, Langley J, et al: Increasing daily walking lowers blood pressure in postmenopausal women. Med Sci Sports Exerc 33:1825–1831, 2001

Muir-Cochrane E: Medical co-morbidity risk factors and barriers to care for people with schizophrenia. J Psychiatr Ment Health Nurs 13:447–452, 2006

Murphy M, Neville A, Neville C, et al: Accumulating brisk walking for fitness, cardiovascular risk, and psychological health. Med Sci Sports Exerc 34:1468–1474, 2002

Nasrallah HA, Meyer JM, Goff DC, et al: Low rates of treatment for hypertension, dyslipidemia and diabetes in schizophrenia: data from the CATIE schizophrenia trial sample at baseline. Schizophr Res 86:15–22, 2006

National Association of State Mental Health Program Directors: Morbidity and Mortality in People With Serious Mental Illness. Edited by Parks J, Svendsen D, Singer P, Foti ME. Alexandria, VA, National Association of State Mental Health Program Directors, October 2006. http://www.nasmhpd.org/general_files/publications/med_directors_pubs/Technical%20Report%20on%20Morbidity%20 and%20 Mortaility%20-%20Final%2011-06.pdf. Accessed August 4, 2009.

National Heart, Lung, and Blood Institute: Morbidity and Mortality: 2007 Chart Book on Cardiovascular, Lung, and Blood Diseases. Bethesda, MD, National Institutes of Health, 2007

O'Day B, Killeen MB, Sutton J, et al: Primary care experiences of people with psychiatric disabilities: barriers to care and potential solutions. Psychiatr Rehabil J 28:339–345, 2005

O'Donnell MP: Definition of health promotion. Am J Health Promot 1:4–5, 1989

Ohlsen RI, Peacock G, Smith S: Developing a service to monitor and improve physical health in people with serious mental illness. J Psychiatr Ment Health Nurs 12:614–619, 2005

O'Sullivan J, Gilbert J, Ward W: Addressing the health and lifestyle issues of people with a mental illness: the Healthy Living Programme. Australas Psychiatry 14:150–155, 2006

Prior P, Hassall C, Cross KW: Causes of death associated with psychiatric illness. J Public Health Med 18:381–389, 1996

Reeves RR, Pendarvis EJ, Kimble R: Unrecognized medical emergencies admitted to psychiatric units. Am J Emerg Med 18:390–393, 2000

Richardson CR, Faulkner G, McDevitt J, et al: Integrating physical activity into mental health services for persons with serious mental illness. Psychiatr Serv 56:324–331, 2005

Rohde P, Lewinsohn PM, Brown RA, et al: Psychiatric disorders, familial factors and cigarette smoking, I: associations with smoking initiation. Nicotine Tob Res 5:85–98, 2003

Rosenberg S, Brunette M, Oxman T, et al: Best practices for blood-borne diseases among clients with serious mental illness. Psychiatr Serv 55:660–664, 2004

Rothman AJ, Baldwin AS, Hertel AW: Self-regulation and behavior change: disentangling behavioral initiation and behavioral maintenance, in Handbook of Self-Regulation: Research, Theory, and Applications. Edited by Baumeister RF, Vohs KD. New York, Guilford, 2004, pp 130–148

Ryan MC, Collins P, Thakore JH: Impaired fasting glucose tolerance in first-episode, drug-naive patients with schizophrenia. Am J Psychiatry 160:284–289, 2003

Sahay TB, Ashbury FD, Roberts M, et al: Effective components for nutrition interventions: a review and application of the literature. Health Promot Pract 7:418–427, 2006

Schyve PM, Smithline F, Meltzer HY: Neuroleptic-induced prolactin level elevation and breast cancer: an emerging clinical issue. Arch Gen Psychiatry 35:1291–1301, 1978

Simons-Morton DG, Calfas KJ, Oldenburg B, et al: Effects of interventions in health care settings on physical activity or cardiorespiratory fitness. Am J Prev Med 15:413–430, 1998

Snyder K, Dobscha SK, Ganzini L, et al: Clinical outcomes of integrated psychiatric and general medical care. Community Ment Health J 44:147–154, 2007

Sokal J, Messias E, Dickerson FB, et al: Comorbidity of medical illnesses among adults with serious mental illness who are receiving community psychiatric services. J Nerv Ment Dis 192:421–427, 2004

Solfrizzi V, Capurso C, D'Introno A, et al: Lifestyle-related factors in predementia and dementia syndromes. Expert Rev Neurother 8:133–158, 2008

Susser E, Valencia E, Berkman A, et al: Human immunodeficiency virus sexual risk reduction in homeless men with mental illness. Arch Gen Psychiatry 55:266–272, 1998

Taylor WC, Hepworth JT, Lees E, et al: Readiness to change physical activity and dietary practices and willingness to consult healthcare providers. Health Res Policy Syst 2:2, 2004

Thomas R, Davies N: Lifestyle during and after cancer treatment. Clin Oncol 19:616–627, 2007

Thommessen MH, Martinsen EW, Arsky GH: Diet and physical activity in Norwegian psychiatric institutions. Tidsskr Nor Laegeforen 125:3297–3299, 2005

Tidey JW, Rohsenow DJ, Kaplan GB, et al: Cigarette smoking topography in smokers with schizophrenia and matched non-psychiatric controls. Drug Alcohol Depend 80:259–265, 2005

Torrey EF: Prostate cancer and schizophrenia. Urology 68:1280–1283, 2006

Tsuang MT: Heterogeneity of schizophrenia. Biol Psychiatry 10:465–474, 1975

Uebelacker LA, Wang PS, Berglund P, et al: Clinical differences among patients treated for mental health problems in general medical and specialty mental health settings in the National Comorbidity Survey Replication. Gen Hosp Psychiatry 28:387–395, 2006

U.S. Department of Health and Human Services: Clinical Practice Guideline: Treating Tobacco Use and Dependence. Atlanta, GA, U.S. Department of Health and Human Services, 2000

U.S. Department of Health and Human Services: The Health Consequences of Smoking: A Report of the Surgeon General. Atlanta, GA, U.S. Department of Health and Human Services, Centers for Disease Control and Prevention, National Center for Chronic Disease Prevention and Health Promotion, Office on Smoking and Health, 2004

Ussher MH, Taylor AH, West R, et al: Does exercise aid in smoking cessation?: a systematic review. Addiction 95:199–208, 2000

Vreeland B: Bridging the gap between mental and physical health: a multidisciplinary approach. J Clin Psychiatry 68 (suppl 4):26–33, 2007

Wadden TA, Brownell KD, Foster GD: Obesity: responding to the global epidemic. J Consult Clin Psychol 70:510–525, 2002

Wan JJ, Morabito DJ, Khaw L, et al: Mental illness as an independent risk factor for unintentional injury and injury recidivism. J Trauma 61:1299–1304, 2006

Wang PS, Walker AM, Tsuang MT, et al: Dopamine agonists and the development of breast cancer. Arch Gen Psychiatry 59:1145–1154, 2002

Warburton DE, Nicol CW, Bredin SS, et al: Health benefits of physical activity: the evidence. CMAJ 174:801–809, 2006

Windgassen K, Wesselman U, Schulze Mönking H: Galactorrhea and hyperprolactinemia in schizophrenic patients on neuroleptics: frequency and etiology. Neuropsychobiology 33:142–146, 1996

World Health Organization: Ottawa Charter for Health Promotion (WHO Publ No WHO/HPR/HEP/95.1). Geneva, World Health Organization, 1986. Available at: http://www.who.int/hpr/NPH/docs/ottawa_charter_hp.pdf. Accessed October 29, 2008.

World Health Organization: Health promotion glossary (WHO Publ No WHO/HRP/HEP/98.1). Geneva, World Health Organization, 1998. Available at: http://www.who.int/hpr/NPH/docs/hp_glossary_en.pdf. Accessed October 29, 2008.

World Health Organization: WHO Global Forum IV on Chronic Disease Prevention and Control—summary report. Geneva, World Health Organization, 2004. Available at: http://www.phac-aspc.gc.ca/publicat/wgf4-fmo4/wgf4-fmo4_sr/toc-eng.php. Accessed October 29, 2008.

Worley NK, Drago L, Hadley T: Improving the physical health–mental health interface for the chronically mentally ill: could nurse case managers make a difference? Arch Psychiatr Nurs 4:108–113, 1990

Ziedonis DM, George TP: Schizophrenia and nicotine use: report of a pilot smoking cessation program and review of neurobiological and clinical issues. Schizophr Bull 23:247–254, 1997

13

Prevention of Cigarette Smoking

Principles for Psychiatric Practice

Rebecca A. Powers, M.D., M.P.H.

Michael T. Compton, M.D., M.P.H.

Despite widespread knowledge of its detrimental effects, cigarette smoking remains a major public health concern. In fact, cigarette smoking is the leading preventable cause of the death in the United States (Mokdad et al. 2004; U.S. Department of Health and Human Services 1994). According to *Healthy People 2010*, which documents the most significant preventable threats to health and establishes national goals to reduce those threats, tobacco-related deaths number more than 430,000 per year among U.S. adults, representing more than 5 million years of potential life lost (U.S. Department of Health and Human Services 2000). Furthermore, according to the Centers for Disease Control and Prevention, from 1995 to 1999 smoking caused approximately $160 billion in annual health-related economic losses (Centers for Disease Control and Prevention 2002).

It was not until the 1950s and 1960s that political interventions pertaining to tobacco control began to take place in light of consistent findings of an association between smoking and cancer and cardiovascular disease. Since then, the recognized detrimental effects of smoking—as well as the adverse effects of secondhand smoke inhaled by those who do not smoke themselves—have led to the prohibition of smoking in countless workplaces and public places such as restaurants, theatres, hospitals, governmental buildings, and even bars. In turn, smoking has become less socially acceptable in many facets of American society. Secondhand smoke, also referred to as *environmental tobacco smoke*, increases the risk of cardiovascular disease and a number of lung conditions, perhaps most importantly asthma and bronchitis in children. Secondhand smoke inhalation is responsible for an estimated 3,000 lung cancer deaths each year among adult nonsmokers (U.S. Department of Health and Human Services 2000). Efforts to reduce secondhand smoke exposure, along with numerous other efforts to prevent or help people quit smoking, have gained increasing public attention in recent years.

The previous chapter (Chapter 12, "Health Promotion and the Prevention of Somatic Illnesses in Psychiatric Settings") provided information for clinicians on changing adverse health behaviors such as poor diet, physical inactivity, and cigarette smoking. In this chapter, without being overly redundant, we focus specifically on the prevention of cigarette smoking among patients seen in psychiatric practice settings. Given the prominent public health burden associated with smoking, and in light of the remarkably high rates of smoking among people with serious mental illnesses (as discussed below), focused attention on the issue of cigarette smoking is warranted.

Smoking as an Efficient Means of Nicotine Delivery

Cigarettes are the most commonly used form of tobacco, followed by cigars, pipes, *bidis* (thin, inexpensive, locally produced, often flavored, Indian cigarettes made of cut tobacco rolled in leaf), and *kreteks* (cigarettes made from Indonesian tobacco and ground clove buds). Cigars are produced through a different process than cigarettes and are quite variable in their chemical characteristics. Bidis and kreteks may be produced with or without filters. Even though such locally produced tobacco products may have less tobacco per piece, they are usually smoked more slowly and with more inhalations, achieving a greater amount of nicotine intake.

Inhaling a small volume of smoke into the mouth or lungs provides highly efficient and rapid delivery of nicotine into the brain. Smokers generally inhale with deeper and more rapid breathing compared with normal tidal breathing, though this varies across smokers. Individuals who smoke obviously differ in terms of body size, but also in smoking behavior, lung morphology, rate of breathing and lung clearance, metabolism, genetics, and physiology related to nicotinic receptors and pathways. In addition, tobacco products vary in nicotine content, as well as gaseous and particulate matter content. The shape and size of inhaled particles affects their distribution in the branching points of the bronchial tree. Despite variability across individuals and in cigarette content, smoking nicotine-containing products is particularly reinforcing due to rapid central effects.

Most regular smokers experience withdrawal symptoms within hours of the last cigarette, and these unpleasant effects are alleviated by smoking the next cigarette. Thus, cigarettes become, for most smokers, the only way to self-medicate withdrawal symptoms, in addition to providing reported calming or pleasurable effects. Satisfaction and a sense of well-being are frequently reported effects, driven by nicotine's actions in central reward pathways in the brain. As noted above, the pulmonary delivery system is efficient, and nicotine can reach the brain in 10–20 seconds. Cigarette smoking is highly addictive in part because of such rapid reinforcement.

Smoking and Disease

Cigarette smoke contains approximately 4,800 identified compounds. About 70 of these agents are known animal carcinogens, and 11 have been proven to be carcinogenic in humans (International Agency for Research on Cancer 1972–2000). Carbon monoxide, ammonia, benzene, toluene, styrene, hydrogen cyanide, lead, hydrogen sulfide, formaldehyde, formic acid, naphthalene, quinines, and phenols are among the most harmful compounds (Hoffmann et al. 2001). The addictive component of tobacco is nicotine, and it is for this reason that a leading form of pharmacological treatment of cigarette smoking/nicotine dependence is nicotine replacement therapy, which increases cessation rates by 1½- to 2-fold (Silagy et al. 2002). Although nicotine replacement therapy helps tremendously with smoking cessation, it does not replace all aspects of smoking behavior, such as sensations in the tongue, nose, mouth, throat, windpipe, and chest, as well as daily routines and habits that are built around frequent smoking.

Cigarette smoking has been linked causally to compromised pulmonary function, chronic obstructive airway diseases such as chronic bronchitis, influenza, pneumonia, asthma, acute myocardial infarction, stroke, atherosclerosis, chronic vascular disease, multiple sclerosis, dementia, and, of course, lung cancer. The risk of lung cancer increases directly with the number of cigarettes smoked and decreases when one successfully quits smoking. Other types of cancers are related to smoking, and excessive alcohol intake in combination with smoking greatly increases the risk of some cancers and other diseases. Smoking results in more deaths each year in the United States than acquired immunodeficiency syndrome; alcohol, cocaine, and heroin use; homicide; suicide; motor vehicle crashes; and fires, combined (U.S. Department of Health and Human Services 2000). For a review of the risks of smoking during pregnancy, see "Smoking Cessation in Pregnancy."

Epidemiology of Cigarette Smoking

Rates of Cigarette Smoking in the General U.S. Population

The Centers for Disease Control and Prevention (2004a) reported the prevalence of adult cigarette smoking in 2002 to be 22.5%. Similar prevalence rates were observed in 2003, using data from the Behavioral Risk Factor Surveillance System (BRFSS), which is a state-based, random-digit, telephone survey that collects data on noninstitutionalized U.S. civilians ages 18 years or older (Centers for Disease Control and Prevention 2004c). In that survey, *current smokers* were defined as those who reported having smoked 100 cigarettes or more during their lifetime and who currently smoke every day or on some days. In 2003, the median prevalence of current cigarette smoking among adults was 22.1% in the 50 states and the District of Columbia (ranging from 12.0% in Utah to 30.8% in Kentucky). Also documented by the 2003 BRFSS, smoking prevalence is higher among men (median, 24.8%) than women (median, 20.3%) in the 50 states and the District of Columbia. It was estimated that 21.9% of high school students smoked in 2003, the lowest rate since 1991 (Centers for Disease Control and Prevention 2004b). However, it should be noted that nearly all initiation of tobacco use occurs before age 18, indicating that ongoing development of effective smoking prevention approaches in children and adolescents is a public health priority (Pérez-Stable and Fuentes-Afflick 1998).

American smokers spent about $400 billion on cigarettes in 2001 (Federal Trade Commission 2003), making smoking tobacco the most expensive addictive behavior in the United States. Tobacco-related health expenses, deaths, and prevention efforts cost billions of dollars. In the mid to late 1990s, life expectancy in male and female smokers was reduced by an average of 13.2 and 14.5 years, respectively (Centers for Disease Control and Prevention 2002).

Rates of Cigarette Smoking Among People With Serious Mental Illnesses

Data from the National Comorbidity Survey revealed that whereas the population prevalence of current smoking among those with no mental illness was 22.5%, a remarkable 41.0% of those reporting a mental illness in the past month were current smokers (Lasser et al. 2000). The research team defined *current smoking* as a response of "in the past month" when participants were asked, "When was the last time you smoked fairly regularly—in the past month, past six months, past year, or more than a year ago?" Based on the survey data, the odds ratio for cigarette smoking among individuals with mental illnesses versus among individuals without such disorders, is approximately 2.7 (95% confidence interval, 2.3, 3.1) (Lasser et al. 2000). Smokers who have a mental illness also appear to consume more cigarettes than smokers who do not have a mental illness; specifically, the National Comorbidity Survey reported that current smokers without a mental illness in the past month had a mean peak consumption of 22.6 cigarettes per day, compared with 26.2 in those with a mental illness. Astonishingly, it was estimated that those with a diagnosable mental disorder in the past month consume approximately 44% of all cigarettes smoked in the United States (Lasser et al. 2000), and this estimate is supported by data from the National Epidemiologic Survey on Alcohol and Related Conditions: in that survey Grant and colleagues (2004) documented that nicotine-dependent individuals with at least one comorbid psychiatric disorder made up 7.1% of the population, yet consumed 34.2% of all cigarettes smoked in the United States.

Extraordinarily high rates of cigarette smoking have been documented among those with severe and persistent mental illnesses, such as schizophrenia (Goff et al. 1992; Lohr and Flynn 1992; Ziedonis et al. 1994). Most studies find prevalence rates of cigarette smoking among individuals with schizophrenia to be about 90% (Williams and Ziedonis 2004), which conveys grave health consequences for people with that disorder. A meta-analysis of 42 studies across 20 countries demonstrated a strong association between schizophrenia and current smoking, and showed that heavy smoking and high nicotine dependence were more frequent in smokers with schizophrenia than in smokers in the general population (de Leon and Diaz 2005). According to Lasser and colleagues (2000), smoking prevalence increases with the number of psychiatric diagnoses. The high prevalence and intensity of tobacco smoking in psychiatric patients undoubtedly translates into adverse health outcomes at higher rates than in the general population.

Thus, cigarette smoking/nicotine dependence is very common among psychiatric patients—yet it is often left out of listed axial diagnoses or problem lists, therefore not receiving the clinical attention that it deserves. Psychiatrists and other mental health professionals should inquire about cigarette smoking in every patient. Understanding some of the mechanisms that influence continued smoking and a desire, or lack thereof, to quit smoking, can help with setting goals for cessation. As noted earlier, nicotine addiction is related to powerful biological reward and reinforcement mechanisms. With its use, neurotransmitters are released that are associated with effects that reinforce the urge to smoke, including enhanced concentration and alertness as well as reduced tension, fatigue, and pain (Pomerleau 1985). Furthermore, for some users it can help control body weight by reducing appetite (Pomerleau and Pomerleau 1984). Nicotine causes no immediate impairment in mental/cognitive functioning; in fact, it can enhance performance on some attentional tasks. For many smokers, including those with serious mental illnesses, these perceived positive attributes of smoking outweigh the known negatives.

The connection between serious mental illnesses and very high rates of cigarette smoking are likely influenced by complex biological factors (e.g., central nicotinic receptors and brain reward pathways), social factors (e.g., social connectedness by smoking together), and psychological factors (e.g., subtle enhancement of cognition and pleasurable effects). Additionally, similar to contemporary notions that serious mental illnesses and addictive disorders may share underlying genetic diatheses, people who are genetically prone to developing serious mental illnesses may be more genetically prone to tobacco exposure and/or nicotine dependence.

In addition to the connection between cigarette smoking and serious mental illnesses like psychotic disorders, there is a high level of comorbidity between cigarette smoking and alcohol use disorders. Smokers are much more likely to consume alcohol and 10 times more likely to develop alcohol dependence than nonsmokers. Some 80%–95% of all individuals with alcohol dependence also smoke cigarettes and 70% are heavy smokers (Campaign for Tobacco-Free Kids 2002). Adolescents who smoke daily have a greater risk of developing an alcohol use disorder later in life. Tobacco use commonly precedes other drug use, thus potentially serving as a "gateway" to the use of alcohol and illicit drugs (Pérez-Stable and Fuentes-Afflick 1998). The greater the level of cigarette smoking, the greater the chance of illicit drug use. A young person who smokes more than 15 cigarettes per day is 10 times more likely to use any illicit drug and 100 times more likely to use cocaine than a nonsmoker (Campaign for Tobacco-Free Kids 2002). Therefore, screening for cigarette smoking, alcohol use, and other drug use should occur in each evaluation, and is imperative in clinical practice with adolescents.

Risk and Protective Factors for Cigarette Smoking

Environmental and social factors clearly play a role in determining who will develop a smoking habit and nicotine dependence. The majority of adolescents will attempt to smoke at least once by the twelfth grade, and experimenting usually begins in the early teenage years. Psychosocial motives are the driving force behind the onset of smoking. The earlier a youth begins to smoke, the more likely that she or he will continue to smoke into adulthood. Most teens tolerate the body's initial physical attempt to reject smoking during their first few trials, because the desired image and unspoken or overt social pressures often override this. Research has shown that predictors of cigarette smoking in adolescents include self-reported smoking susceptibility (i.e., how certain the adolescent feels about smoking or not smoking in the future), peer smoking (i.e., how many of the adolescent's closest friends smoke), lower grade-point averages, and greater risk-taking attitudes (Pérez-Stable and Fuentes-Afflick 1998). Even though in the first years of smoking adolescents may not inhale as deeply as adult smokers do, their smoking behavior quickly becomes comparable to that of adults, and they can experience the same types of cravings and withdrawal symptoms. By the age of 20 years, 80% of young smokers regret having ever started (Jarvis 2004).

It is important to understand the reasons that adolescents and young adults develop a smoking habit if one wants to promote prevention. Such risk factors include the following (Turner et al. 2004):

- The presence of a smoker in the household
- A single-parent home and/or a strained relationship with a parent
- A comorbid psychiatric disorder
- A low level of expressed self-esteem or self-worth
- Poor academic performance
- High levels of aggression and rebelliousness in boys
- Preoccupation with weight and body image in girls
- An adolescent's perception that parents do not disapprove of smoking
- Affiliation with peers who smoke
- Availability of cigarettes

In addition to these risk factors, studies of twins show genetic links to both smoking and nicotine dependence. Thus, clinicians must be aware of the aforementioned risk factors, as well as the patient's family history of cigarette smoking, when assessing risk of the initiation or escalation of tobacco use.

Mass media contribute greatly to the learning of cigarette smoking, especially in the young. Advertisements have focused on the association between smoking and fun, excitement, social norms, power, sex, wealth, and a means of displaying rebellion and independence. One of the most potent forms of marketing is the portrayal of smoking in the movies. A sponsor's involvement in movies is often hidden from the audience, which is exposed to "a more powerful force than overt advertising" (Glantz 2003). The movie industry still portrays smoking as a relaxing solution to stress and an acceptable social activity, whereas the television industry has taken a more responsible stand on the subject in recent years. Regarding the connection between a child's favorite movie star and that star's on-screen use of cigarettes, "a clear relation between on-screen use and the initiation of smoking in the adolescents who admire them" has been reported (Tickle et al. 2001, p. 20). Tobacco use actually increased in the movies in the 1990s, after decreasing in the 1970s and 1980s. Unfortunately, that increase mirrored the amount of smoking displayed in the 1950s, when it was twice as prevalent in society compared with its prevalence in 2002 (Glantz et al. 2004). R-rated movies contain the most tobacco use, and are the ones most likely to show a major character smoking. It is estimated that only 6% of actors shown smoking in films depict a negative reaction to cigarette smoking, such as coughing, comments about health, or other gestures of disapproval (Dalton et al. 2002). In May 2007, the Motion Picture Association of America announced that smoking content would become a factor in the rating of films, and that context, glamorization, and pervasiveness would enter into the decision about ratings (Dalton et al. 2002).

Prevention of Cigarette Smoking

Every day, an estimated 3,000 youths start smoking. The vast majority of adult smokers tried their first cigarette before the age of 18 years, and more than half became daily smokers before this age (U.S. Department of Health and Human Services 2000). Almost half of adolescents who continue smoking regularly will eventually die from a smoking-related illness. For these reasons, it is critical that prevention efforts target youths. Prevention efforts have been helpful in that a slight but steady decline in both adult and adolescent smoking prevails. Young children are often targeted in prevention programs because the mean age of onset of smoking is 16 years, and resistance training skills are helpful to reduce smoking initiation in nonsmokers whether they are at high or low risk (Evans 1988).

Prevention efforts focus on encouraging youths to not learn the behavior of smoking in the first place, and on teaching them how to resist social pressures to smoke (primary prevention of cigarette smoking). Social influences play the largest role in determining who will begin to smoke, who will become dependent, and who will quit. This is evident even in animal models—when researchers tried to train rhesus monkeys to begin smoking and discovered that it was very difficult, they concluded that "environmental factors play the primary role in developing smoking behavior" (Bandura 1965). Therefore, intervening with psychosocial prevention modalities is likely to be the most effective approach given that psychosocial motives lead to experimentation in the early teenage years. The symbolic expression of autonomy and independence often causes the first-time user to light a cigarette. Most adolescents (nearly 60%) attempt this at least once by the twelfth grade, even though they are aware of smoking's harmful effects.

The prevalence of cigarette smoking is likely even higher among adolescents and young adults who have, or who go on to develop, a serious mental illness. For example, in a recent study of 109 older adolescents and young adults (mean age, 23.1 ± 4.7 years) hospitalized for a first episode of nonaffective psychosis, Stewart and colleagues (in press) found that 73.4% had smoked cigarettes at least at one point in their lives (mean age at first use, 15.5 ± 4.0 years), 58.7% smoked on a weekly basis (mean age when weekly use began, 16.9 ± 3.7 years), and 48.6% smoked daily (mean age when daily use began, 17.6 ± 4.0 years). The prevention of cigarette smoking is an important public health goal, and the prevention of cigarette smoking among patients with psychiatric illnesses and in adolescents and young adults who may be developing, or are at risk for developing, a psychiatric illness is of utmost importance.

The *primary prevention* of cigarette smoking involves efforts to reduce the incidence of smoking initiation. Thus, as emphasized in the foregoing discussion, primary prevention efforts must target youths. Many smoking prevention programs have been implemented and studied in school settings (Pérez-Stable and Fuentes-Afflick 1998). Health policy interventions, including greater enforcement of existing laws and increasing the cost of cigarettes by taxation, are also effective universal preventive interventions. *Secondary prevention* of cigarette smoking (Haustein 2003) entails the early detection of and interventions for youths and young adults who have recently begun cigarette smoking or are in the early phases of regular use or even nicotine dependence. *Tertiary prevention* involves the treatment of cigarette smoking and nicotine dependence—with the goal of smoking cessation—to reduce long-term morbidity and mortality. Guidelines are available for the treatment of nicotine dependence in clinical practice settings (Agency for Health Care Policy and Research 1996) and in specialty mental health care settings (Hughes et al. 1996). Treatment modalities include the use of various forms of nicotine replacement therapy and other pharmacological approaches as well as psychosocial approaches (see "Assisting Patients With Smoking Cessation").

In addition to categorizing the prevention of cigarette smoking based on the traditional public health classification of primary, secondary, and tertiary prevention, tobacco prevention and control efforts can be categorized based on knowledge of epidemiological trends, statistics on cessation and treatment, levels of exposure to secondhand smoke, and social and environmental changes. In general, the nation's overall health goal pertaining to tobacco use is to reduce illnesses, disability, and deaths related to tobacco use and exposure to secondhand smoke (U.S. Department of Health and Human Services 2000). This goal can be accomplished by focusing on a broad array of tobacco-related objectives, as shown in Table 13–1.

Recommendations for Clinical Practice

Screening for Cigarette Smoking and the Five *As*

The Veterans Administration and Department of Defense assert that screening for tobacco use in primary care should occur at least three times per year, and screening for tobacco use in other health care specialties or disciplines should be done at least once per year (National Guideline Clearinghouse 2004). Given the high prevalence of cigarette smoking in psychiatric populations, it may be advisable to screen for cigarette smoking much more frequently (e.g., at least quarterly) in mental health care settings.

Because of the importance of smoking as a risk factor for so many physical illnesses, screening for cigarette smoking should be considered another vital sign that receives regular assessment by health care professionals. Some clinical practice guidelines recommend "the five *As*" for health care professionals to use as a brief intervention with patients who smoke (Fiore et al. 2000). It is better to ask open-ended questions rather than questions that simply elicit yes

Table 13–1. A summary of the Healthy People 2010 U.S. health objectives pertaining to cigarette smoking

Tobacco use in population groups

Reduce cigarette smoking by adults ages ≥18 years from a baseline of 24% to 12%

Reduce past-month cigarette smoking by students in grades 9–12 from a baseline of 35% to 16%

Increase the average age of first tobacco use among adolescents ages 12–17 years from a baseline of 12 years to 14 years

Increase the average age of first tobacco use among young adults ages 18–25 years from a baseline of 15 years to 17 years

Cessation and treatment

Increase smoking cessation attempts by adult smokers from 41% to 75% (at baseline, 41% of adult smokers ages ≥18 years stopped smoking for ≥1 day because they were trying to quit; data age-adjusted to the year 2000 standard population)

Increase smoking cessation during pregnancy from 14% to 30% (at baseline, 14% of females ages 18–49 years stopped smoking during the first trimester of their pregnancy)

Increase tobacco use cessation attempts by adolescent smokers from 76% to 84% (at baseline, 76% of persons in grades 9–12 who had ever been daily smokers had tried to quit smoking)

Increase insurance coverage of evidence-based treatment for nicotine dependence from 75% to 100% for managed care organizations, and from 24% to 51% for Medicaid programs

Exposure to secondhand smoke

Reduce the proportion of children who are regularly exposed to tobacco smoke at home from 27% to 10% (27% of children ages ≤6 years lived in a household where someone smoked inside the house ≥4 days per week in 1994)

Reduce the proportion of nonsmokers exposed to environmental tobacco smoke from 65% to 45% (65% of nonsmokers ages ≥4 years had a serum nicotine level >0.10 ng/mL in 1988–1994; data age-adjusted to the year 2000 standard population)

Increase smoke-free and tobacco-free environments in schools, including all school facilities, property, vehicles, and school events from 37% to 100% (37% of middle, junior high, and senior high schools were smoke free and tobacco free in 1994)

Increase the proportion of worksites with ≥50 employees with formal smoking policies that prohibit smoking or limit it to separately ventilated areas from a baseline of 79% to 100%

Establish laws on smoke-free indoor air that prohibit smoking or limit it to separately ventilated areas in public places and worksites to 51% (e.g., in restaurants, from 3% at baseline to 51%; in public transportation, from 16% to 51%; and in retail stores from 4% to 51%)

Table 13–1. A summary of the Healthy People 2010 U.S. health objectives pertaining to cigarette smoking *(continued)*

Social and environmental changes

Reduce the illegal sales rate to minors through enforcement of laws prohibiting the sale of tobacco products to minors (i.e., increase the percentage of jurisdictions that have a ≤5% illegal sales rate to minors, from 0% at baseline to 51%)

Increase the number of states that suspend or revoke state retail licenses for violations of laws prohibiting the sale of tobacco to minors, from 34 states to all states

Increase adolescents' disapproval of smoking (e.g., from 80% at baseline to 95% in the eighth grade, and from 69% at baseline to 95% in the twelfth grade)

Eliminate laws that preempt stronger tobacco control laws from 30 states that had preemptive tobacco control laws in the areas of clean indoor air, minors' access laws, or marketing, to no states
TRY THIS: Reduce/Eliminate the number of states that
OR: Eliminate laws that….(currently existing in 30 states)….

Increase the average federal and state tax on tobacco products from $0.63 for cigarettes at baseline to $2.00 (based on a 24-cent federal tax and 39-cent average state tax in 1998)

Note. Baseline statistics, unless otherwise indicated, generally pertain to the year 1998. Targets for health objectives pertain to 2010. Developmental objectives are not shown. Mention of *states* include the District of Columbia.
Source. Adapted from U.S. Department of Health and Human Services 2000.

or no answers, as it increases disclosure of smoking substantially. The five *A*s are as follows:

- Ask about smoking status.
- Advise the patient to quit.
- Assess the patient's willingness to quit.
- Assist by suggesting and encouraging the use of problem-solving methods and skills for cessation.
- Arrange for follow-up contacts to maximize the chances of relapse prevention.

Assisting Patients With Smoking Cessation

If the physician or other health care provider finds that a patient who smokes is currently uninterested in or unwilling to quit at the time, the clinician should help the patient realize the immediate and long-term risks of continuing to smoke, the benefits of quitting sooner rather than later, and the patient's perceived barriers to quitting. These issues should be personalized as much as possible to the particular patient. If the patient is willing to quit at the time, assistance should be provided, such as:

- Helping the patient choose a target quitting date
- Enhancing social support
- Suggesting and prescribing appropriate pharmacotherapy
- Advising about withdrawal symptoms
- Recommending behavioral and cognitive coping responses and techniques
- Possibly even referring the patient to an intensive behavioral counseling program in the area

The last of the five *A*s is extremely important because evidence shows that the total contact time with a health care professional predicts treatment outcome. Follow-up contact—by phone, mail, direct visit, or written materials—communicates the importance of smoking cessation, gives the patient additional support, and provides an opportunity for discussion of any issues that arise along the process of quitting.

Some characteristics of people who successfully quit smoking, compared with those who do not succeed with quitting, are as follows: confidence in the ability to remain abstinent, lighter smoking before quitting, smoking for fewer years, being governed less by habit and need for stimulation provided by smoking, and having quit for longer periods during previous attempts to discontinue cigarette use (Mothersill et al. 1988). It is helpful for some patients to consider the fact that most people actually "quit" when they go to bed at night, suggesting that quitting is, in fact, physiologically and psychologically possible. It should be noted that depression and poor coping lead to more withdrawal symptoms and higher relapse rates relative to the process of quitting in nondepressed smokers (Hall 1988).

Diverse treatment modalities are available, including nicotine replacement therapy in the form of nasal sprays, lozenges, inhalers, gums, and transdermal patches (Haustein 2003); hypnosis; aversive therapy; acupuncture; and a number of other pharmacological and psychosocial approaches, including motivational interviewing and supportive psychotherapy with goal setting and close follow-up. Systemic nicotine administration and behavioral counseling can sustain abstinence in 60% of patients (Haustein 2003). Bupropion at dosages of 300 mg per day increases the quitting rate of smokers with and without depression (Hurt et al. 1997). In smokers without depression, a double-blind, placebo-controlled study found that over weeks from the target quitting date, the success rate of continuous abstinence with placebo was only 10.5%, whereas success rates with sustained-release bupropion at dosages of 50 mg twice daily, 150 mg once daily, and 150 mg twice daily were 13.7%, 18.3%, and 24.4%, respectively (Hurt et al. 1997). After 1 year, continued benefits in terms of ongoing smoking cessation were seen in the groups treated with 150 mg or 300 mg of bupropion. Another pharmacological agent for smoking cessation is varenicline, a partial agonist selective for nicotinic acetylcholine receptor subtypes. Varenicline is available in monthly dosage packs and is approved for a 12-week course of treatment, though if continued for another 12 weeks the likelihood of long-term cessation is even greater. In a large study involving more than 1,200 participants, continuous abstinence rates in the varenicline-treated group and the group receiving placebo were 70.5% and 49.6%, respectively, after 24 weeks of treatment, and 43.6% and 36.9% at the 52-week follow-up (Tonstad et al. 2006).

The use of nicotine replacement therapy or any medication without behavioral support is not likely to be successful. All medications and treatments used for smoking cessation are more successful when used with behavioral measures. Regarding behavioral treatments alone, even though effective, few smokers are interested in attending specific smoking cessation classes. Simple computer-tailored behavioral support systems that are available through manufacturers of smoking cessation products have been found to double cessation rates for some (Thompson et al. 1988). Technology-facilitated modalities, such as so-called *Web-assisted tobacco interventions*, may be helpful. For example, a recent study demonstrated the efficacy of a smoking cessation Web site for college students that incorporated both individually tailored feedback and peer e-mail support (An et al. 2008; Klatt et al. 2008).

When helping patients to quit smoking, psychiatrists and other mental health professionals should be aware that initiation or discontinuation of smoking can affect blood levels of multiple medications. For instance, abstinence from smoking, perhaps while a patient is hospitalized and not allowed to smoke, can increase the blood concentrations of clozapine, desipramine, fluvoxamine, imipramine, haloperidol, and olanzapine. Higher concentrations may be associated with greater side effects. Similarly, resuming or beginning smoking can cause lowering of therapeutic levels of these agents, which may be associated with a poor response to medication.

Smoking Cessation in Adolescence

Ideally, mental health care providers will be able to identify early smoking behaviors in adolescent patients and work closely with them to quit and abstain completely. It is critical that cigarette smoking prevention efforts be thorough and ongoing for adolescents identified as being at high risk for nicotine dependence by virtue of a strong family history of cigarette smoking, an accumulation of psychosocial risk factors, or early or experimental use of tobacco products. Because most nicotine-dependent adults began smoking in adolescence, this is a critical developmental age for the prevention of cigarette smoking.

Smoking Cessation in Pregnancy

The prevention of cigarette smoking during pregnancy, and immediate assistance for pregnant patients who do smoke cigarettes, deserves special attention. Smoking at any time during pregnancy increases the risk of miscarriage, placenta previa, placental abruption, neonatal mortality, premature delivery, low birth weight, and sudden infant death syndrome in the newborn. Fetal lung and heart development are significantly affected by cigarette smoking. Fetal nicotine exposure can also result in changes in central dopaminergic and cholinergic signaling, decreased hippocampal cell size, and other central nervous system effects that may be associated with long-lasting structural and functional impairments. In addition, fetuses of mothers who smoke are exposed to tobacco-related carcinogens, some of which have been shown to cause genomic and transcriptional alterations in the developing fetal liver in hamsters (Correa et al. 1990).

Cognitive functions such as learning and memory can be adversely affected by prenatal smoking (Roy et al. 2002). Maternal smoking substantially increases the risk of learning disabilities and behavioral problems in children. Scores on cognitive functioning tests are lower in children of mothers who smoked during pregnancy compared with scores in children whose mothers did not smoke. Externalizing behaviors—oppositionality, aggression, overactivity, and even diagnosable conduct disorder and attention-deficit/hyperactivity disorder—are related to maternal smoking (Thapar et al. 2003).

Measures found to be effective and cost-beneficial for pregnant smokers in public health maternity clinics include personal counseling, referrals to smoking cessation clinics, behavioral modification techniques, and antismoking pamphlets (Windsor et al. 1993). The five *A*s presented earlier represent an easy-to-use, evidence-based clinical counseling approach for assessment. Their use can double or even triple the quitting success rate among pregnant smokers, even in low-income or socioeconomically disadvantaged patients, who are especially likely to smoke during this critical time (Ross et al. 2002). Counseling for this population needs to be targeted to the particular individual and this particular situation (i.e., pregnancy), given that the choice to smoke is affecting not only the woman but also the fetus. Because there is such a high rate of relapse, follow-up visits with specific assessment and treatment of smoking are crucial, especially in the postpartum period, when the focus is often on the new baby and the mother's struggle with smoking could be inadvertently overlooked or forgotten.

Preventing Relapse

Relapse commonly occurs in the context of cyclical episodes of smoking and discontinuation in regular smokers. Roughly 75%–80% of quitters who are initially successful resume smoking within 6 months (Cohen et al. 1989). However, if a person can remain abstinent for 60 months the risk of relapse is negligible (U.S. Department of Health and Human Services 1989). Smoking relapse is often triggered by nicotine withdrawal symptoms such as cravings, tension, aggressiveness, depression, difficulty concentrating, irritability, hunger, and restlessness. It is also triggered by stress and environmental cues such as being in the presence of someone who is smoking. Negative affects like sadness, anger, and anxiety, brought on by various situations, increase the risk of relapse. Relapse is particularly common in the context of alcohol use, boredom, meal times, and hunger (Brownell et al. 1986).

Helpful relapse prevention strategies include identifying and modifying situations and circumstances that could lead to relapse, anticipating those situations before they occur, and identifying and utilizing coping strategies so they can become automatic when there is an urge to smoke. One must practice antiaddictive thinking and thus stop reinforcing ideas such as "I need a cigarette to relax" or "I will gain weight if I quit smoking." One must practice effective management of negative mood states, interpersonal conflict, stress, and boredom. Social support is also helpful whether a person quits in a group therapy setting or individually. A well-balanced lifestyle is imperative so that one finds healthy ways of enjoying life, social support, and acceptance among peers.

Conclusion

Given the importance of tobacco use as a risk factor for so many illnesses, screening for it should be another vital sign and requires regular assessment by health care professionals. Simply asking about smoking is a step toward a preventive strategy. If someone is not already smoking or has in the past, this questioning alerts the patient to the importance of abstinence.

Key Points

- Cigarette smoking is a major public health concern deserving focused attention in all health care settings, but particularly in mental health care settings given the very high rates of cigarette smoking and nicotine dependence among people with other substance use disorders and mental illnesses.

- The prevention of cigarette smoking among patients with psychiatric illnesses and in adolescents and young adults who may be developing, or are at risk for developing, a psychiatric illness is of utmost importance.

- Whereas the prevalence of cigarette smoking is approximately 22% in the general U.S. population, rates of smoking are much higher among people with mental illnesses, and may be as high as 90% in people with serious mental illnesses like schizophrenia.

- Although cigarette smoking/nicotine dependence is very common among psychiatric patients, it is often left out of listed axial diagnoses or problem lists, therefore not receiving the clinical attention that it deserves. Psychiatrists and other mental health professionals should inquire about cigarette smoking in every patient.

- Given the importance of smoking as a risk factor for so many physical illnesses, screening for cigarette smoking should be considered another vital sign that receives regular assessment by health care professionals. The 5 *A*s can be used for a brief intervention by health care professionals with patients who smoke: **A**sk about smoking status, **A**dvise to quit, **A**ssess willingness to quit, **A**ssist by suggesting and encouraging the use of problem-solving methods and skills for cessation, and **A**rrange follow-up contacts and relapse prevention.

• Adolescence and pregnancy are two especially critical developmental periods in which smoking prevention efforts should be emphasized.

References

The Agency for Health Care Policy and Research Smoking Cessation Clinical Practice Guideline. JAMA 275:1270–1280, 1996

An LC, Klatt C, Perry CL, et al: The RealU online cessation intervention for college smokers: a randomized controlled trial. Prev Med 47:194–199, 2008

Bandura A: Influence of models' reinforcement contingencies on the acquisition of imitative responses. J Abnorm Psychol 66:575–582, 1965

Brownell KD, Marlatt GA, Lichtenstein E, et al: Understanding and preventing relapse. Am Psychol 41:765–782, 1986

Campaign for Tobacco-Free Kids: Smoking and other drug use. January 2002. Available at: http://tobaccofreekids.org/research/factsheets/pdf/0106.pdf. Accessed December 18, 2008.

Centers for Disease Control and Prevention: Annual smoking-attributable mortality, years of potential life lost, and economic costs—United States, 1995–1999. MMWR Morb Mortal Wkly Rep 51:300–303, 2002

Centers for Disease Control and Prevention: Cigarette smoking among adults—United States, 2002. MMWR Morb Mortal Wkly Rep 53:427–431, 2004a

Centers for Disease Control and Prevention: Cigarette smoking among high school students—United States, 1991–2003. MMWR Morb Mortal Wkly Rep 53:499–502, 2004b

Centers for Disease Control and Prevention: State-specific prevalence of current cigarette smoking among adults—United States, 2003. MMWR Morb Mortal Wkly Rep 53:1035–1037, 2004c

Cohen S, Lichtenstein E, Prochaska JO, et al: Debunking myths about self-quitting: evidence from 10 prospective studies of persons quitting smoking by themselves. Am Psychol 44:1355–1365, 1989

Correa E, Joshi PA, Castonguay A, et al: The tobacco-specific nitrosamine 4-(methyl-nitrosamino)-1-(3-pyridyl)-1-butanone is an active transplacental carcinogen in Syrian golden hamsters. Cancer Res 50:3435–3438, 1990

Dalton M, Tickle J, Sargent J, et al: The incidence and context of tobacco use in popular movies from 1988 to 1997. Prev Med 34:516–523, 2002

de Leon J, Diaz FJ: A meta-analysis of worldwide studies demonstrates an association between schizophrenia and tobacco smoking behaviors. Schizophr Res 76:135–157, 2005

Evans RI: How can health lifestyles in adolescents be modified?: some implications from a smoking prevention program, in Handbook of Pediatric Psychology. Edited by Routh DK. New York, Guilford, 1988, pp 321–331

Federal Trade Commission: Federal Trade Commission Cigarette Report for 2001. Washington, DC, Federal Trade Commission, 2003

Fiore MC, Bailey WC, Cohen SJ, et al: Clinical Practice Guideline: Treating Tobacco Use and Dependence. Rockville, MD, U.S. Department of Health and Human Services, 2000

Glantz S: Smoking in movies: a major problem and a real solution. Lancet 362:258–259, 2003

Glantz SA, Kacirk KW, McCulloch C: Back to the future: smoking in movies in 2002 compared with 1950 levels. Am J Public Health 94:261–263, 2004

Goff DC, Henderson DC, Amico E: Cigarette smoking in schizophrenia: relationship to psychopathology and medication side effects. Am J Psychiatry 149:1189–1194, 1992

Grant BF, Hasin DS, Chou SP, et al: Nicotine dependence and psychiatric disorders in the United States: results from the national epidemiologic survey on alcohol and related conditions. Arch Gen Psychiatry 61:1107–1115, 2004

Hall SM: Smoking, sweets, and sadness: dependence, treatment failure, and regulatory systems. Paper presented at the annual meeting of the American Psychological Association, Atlanta, GA, 1988

Haustein KO: What can we do in secondary prevention of cigarette smoking? Eur J Cardiovasc Prev Rehabil 10:476–485, 2003

Hoffmann D, Hoffmann I, El-Bayoumy K: The less harmful cigarette: a controversial issue: a tribute to Ernst L. Wynder. Chem Res Toxicol 14:767–790, 2001

Hughes JR, Fiester S, Goldstein MG, et al: American Psychiatric Association practice guideline for the treatment of patients with nicotine dependence. Am J Psychiatry 153 (suppl 10):S1–S31, 1996

Hurt RD, Sachs DP, Glover ED, et al: A comparison of sustained-release bupropion and placebo for smoking cessation. N Engl J Med 337:1195–1202, 1997

International Agency for Research on Cancer: IARC Monographs on the evaluation of carcinogenic risks of chemicals to humans, 1972–2000, Vol 1–77. Available at: http://monographs.iarc.fr/ENG/Monographs/PDFs/index.php. Accessed December 22, 2008.

Jarvis MJ: Why people smoke. BMJ 328:277–279, 2004

Klatt C, Berg CJ, Thomas JL, et al: The role of peer e-mail support as part of a college smoking-cessation website. Am J Prev Med 35 (suppl 6):S471–478, 2008

Lasser K, Boyd JW, Woolhandler S, et al: Smoking and mental illness: a population-based prevalence study. JAMA 284:2606–2610, 2000

Lohr JB, Flynn K: Smoking and schizophrenia. Schizophr Res 8:93–102, 1992

Mokdad AH, Marks JS, Stroup DF, et al: Actual causes of death in the United States, 2000. JAMA 291:1238–1245, 2004

Mothersill KJ, McDowell I, Rosser W: Subject characteristics and long-term post-program smoking cessation. Addict Behav 13:29–36, 1988

National Guideline Clearinghouse: VA/DoD clinical practice guideline for the management of tobacco use, 2004. Available at: http://www.guidelines.gov/summary/summary.aspx?doc_id=6107. Accessed December 17, 2008.

Pérez-Stable EJ, Fuentes-Afflick E: Role of clinicians in cigarette smoking prevention. West J Med 169:23–29, 1998

Pomerleau OF: The "why" of tobacco dependence: underlying reinforcing mechanisms in nicotine self-administration, in The Pharmacologic Treatment of Tobacco Dependence: Proceedings of the World Congress, November 4–5, 1985. Edited by Ockene JK. Cambridge, MA, Institute for the Study of Smoking Behavior and Policy, 1985, pp 32–47

Pomerleau OF, Pomerleau CS: Neuroregulators and the reinforcement of smoking: toward a biobehavioral explanation. Neurosci Biobehav Rev 8:503–513, 1984

Ross JA, Swensen AR, Murphy SE: Prevalence of cigarette smoking in pregnant women participating in the special supplemental nutrition programme for Women, Infants and Children (WIC) in Minneapolis and Saint Paul, Minnesota, USA. Paediatr Perinat Epidemiol 16:246–248, 2002

Roy TS, Seidler FJ, Slotkin TA: Prenatal nicotine exposure evokes alterations of cell structure in hippocampus and somatosensory cortex. J Pharmacol Exp Ther 300:124–133, 2002

Silagy C, Lancaster T, Stead L, et al: Nicotine replacement therapy for smoking cessation. Art No: CD000146. DOI: 10.1002/14651858.CD000146.pub2, 2002

Stewart T, Goulding SM, Pringle M, et al: A descriptive study of nicotine, alcohol, and cannabis use in urban, socially disadvantaged, predominantly African American patients with first-episode nonaffective psychosis. Clinical Schizophrenia and Related Psychoses (in press)

Thapar A, Fowler T, Rice F, et al: Maternal smoking during pregnancy and attention deficit hyperactivity disorder symptoms in offspring. Am J Psychiatry 160:1985–1989, 2003

Thompson RS, Michnich ME, Friedlander L, et al: Effectiveness of smoking cessation interventions integrated into primary care practice. Med Care 26:62–76, 1988

Tickle JJ, Sargent JD, Dalton MA, et al: Favorite movie stars, their tobacco use in contemporary movies, and its association with adolescent smoking. Tob Control 2001 10:16–22, 2001

Tonstad S, Tønnesen P, Hajek P, et al; Varenicline Phase 3 Study Group: Effect of maintenance therapy with varenicline on smoking cessation: a randomized controlled trial. JAMA 296:64–71, 2006

Turner L, Mermelstein R, Flay B: Individual and contextual influences on adolescent smoking. Ann N Y Acad Sci 1021:175–197, 2004

U.S. Department of Health and Human Services: Reducing the Health Consequences of Smoking: 25 Years of Progress: A Report of the Surgeon General. Washington, DC, US Government Printing Office, 1989

U.S. Department of Health and Human Services: Reducing Tobacco Use: A Report of the Surgeon General. Washington, DC, Government Printing Office, 1994

U.S. Department of Health and Human Services: Healthy People 2010. U.S. Department of Health and Human Services, Office of Disease Prevention and Health Promotion, 2000. Available at: http://www.healthypeople.gov. Accessed December 16, 2008.

Williams JM, Ziedonis D: Addressing tobacco among individuals with a mental illness or an addiction. Addict Behav 29:1067–1083, 2004

Windsor RA, Lowe JB, Perkins LL, et al: Health education for pregnant smokers: its behavioral impact and cost benefit. Am J Public Health 83:201–206, 1993

Ziedonis DM, Kosten TR, Glazer WM, et al: Nicotine dependence and schizophrenia. Hosp Community Psychiatry 45:204–206, 1994

Index

*Page numbers printed in **boldface** type refer to tables or figures.*

"A" (Adderall), 183
Abecedarian Project, 41
Abuse-focused cognitive-behavioral therapy (AF-CBT), 254
Abusive Men Exploring New Directions (AMEND), **259, 260**
Academic self-efficacy, 62
Acamprosate, 193
ACTIVE. *See* Advanced Cognitive Training for Independent and Vital Elderly trial
Adderall ("A"), 183
ADH. *See* Alcohol dehydrogenase
ADHD. *See* Attention-deficit/hyperactivity disorder
Adolescents, 40. *See also* Peers
    cognitive and social development, 64–65
    conduct disorder, 274, 276
        delinquency and, 279, 281
        DSM-IV-TR criteria, **278–279**
        epidemiology and public health impact, 276
        preventive interventions, 277–284
            primary, 279–281
            secondary, 282–283
            tertiary, 283–284
    protective factors and health promotion interventions, 284–289
    risk factors, 276–277
    depression and, 14
    developmental assets, **285–287**, 291
    normal, 274
    pregnancy and, 19
    prevention principles in psychiatric practice, 273–206
    recommendations for prevention of harm and promotion of strength in youth, 290, **291**
    smoking and, 371, 380
    stages of development, **275**
    substance abuse and, 181–191
    suicidal behavior and, 231–232
    transition to adulthood, 289
Adolescent Training and Learning to Avoid Steroids (ATLAS), 190–191
Advanced Cognitive Training for Independent and Vital Elderly (ACTIVE) trial, 320
Adversity, as risk factor for suicide, 216
AF-CBT. *See* Abuse-focused cognitive-behavioral therapy
African American mothers, 63

387

Age. *See also* Adolescents; Children;
    Elderly
  as risk factor for dementia, 311
Age-related macular degeneration
    (AMD), 306
Agoraphobia, 85
Alanine transaminase (ALT) marker,
    209
Alcohol, 17
  dependence, 172–177
    death and, 167
    definition, 178–179
    mental health professionals
        assessment and advice to
        patients about problematic
        alcohol use, 177–179
    preventive interventions,
        175–177
      indicated, 176–177
      selective, 176
      universal, 175–176
    protective factors, 174–175
    relapse prevention, 191–193
    risk and protective factors,
        172–175
      genetics and alcohol
          dependence, 172–173
      social/environmental and
          psychological risk
          factors, 173–174
    screening tests, 204–209
  dry drunk, 179
  prevention of abuse, 163–210
  prevention paradox, 164
  problem and benefit, 164–169,
      167, 168–169
  screening for use disorders, 19–20
  tests for use, 209
    chronic, 209

    less recent use, 209
    recent use, 209
Alcohol abuse, definition, 178
Alcohol dehydrogenase (ADH),
    167–168
Alcohol Use Disorders Identification
    Test (AUDIT), 177, 205–207
ALT. *See* Alanine transaminase marker
Alzheimer's disease. *See also* Elderly
  antioxidants and, 313
AMD. *See* Age-related macular
    degeneration
AMEND. *See* Abusive Men Exploring
    New Directions
American Indians, 173, 213
Amphetamines, 183
Antidepressants
  for management of late-life
      depression, 302–303
  for mood disorders, 67
  for prevention of suicidal behavior,
      220–222
Antioxidants, Alzheimer's disease and, 313
Antipsychotics, 331
  for prevention of suicidal behavior,
      223–224
Anxiety disorders, 13
  complementary and alternative
      medicine in prevention,
      105–123
  DSM-III-R definition, 109
  epidemiology, 84–85
  onset, 85
  prevention, 83–103
    costs, 97–98
    intervention strategies, delivery
        formats, and settings, 97
    during life course, 94–95
    targeted efforts, 95–96, **96**

prevention studies, 87–92
  indicated preventive
        interventions, 87–88
  selective preventive
        interventions, 88–91
  universal preventive
        interventions, 91–92
  public and provider education,
        92–93
  risk factors, 85–87
    demographic factors, 85–86
    environmental factors, 86–87
    genetics/family history, 86
    personality/temperament, 86
  treatment, 84–85
Asian and Pacific Islanders, 173, 213
Aspartate transaminase (AST) marker,
      209
AST. *See* Aspartate transaminase marker
ATLAS. *See* Adolescent Training and
      Learning to Avoid Steroids
Attention-deficit/hyperactivity disorder
      (ADHD), 19–20, 185
  alcohol use and, 173–174
Attitude, pessimistic, 90–91
AUDIT. *See* Alcohol Use Disorders
      Identification Test

Beck Depression Inventory, 110
Behavior, adverse, 17–18
  prevention, 12
Behavioral Risk Factor Surveillance
      System (BRFSS), 368, 369
Benzodiazepines, 117, 170
Bereavement, 302. *See also* Death
Bidis, 366. *See also* Smoking
Biological traits, as risk factor for
      suicide, 216

Biomarkers, as risk factor for mild
      cognitive impairment, 318
Bipolar disorder, 52. *See also* Thyroid
      disease
  collaborative care approach, 71
  environmental factors, 58–59
  general medical illnesses and, 59
  genetic vulnerability, 54–55
  pharmacotherapy and, 69
  secondary prevention, 67
  sleep disturbances and, 58–59
  sociodemographic characteristics,
        56–57
Blacks, 213
BMI. *See* Body mass index
Body mass index (BMI), 336
Box, George, 211
Brahmi, 106
BRFSS. *See* Behavioral Risk Factor
      Surveillance System
Bullying, 17–18, 19
Buprenorphine, 192–193
Bupropion, 221, 378–379

CAGE (cut down, annoyed, guilt, and
      eye opener) questions, 204–205
CAM. *See* Complementary and
      alternative medicine
Campaign for Tobacco-Free Kids, 371
Cancer, 333
Cannabis spp., 135, 179
  prevention, 192
CAPS. *See* Coping and Promoting
      Strength program
Carbohydrate-deficient transferrin
      (CDT) test, 209
Cardiovascular disease, 336–337
  depression and, 59

CATIE study, 332
CBT. *See* Cognitive-behavioral therapy
CDT. *See* Carbohydrate-deficient
transferrin test
Center of Epidemiologic Studies
Depression Scale (CES-D), 305
CES-D. *See* Center of Epidemiologic
Studies Depression Scale
Child-Parent Psychotherapy for Family
Violence (CPP-FV), 258,
259–260, **259**
Child physical abuse, 216, 250–255
outcomes, **251**
primary prevention, 250–253, **251**
risk factors, **249**
secondary prevention, 253–254
tertiary prevention, 254–255
Children
cognitive and social development,
64–65
of depressed mothers, 14
drug abuse and, 181–191
preventive interventions,
187–191
risk and protective factors,
183–187
substance abuse and, 181–191
Child sexual abuse, 255–256
outcomes, **251**
primary prevention, 255–256
tertiary prevention, 256
Child Witness to Violence Project, 260
Choose Respect, 257
CHR. *See* Clinical high risk status
Citalopram, 221
Clinical high risk (CHR) status, 141
Clinical practice. *See also* Mental health
professionals
collaborative care approach, 70–71

complementary and alternative
medicine and, 115–117
education for early detection of
suicidal behavior, 219
empirical and clinical implications,
37–41
cause, correlate or consequence,
38
process-oriented research and
developmental timing,
38–40
risk- and resilience-informed
intervention, 40–41
identification and understanding of
risk factors and protective
factors, 29–48
mental health professionals
assessment and advice to
patients about problematic
alcohol use, 177–179
prevention advice, 146–148,
232–235
prevention principles for adolescents
in psychiatric practice,
273–296
primary care psychiatrist, 348
principles of family violence
prevention, 261–267
primary prevention, 261–262
secondary prevention, 262–263
tertiary prevention, 264–267
promotion of prevention of mood
disorders, 70–72
protective factors to promote
positive development and
health, 34–37
risk factors to predict
maladjustment and pathology,
30–34

role in prevention of anxiety
disorders, 93
for smoking prevention, 375–382
split treatments for suicide
prevention, 234
Clozapine, 223–224, 331, 345
Cognitive-behavioral therapy (CBT),
190, 319–320
for prevention of mood disorders,
67
for treatment of anxiety disorders,
87
Cognitive reserve hypothesis, 314
Collaborative care, 70–71
Communities That Care, 16–17, 281
Community
in mental health prevention, 16–17
preventive interventions for
substance abuse and, 187–188
Community Advocacy Project, 258
Compensatory factors, 34
Competencies, 37
Complementary and alternative
medicine (CAM)
background, 111–113
definition, 105–107
distinction between, 107
exercise, 110, 114–115
herbs, 106–107
integrative medicine, 106
meditation, 113–114
mental health practitioners and,
115–117
mental illness treatment and,
108–110
efficacy, 109–110
overview, 108–109
in prevention of depression and
anxiety, 105–123

in the United States, 107–108
yoga, 110, 114
Composite International Diagnostic
Interview, 109
Conduct disorder, 17–18, 274, 276
DSM-IV-TR criteria, **278–279**
epidemiology and public health
impact, 276
preventive interventions, 277–284
primary, 279–281
secondary, 282–283
tertiary, 283–284
risk factors, 276–277
Coping
active, 61
approach, 61
styles, 61
Coping and Promoting Strength
(CAPS) program, 90, 95
model, **96**
Coping with Depression Course,
68–69
Cough medicine, 183
CPP-FV. *See* Child-Parent
Psychotherapy for Family Violence
Crisis hotlines, 226–227
for domestic violence, 258

DAIP. *See* Domestic Abuse Intervention
Project (DAIP)
DARE. *See* Drug Abuse Resistance
Education
DCM. *See* Depression care management
Death
associated with alcohol dependence,
167
bereavement and, 302
rates, 328–329
Delinquency, 17–18, 279, 281

DELTA. *See* Domestic Violence
        Prevention Enhancement and
        Leadership Through Alliances
Dementia, 309–316
    clinical characteristics, 309,
        319–311
    epidemiology, 309, 311
    prevention, 315–316
        primary, 315–316
        secondary, 315–316
        tertiary, 316
    risk factors, 311–314
        age, 311
        dietary and nutritional factors,
            313
        educational level, 314
        genetic factors, 312
        physical inactivity, 313
        presence of mild cognitive
            impairment, 311–312
        social/network/leisure activities,
            313
        systemic inflammation, 313
        vascular risk factors and
            disorders, 312–313
    treatment, 314–315
Depression, 49. *See also* Mood disorders
    in adolescents, 14
    bipolar, 49
    complementary and alternative
        medicine in prevention,
        105–123
    description, 50
    environmental factors, 57–58
    general medical illnesses and, 59
    late-life, 299–308
    major, 49
    marital status and, 55
    mortality and, 50–51

mothers and children and, 14
    prevalence, 55–56
    as risk factor for suicide, 219
    secondary, 223
    sociodemographic characteristics,
        55–56
    studies, 221
    symptoms, 300
    trauma and, 58
    twin studies and, 57–58
    unipolar, 49, 50
Depression care management (DCM),
        307–308
Development
    theories and norms, 39
    timing, 38–41
Dextroamphetamine, 183
Diabetes, 331, 336
*Diagnostic and Statistical Manual of
    Mental Disorders* (DSM), 3
    course specifiers for schizophrenia,
        131–132
    definition of alcohol abuse, 178
    definition of anxiety disorders,
        109
    diagnostic criteria for alcohol abuse,
        165–166, **167**
    diagnostic criteria for conduct
        disorder, **278–279**
    diagnostic criteria for dementia,
        310–311
    diagnostic criteria for major
        depressive episode, 50, **51**
    diagnostic criteria for manic
        episode, 52, **53**
    diagnostic criteria for schizophrenia,
        129, **130–131**
    diagnostic criteria for substance
        dependence, **168–169**

Diet, 13
    health promotion and, 338
    as risk factor for dementia, 313
Dinosaur School, 18
Disulfiram, 193
Divalproex, for prevention of
        recurrence of mania and
        depression in bipolar disorder, 69
Domestic Abuse Intervention Project
        (DAIP), **259**, 260
Domestic violence, 256–260
    counseling, 260
    hotlines, 258
    legislation, 256–257
    primary prevention, 256–257
    risk factors, **250**
    secondary prevention, 257
    shelters, 258
    tertiary prevention, 257–260, **259**
Domestic Violence Home Visit
        Intervention, 260
Domestic Violence Prevention
        Enhancement and Leadership
        Through Alliances (DELTA),
        256–257
Donepezil, for treatment of dementia,
        314
Dopamine, 115
Drug abuse
    prevention, 163–210
        in children and adolescents,
            181–191
            preventive interventions,
                187–191
            risk and protective factors,
                183–187
        relapse prevention, 191–193
Drug Abuse Resistance Education
        (DARE), 180–181

Dry drunk, 179
DSM. *See Diagnostic and Statistical
    Manual of Mental Disorders*
Duloxetine, 221
DUP. *See* Duration of untreated
    psychosis
Duration of untreated psychosis
    (DUP), 128, 144–145

ECA. *See* Epidemiologic Catchment
    Area
ECG. *See* Electrocardiogram
Ecstasy (methylenedioxymethamphet-
    amine; MDMA), 182–183
ECT. *See* Electroconvulsive therapy
Education. *See also* Schools
    for anxiety disorders, 92–93
    of health care professionals, 219
    for prevention of mood disorders,
        65
    as risk factor for dementia, 314
    for suicidal behavior, 218
Elderly, 17. *See also* Alzheimer's disease
    contact for prevention of suicidal
        behavior, 227–228
    dementia, 309–316
        clinical characteristics, 309,
            310–311
        epidemiology, 309, 311
        prevention, 315–316
            primary, 315–316
            secondary, 316
            tertiary, 3316
        risk factors, 311–314
            age, 311
            dietary and nutritional
                factors, 313
            educational level, 314
            genetic factors, 312

Elderly *(continued)*
  dementia *(continued)*
    risk factors *(continued)*
      physical inactivity, 313
      presence of mild cognitive
          impairment, 311–312
      social/network/leisure
          activities, 313
      systemic inflammation, 313
      vascular risk factors and
          disorders, 312–313
    treatment, 314–315
  late-life depression, 299–308
    clinical characteristics,
        299–300
    epidemiology, 300–301
    prevention, 303–308
      primary, 304–307
      secondary, 307–308
      tertiary, 308
    risk factors, 301–302
      biological, 301
      psychosocial, 302
    treatment, 302–303
  mild cognitive impairment,
      316–320
    clinical characteristics, 317
    epidemiology, 317
    prevention, 319–320
      primary, 319–320
      secondary, 320
      tertiary, 320
    risk factors, 318
      biomarkers, 318
      genetics, 318
    treatment, 318–319
  prevention principles, 297–326
Electrocardiogram (ECG), 345
Electroconvulsive therapy (ECT)
  for management of late-life
      depression, 302, 303
  for prevention of suicidal behavior,
      224–225
Employee Assistance Programs, 16
Environment
  alcohol dependence risk factors and,
      173–174
  preventive interventions for
      substance abuse and, 187–188
  risk factors
    for anxiety disorders, 86–87
    for bipolar disorder, 58–59
    for depression, 57–58
    for mood disorders, 57–59
    for suicide, 217
  secondhand smoke, 366, **376**
Epidemiologic Catchment Area (ECA),
    50–51
  in anxiety disorders, 84–85
Epidemiology
  in mental health prevention, 9–10
  of mood disorders, 49–50
  of suicide, 212–213
    in the United States, 212–213
    worldwide, 212
Escitalopram, 221
Exercise, 13, 21, 110, 114–115,
    341–342. *See also* Physical inactivity
  health promotion and, 337–338

Families and Schools Together
    Program, 64
Family
  genetic vulnerability to mood
      disorders, 54
  history
    as risk factor for anxiety
        disorders, 86

as risk factor for suicide, 215
identification of at risk family
members for prevention of
suicidal behavior, 230
of mental health patients, 13–14
preventive interventions for
substance abuse and, 187
protective factors, 34, **35**
risk factors and, 31, **31**, 32
Family violence, prevention, 243–272.
See also Parents
child maltreatment, 250–256
child physical abuse and neglect,
250–255
primary prevention,
250–253, **251**
secondary prevention,
253–254
tertiary prevention, 254–255
child sexual abuse, 255–256
primary prevention,
255–256
tertiary prevention, 256
domestic violence, 256–260
primary prevention, 256–257
secondary prevention, 257
tertiary prevention, 257–260,
259
etiologies, 246–250, **247**
family (mesosystem) risks,
247–248
individual (microsystem) risks,
246–247
interaction of risk and protective
factors, 248–250, **249**, 250
society (macrosystem) risks,
248
mental health care for the victim,
266–267

physical health care of the victim,
265–266
prevalence, 244–245
principles of prevention for mental
health professionals, 261–267
primary prevention, 261–262
secondary prevention, 262–263
tertiary prevention, 264–267
safety plan, 264–265
Family Violence Prevention and
Services Act, 256
FDA. *See* U.S. Food and Drug
Administration
FEAR plan, 87–88
Fetal alcohol syndrome, 166
Fluoxetine, 221
Fluphenazine, 223
Fluvoxamine, 221
FRIENDS skills, 91–92

GAD. *See* Generalized anxiety
disorder
Galantamine, for treatment of
dementia, 314
Gamma-glutamyltransferase (GGT)
test, 209
Gatekeeper programs
for adolescents in suicide
prevention, 232
education, 218
training in mental health
prevention, 15
GBG. *See* Good Behavior Game
Generalized anxiety disorder (GAD),
85
Genetics, 36
alcohol dependence and, 172–173
implications for prevention of mood
disorders, 60

Genetics *(continued)*
   as risk factor
      for anxiety disorders, 86
      for dementia, 312
      for mild cognitive impairment,
         318
   schizophrenia and, 135
   suicidal behavior and, 216
   vulnerability to mood disorders,
      54–55
Geriatric Mental State AGECAT
    (Automated Geriatric Examina-
    tion for Computer Assisted
    Taxonomy) system, 306–307
GGB. *See* Good Behavior Game
GGT. *See* Gamma-glutamyltransferase
    test
Ginseng (*Panax* spp.), 117
Glucose challenge test, 209
Good Behavior Game (GGB), 14–15

Haloperidol, 223
Hamilton Anxiety Scale, 110
Hamilton Rating Scale for Depression,
    224
HDL. *See* High-density lipoprotein
    cholesterol
Head Start program, 18, 41
Health care
   barriers, 333–334
   disparities, 331–333
   promotion, 284–289, 328–334
   public, 276
Health promotion, 20
   in clinical practice, 34–37, **35**
   definition, 334–335
Healthy Families America, 252–253
Healthy People 2010, 139, 365,
    376–377

Herbs, 106–107. *See also*
    Complementary and alternative
    medicine
High-density lipoprotein (HDL)
    cholesterol, 169, 336
High/Scope Perry Preschool Program,
    18
Hispanics, 213
HIV. *See* Human immunodeficiency
    virus
Human immunodeficiency virus
    (HIV), 185–186, 329, 344
Hydrocodone (Vicodin), 183
Hypercholesterolemia, 345
Hyperglycemia, 331
Hypericin, 117
Hypericum perforatum (St. John's wort),
    107, 110, 117
Hyperlipidemia, 345
Hypertension, 336

Ideation, 226, 233
Incredible Years program, 18
Individual characteristics, as risk factor
    for suicide, 216–217
Inhalants, 183
Injuries, 19–20
Insel, Dr. Thomas, 8
Institute of Medicine (IOM), 2
   classification, 6–9, 7
     of prevention, 7
   selective preventive interventions, 6,
     8
   target population addressed, 6
   universal preventive interventions, 6
Integrative medicine, 106. *See also*
    Complementary and alternative
    medicine
Internalizing, 84

Interventions
    evidence-based, 11–12
    indicated preventive, 7, 8, 176–177,
        299
    multilevel programs for suicidal
        behavior, 219–220
    preemption, 8
    selective preventive interventions, 6,
        7, 8, 176, 299
    target population addressed, 6
    universal preventive interventions,
        6, 7,175–176, 299
IOM. *See* Institute of Medicine
IQ level, 31, 35

Kapikacchu, 106
Kava (*Piper methysticum*), 107, 110
Keeping Families Strong, 14
Kids' Club, 258, **259**
Kraepelinian schizophrenia, 129
Kreteks, 366. *See also* Smoking

Late-life depression, 299–308
    clinical characteristics, 299–300
    epidemiology, 300–301
    prevention, 303–308
        primary, 304–307
        secondary, 307–308
        tertiary, 308
    risk factors, 301–302
        biological, 301
        psychosocial, 302
LDL. *See* Low-density lipoprotein
Legislation
    against domestic violence, 256–257
    in mental health prevention, 17
    suicide rates and, 228
Life Skills Training, 190, 194
Lifestyle, 337

Lifestyle Management Class, 176
Lithium
    for prevention of recurrence of
        mania and depression in
        bipolar disorder, 69
    for prevention of suicidal behavior,
        222
Liver function tests, 177, 209
Low-density lipoprotein (LDL), 312,
    336

Mania
    DSM-IV-TR diagnostic criteria, 52,
        53
    symptoms, 52
Marijuana. *See Cannabis* spp.
Marital status, depression and, 55
Masai infants, 37
MAST. *See* Michigan Alcohol Screening
    Test
MCI. *See* Mild cognitive impairment
MCV. *See* Mean cell volume
MDMA (methylenedioxymethamphet-
    amine; ecstasy), 182–183
Mean cell volume (MCV), 209
Media campaigns, for prevention of
    suicidal behavior, 229
Medicaid, 331–332
Medications, safer use of, 229
Meditation, 113–114
Memantine, for treatment of dementia,
    314
Mental health prevention
    classifications, 2–9
        Institute of Medicine, 6–9, 7
        traditional public health, 3–6, 4
    integrated with substance abuse
        disorders, 193–194
    legislation, 17

Mental health prevention *(continued)*
overview, 1–28
prevention-minded clinical practice,
12, 21–22
principles, 9–21
of relapse, 12
versus treatment, 3
Mental health professionals. *See also*
Clinical practice
goals, 17–20
promotion of mental health, health,
and wellness, 20–21
Mental health promotion, definition, 20
Mentors, 62–63
Methadone, 192–193
Methylphenidate (Ritalin), 183
Michigan Alcohol Screening Test
(MAST), 176, 207–208
Mild cognitive impairment (MCI),
316–320
clinical characteristics, 317
epidemiology, 317
prevention, 319–320
primary, 319–320
secondary, 320
tertiary, 320
as risk factor for dementia, 311–312
risk factors, 318
biomarkers, 318
genetics, 318
treatment, 318–319
Mind-body medicine, 106. *See also*
Complementary and alternative
medicine
Mirtazapine, 221
Moms Empowerment, 258–259, **259**
Mood disorders, 13. *See also* Depression
description, 50
development, 52

DSM-IV-TR diagnostic criteria
for major depressive episode, **51**
for manic episode, **53**
environmental factors, 57–59
epidemiology, 50–52
general medical illnesses and, 59
genetic vulnerability, 54–55
prevention, 49–81
implications, 59–60
primary, 63–65
secondary, 65–67
tertiary, 67–70
promotion of prevention in routine
clinical practice, 70–72
protective factors and implications
for prevention, 60–63
risk factors and implications for
prevention, 52–60
sociodemographic characteristics,
55–57
Mood stabilizers, for prevention of
recurrence of mania and
depression in bipolar disorder, 69
Mortality, depression and, 50–51, 59

Naltrexone, 192–193
NAPLS. *See* North American Prodrome
Longitudinal Study
National Advisory Mental Health
Council's Clinical Treatment and
Services Research Workgroup, 71
National Center for Complementary
and Alternative Medicine
(NCCAM), 105–106
National Child Traumatic Stress
Network, 254
National Comorbidity Survey (NCS),
50–51, 369
National Domestic Violence Hotline, 258

National Epidemiologic Survey on Alcohol and Related Conditions, 370

National Health Interview Survey, 107

National Institute of Mental Health Strategic Plan for Mood Disorders, 71

National Institute on Alcohol Abuse and Alcoholism, 167

National Institute on Drug Abuse, 167

National Longitudinal Study on Adolescent Health, 174–175

National Task Force on Fetal Alcohol Syndrome/Fetal Alcohol Effects, 166

NCCAM. *See* National Center for Complementary and Alternative Medicine

NCS. *See* National Comorbidity Survey

NCS-R. *See* U.S. National Comorbidity Survey Replication

Nefazodone, 221

Neuroleptic dysphoria, 223

Nicotine. *See* Smoking

Nonsteroidal anti-inflammatory drugs (NSAIDS), 313, 315

Noradrenalin, 115

Norepinephrine, 302–303

North American Prodrome Longitudinal Study (NAPLS), 144

NSAIDS. *See* Nonsteroidal anti-inflammatory drugs

Nurse-Family Partnership (Nurse Home Visitation Program), 252–253

Nurse Home Visitation Program (Nurse-Family Partnership), 252–253

Nutrition, as risk factor for dementia, 313

Obesity, 21, 336

Obsessive-compulsive disorder, 85

ODD. *See* Oppositional defiant disorder

"ODD: A Guide for Families," 282

Olanzapine, 223–224, 331, 345

Older adults. *See* Elderly

Olweus program, 19

Opiate analgesics, 170

Oppositional defiant disorder (ODD), 282

Ottawa Charter for Health Promotion, 20

Oxycodone (OxyContin), 183

OxyContin (oxycodone), 183

PACE. *See* Personal Assistance and Crisis Evaluation clinic

Panax spp. (ginseng), 117

Panic disorder, 85

Paracetamol, 228

Parent-child interaction therapy (PCIT), 255

Parents. *See also* Family violence, prevention
  African American, 63
  with history of anxiety disorder, 89–90
  parent-child relationships, 244
  positive, 289
  quality of, 34, 35
  restrictive, 37

Paroxetine, 221

PCIT. *See* Parent-child interaction therapy

PEARLS. *See* Program to Encourage
    Active, Rewarding Lives for
    Seniors
PeerCare, 16
Peers, 40. *See also* Adolescents
    preventive interventions for
        substance abuse and, 187
    sexual behavior and, 185–186
    substance abuse and, 185–186
Perceived self-efficacy, 62
Personal Assistance and Crisis
    Evaluation (PACE) clinic,
    141–142
Personality
    alcohol abuse and, 173
    as risk factor for anxiety disorders,
        86
    suicidal behavior and, 216–217
Personality disorder, schizotypal, 135–136
Pharmacotherapy
    for prevention of mood disorders,
        67–68
    for prevention of recurrence of
        mania and depression in
        bipolar disorder, 69
    for prevention of suicidal behavior,
        220–224
    side effects, 68
Phobias, 85
Physical abuse. *See* Child physical abuse
Physical health, 13
Physical inactivity. *See also* Exercise
    as risk factor for dementia, 313
Piper methysticum (kava), 107, 110
Posttraumatic stress disorder, 85
Pregnancy. *See also* Women
    home-visit programs, 64
    smoking and, 380–381
    teenage, 19

Prenatal/Early Infancy Project, 64
Preventing Depression in AMD Trial,
    306
Prevention
    of alcohol and drug abuse, 163–210
    of anxiety disorders, 83–103
    based on epidemiological findings,
        9–10
    of cigarette smoking, 365–386
    complementary and alternative
        medicine in depression and
        anxiety, 105–123
    costs, 97–98
    family members of patients and,
        13–14
    of family violence, 243–272
    goals for mental health
        professionals, 17–20
    health promotion, 327–364
    Institute of Medicine classification, 7
    of mood disorders, 49–81
    principles, 9–21
        for adolescents in psychiatric
            practice, 273–296
        for older adults, 297–326
    of relapse, substance abuse, suicide,
        and adverse behaviors, 12–13
    risk factors and protective factors in
        clinical practice, 29–48
    in schizophrenia and other
        psychotic disorders, 125–161
    in schools, workplace, and
        community settings, 14–17
    of somatic illnesses in psychiatric
        settings, 327–364
    studies for anxiety disorders, 87–92
    of suicide, 211–242
    understanding risk factors and
        protective factors, 10–11

Prevention of Mental Disorders: Effective Interventions and Policy Options, 2
Prevention paradox, 164
Prevention psychiatry, 2
Primary prevention
    of child physical abuse and neglect, 250–253, **251**
    of child sexual abuse, 255–256
    definition, 3, 4, 5
    of dementia, 315–316
    of domestic violence, 256–257
    examples in medicine and psychiatry, **4**
    of family violence for mental health practitioners, 261–262
    of late-life depression, 304–307
    of mild cognitive impairment, 319–320
    of mood disorders, 63–65
    of smoking, 374
    of suicidal behavior, 217–220
PRIME (Prevention Through Risk Identification Management and Education) study, 143
Process-oriented research, 38–41
Prodrome concept, of schizophrenia, 128
Program to Encourage Active, Rewarding Lives for Seniors (PEARLS), 308
Project STAR (Students Taught Awareness and Resistance), 188, 194
Promoting Mental Health: Concepts, Emerging Evidence, Practice, 2
Promotive factors, 34
Protective factors, 11, 34
    examples in multiple contexts, 34, **35**
    family-level, 34, **35**
    individual-level, 34, **35**

    for mood disorders and implications for prevention, 60–63
    for smoking, 371–373
    sociocultural level, 34, **35**
    suicide and, 217
PsyCE, 348
Psychiatric illness, as risk factor for suicide, 214–215
Psychiatrist, primary care, 348
Psychosocial interventions, for prevention of mood disorders, 69
Psychotherapy
    for prevention of mood disorders, 67
    for prevention of suicidal behavior, 225–226
Psychotic disorders. *See also* individual psychotic disorders
    prevention principles, 125–161
Public health, impact of adolescent conduct disorder and, 276

QPR. *See* Question, Persuade, and Refer program
Quality of life, 67, 336
Question, Persuade, and Refer (QPR) program, 15–16, 232

RBC. *See* Red blood cell count
Reconnecting Youth program, 189
Red blood cell (RBC) count, 209
Reducing Risks for Mental Disorders: Frontiers for Preventive Intervention Research, 2
Relapse, 12
    prevention of alcohol dependence, 191–193

Relapse *(continued)*
  prevention with drug abuse
      disorders, 191–193
  prevention with substance abuse
      disorders, 191–193
Resilience, 34
  definition, 288–289
Rimonabant, 193
Risk factors
  causal, 10
  in children and adolescents for drug
      abuse, 181–191
  of conduct disorder, 276–277
  for dementia, 311–314
  examples in multiple contexts, 31,
      31
  family-level, 31, **31**, 32
  for family violence prevention,
      246–250, **247**
  high-risk individuals, 30
  individual-level, 31, **31**
  for late-life depression, 301–302
      biological, 301
      psychosocial, 302
  malleable/nonmalleable, 10–11
  for mild cognitive impairment, 318
  in prediction of maladjustment and
      pathology, 30–34
  in prevention of anxiety disorders,
      85–87
  in prevention of mental health,
      10–11
  proxy, 10
  for schizophrenia, 132–136, **133**
  for smoking, 371–373
  sociocultural level, 31, **31**
  of suicide, 213–217, **214**, **215**
Risk gradients, 32–33

Risk markers, for schizophrenia,
      136–138, **136**
Ritalin (methylphenidate), 183
Rivastigmine, for treatment of
      dementia, 314
Role models, 62–63

Salicylate analgesics, 228
Schizophrenia, 32
  antipsychotics and, 223–224
  applications of prevention
      principles, 141–146
      conversion from prodrome to
          psychosis, 141–144
      illness detection and treatment,
          144–145
      prevention of relapse,
          nonadherence, substance
          abuse, physical morbidity,
          and suicide, 145–146
  clinical high risk status, 141
  course, 127–129
  course specifiers, 131–132
  diagnostic criteria and course
      specifiers, 129–132,
      130–131
  epidemiology, 126–127
  Kraepelinian, 129
  lifetime prevalence, 127
  onset, 127–129
  phenomenology, 127–129
  prevention principles, 125–161
  primary, secondary, and tertiary
      prevention, 138–139
  risk factors, 132–136, **133**
  risk markers, 136–138, **136**
  smoking and, 370
  symptoms, 127–129

universal, selective, and indicated preventive interventions, 139–141

Schizotypal personality disorder, 135–136

Schools. *See also* Education
  in mental health prevention, 14–16
  preventive interventions for substance abuse and, 187

Seattle Social Development Project, 189

Secondary prevention, 5
  of child physical abuse and neglect, 253–254
  definition, **4**
  of dementia, 316
  of domestic violence, 257
  examples in medicine and psychiatry, **4**
  of family violence for mental health practitioners, 262–263
  of late-life depression, 307–308
  of mild cognitive impairment, 320
  of mood disorders, 65–67
  of smoking, 374–375
  of suicidal behavior, 220–229

Selective serotonin reuptake inhibitors (SSRIs), 117
  for management of late-life depression, 302–303
  for prevention of suicidal behavior, 220–221

Self-efficacy, 62
  academic, 62

Separation anxiety disorder, 85

Serotonin, 115

Sertraline, 221

Sexual abuse. *See* Child sexual abuse

Sexual behavior, 185–186

Shelters, 258

Signs of Suicide (SOS), 15, 231–232

Sleep
  bipolar disorder and, 58–59
  hygiene, 21

Smoking, 12, 184
  cessation, 342, **376,** 377–381
    in adolescence, 371, 380
    in pregnancy, 380–381
  costs, 369
  disease and, 367–368
  epidemiology, 368–371
    rates among people with serious mental illnesses, 369–371
    rates in the United States, 368–369
  health promotion and, 338–340
  as a means of nicotine delivery, 366–367
  nicotine as illicit drug, 170
  prevention, 365–386, 373–375, **376–377**
    primary, 374
    secondary, 374–375
    tertiary, 375
  recommendations for clinical practice, 375–382
  screening, 375, 377
  relapse prevention, 381–382
  risk and protective factors, 371–373
  schizophrenia and, 370
  secondhand, 366, **376**
  treatment, **376**

Sociocultural level
  alcohol abuse risk factors and, 173–174
  for prevention of suicidal behavior, 226–229

Sociocultural level *(continued)*
  preventive interventions for
      substance abuse and, 187
  protective factors, 34, **35**
  risk factors, 31, **31**
Social phobia, 85
Social support, 62
Somatic illnesses, prevention in
    psychiatric settings, 327–364
  barriers to health care, 333–334
  costs, 334
  death rates, 328–329
  future directions, 349–352
  health behaviors and other illness-
      and medication-related factors,
      329–331
  health care disparities, 331–333
  health promotion
    within the general population,
        335–340
      diet, 338
      physical activity, 337–338
      tobacco use, 338–340
    illness prevention, 334–335
    overview, 328–334
  in people with serious mental
      illnesses, 340–349
    consumer, 341–343
    provider, 343–347
    the system, 347–349
SOS. *See* Signs of Suicide
SSRIs. *See* Selective serotonin reuptake
    inhibitors
St. John's wort (*Hypericum perforatum*),
    107, 110, 117
STIRR (screen, test, immunize, reduce
    risk, and refer), 348
Strengthening Families Program,
    188–189, 194

Substance abuse disorders (SUDs), 12.
    See also Alcohol; Drug abuse
  costs, 170
  integrated with mental health
      treatment, 193–194
  mental health care and, 13
  relapse prevention, 191–193
Sudarshan kriya program, 114
SUDs. *See* Substance abuse disorders
Suicide, 11, 12
  adolescent, 231–232
  assessment, 233
  clinical trials, 230
  epidemiology, 212–213
    in the United States, 212–213
    worldwide, 212
  ideation, 226, 233
  prevention, 211–242
    advice for clinical practitioners,
        232–235
  primary prevention of suicidal
      behavior, 217–220
    early detection and treatment of
        depression, 219
    education of health
        professionals, 219
    gatekeeper education, 218
    multilevel intervention
        programs, 219–220
    public education, 218
  protective factors, 217
  risk factors, 213–217, **214, 215**
    biological traits, 216
    early life adversity, 216
    environmental, 217
    family history, 215
    individual characteristics, 216–217
    psychiatric illnesses and
        comorbidity, 214–215

secondary prevention of suicidal
behavior, 220–229
electroconvulsive therapy,
224–225
pharmacotherapy, 220–224
antidepressants, 220–222
antipsychotics, 223–224
lithium, 222
psychotherapy, 225–226
societal interventions, 226–229
contact with high-risk elderly
individuals, 227–228
crisis hotlines, 226–227
media campaigns, 229
restriction of means, 228
stress-diathesis model, 214, **215**
tertiary prevention of suicidal
behavior, 229–230
follow-up, 229–230
identification of family members
at risk, 230
use of safer medications, 229
Surgeon General's Workshop on
Violence and Public Health, 261
Systemic inflammation, as risk factor
for dementia, 313

T-ACE (tolerance, others annoyed,
control, eye opener), 176
Tele-Check, 228
Tele-Help, 227–228
Temperament
inhibited, 88–89
as risk factor for anxiety disorders,
86
Tertiary prevention, 5–6
of child physical abuse and neglect,
254–255

of child sexual abuse, 256
definition, 4
of dementia, 316
of domestic violence, 257–260, **259**
examples in medicine and
psychiatry, 4
of family violence for mental health
practitioners, 264–267
of late-life depression, 308
of mild cognitive impairment, 320
of mood disorders, 67–70
of smoking, 375
of suicidal behavior, 229–230
Tests
for alcohol dependence screening,
204–209
for smoking screening, 375, 377
TF-CBT. *See* Trauma-focused
cognitive-behavioral therapy
Thiothixene, 223
Thyroid disease, 59. *See also* Bipolar
disorder
Trauma, depression and, 58
Trauma-focused cognitive-behavioral
therapy (TF-CBT), 256
Treatment, versus mental health
prevention, 3
Tricyclic antidepressants, 302–303
TWEAK (tolerance, worried, eye
opener, amnesia, "kut down")
questions, 177
Twins, depression and, 57–58

University of Colorado Separation and
Divorce Program, 65
U.S. Air Force, 218
U.S. Department of Veterans Affairs,
330, 347

U.S. Food and Drug Administration
(FDA), 193, 221
U.S. National Comorbidity Survey
Replication (NCS-R), 84
U.S. Preventive Services Task Force's
Guide to Clinical Preventive
Services, 65–66, 179

Vacha, 106
Vascular risk factors and disorders, as
risk factor for dementia, 312–313
Venlafaxine, 221
VicHealth. *See* Victorial Health
Promotion Foundation
Vicodin (hydrocodone), 183
Victorial Health Promotion
Foundation (VicHealth), 20
Vitamin B$_6$, 313
Vitamin B$_{12}$, 313
Vitamin C, 313
Vitamin E, 313
Vulnerability factors, 30

Wellness, 342
programs, 176
promotion, 20–21
WHO. *See* World Health
Organization
Widows to Widows Program, 17
Women. *See also* Domestic violence;
Family violence, prevention;
Pregnancy
African American mothers, 63
depressed mothers, 14
depression and, 58
as victims of domestic violence,
245
Workplace, in mental health
prevention, 16
World Health Organization (WHO),
20, 298, 335
Composite International Diagnostic
Interview, 109

Yoga, 110, 114